Forensic Medicine for Lawyers

The second edition of this book is dedicated to the memory of
Elizabeth Hope Mason
who really enjoyed being associated with forensic medicine

Forensic Medicine for Lawyers

J. K. Mason, CBE, MD, LLD, FRCPath, DMJ
Regius Professor (Emeritus) of Forensic Medicine, University of Edinburgh

With chapters by
A. K. M. Macrae, MB, FRCPE, FRCPsych
Emeritus Professor of Forensic Psychiatry, University of Edinburgh

J. S. Oliver, BSc, PhD, CChem, MRSC
Lecturer in Forensic Medicine (Toxicology), University of Glasgow

A. T. Proudfoot, BSc, MB, MRCPE
Consultant in Charge of the Regional Poisoning Treatment Centre,
The Royal Infirmary, Edinburgh

Butterworths
London   Boston   Singapore   Sydney   Toronto   Wellington

First edition 1978 (J. Wright & Sons)
(Awarded the Swiney Prize in Jurisprudence)

Second edition 1983
Revised reprint 1986
Reprinted 1988

© Butterworths & Co (Publishers) Ltd, 1983

British Library Cataloguing in Publication Data

Mason, J. K.
    Forensic medicine for lawyers.—2nd ed.
    1. Medical jurisprudence—Great Britain
    I. Title
    614′.19′02434   RA1051

    ISBN 0–407–01370–9

Photoset by Butterworths Litho Preparation Department
Printed in Great Britain by Anchor Brendon Ltd, Tiptree, Essex

Preface to the Second Edition

The first edition of this book was surprisingly well received and is seen embarrassingly often in the hands of Counsel. There has been no slackening in world-wide production of books on forensic medicine and it is with gratitude that I acknowledge the courage of the publishers in chancing the success of a second edition of this one.

There have been many changes in the medico-legal world in the last 5 years and these have dictated an update in my text. With some exceptions—e.g. in the curtailment of the powers of the Coroner or the introduction of new drug regulations—these changes have been mainly in the field of medical jurisprudence. As I suggested back in 1974, many of the old corner-stones of forensic pathology have now become moral and ethical issues. The cause of death of an infant with spina bifida is of less importance than are the rights and wrongs of the death being allowed to occur; the academic forensic doctor must now read the *Journal of Forensic Sciences* in parallel with the *Journal of Medical Ethics*.

Society's acceptance or rejection of an ethos is reflected in the attitudes of the Courts. Current deontological problems are making their own law and are of major concern to the lawyer. I make no apology, therefore, for the fact that the major alterations and additions in the second edition are in this field. The Chapter on death and transplantation, for example, has been completely rewritten and subjects such as consent to treatment, medical negligence and euthanasia have been greatly expanded.

Many friends have been kind enough to point out errors or shortcomings in the original text, and I hope I have incorporated all the important criticisms. I have had the most willing assistance from members of the Faculties of Law and Medicine at the University of Edinburgh and particularly acknowledge the help of Mr J. W. Blackie and Dr R. A. A. McCall Smith of the Departments of Scots and Civil Law, University of Edinburgh; together we have mounted an Honours Course in Medical Jurisprudence and they have done their utmost to keep me on the right lines. I have been increasingly conscious of my deficiencies in English law and I acknowledge with pleasure the painstaking review made from this angle by Professor Richard Card of Trent Polytechnic, Nottingham; once again, however, I stress that the responsibility for any shortcomings is mine alone. My grateful thanks also go to my secretary, Mrs E. A. MacDonald, who has worked on the project with great good spirit.

Miss Daphne Lytton was responsible for the preparation of *Figures 2.1–2.5, 3.1, 11.1, 18.2 and 19.1*; and Mr Ian Lennox for *Figure 10.1*.

It will be noted that I have changed publishers. I wish to thank John Wright's for their unfailing help and courtesy in getting the original book off the ground and Butterworths for similar kindly co-operation over the last year.

Preface to the First Edition

In my inaugural address to the University,* I defined forensic medicine as 'medicine applied to the protection and assistance of individuals in relation to the community'. This concept was based on the 'forum' as being a public place in which those responsible to the public in many spheres argued and defended their views rather than being limited to the criminal court.

It seemed to me that forensic medicine should be taught to medical students in this wide spirit whereas, paradoxically, it was the law students who, in having to decipher and understand the reports of their expert medical witnesses, needed the greater exposure to the details of pathology despite the fact that they had no medical background. I could find no textbook extant which would satisfy their particular needs; what follows is an attempt to fill the gap. One of the main difficulties has been to find the right pitch of knowledge and the book has, in the process of writing, settled into an outline of the LL.B. Course in Forensic Medicine presently given at Edinburgh University. It is, however, hoped that it will still be found useful by practising advocates, solicitors, Procurators Fiscal and Coroners.

I recently read a review which stated that 'the day of the single-author textbook has gone', and it is certain that multiple authorship ensures that each facet of the work is covered by an expert practising in that sphere; the single author attempting a wide range must lose a sense of immediacy.

In an effort to compensate for this, I have shown drafts of the majority of chapters to persons particularly well qualified to criticize and advise. Helpful criticism does not, however, necessarily mean approval and, lest naming one's reviewers might be taken as implying their shared responsibility for, and satisfaction with, the end result, I intend to express my thanks anonymously to the many members of the forensic fraternity, the academic staff of the Faculties of Medicine and of Law in Edinburgh University, the NHS officials, the Government and Local Authority officers and others who have responded so kindly to my calls for help; my gratitude loses no sincerity in its generality.

Three special personal acknowledgements are, however, called for. Professor Keith Simpson and Mr Alistair R. Brownlie have been good enough to read the whole manuscript from the point of view of the forensic pathologist and of the lawyer respectively. They have given invaluable advice although, again, it should be stres-

* *Ambitions for a Motley Coat* (1974), Inaugural Address No. 56, University of Edinburgh.

sed that their participation does not necessarily imply agreement with the views expressed. Mr Charles N. Stoddart has reviewed the text with particular reference to the legal technicalities. In doing so, he has not only improved the book's acceptability to lawyers but has also offered many helpful criticisms; he has my sincere thanks for undertaking a most time-consuming task.

I owe my secretarial assistant, Mrs Gladys Hamilton, a debt of gratitude for unstinting co-operation and much encouragement. A number of temporary assistants have had a hand in the typing but the great bulk of this has been undertaken by Miss Iris Falconer with great skill and good heart.

Finally, I have to thank my wife for letting it happen. At a time of our lives which was, for several reasons, difficult, she spent many lonely hours of televiewing without complaint; I hope this book is worthy of her memory.

J.K.M.

Contents

x   Contents

xii   Contents

Some terms used in medical evidence

The basic intention of this textbook is to give the lawyer a better understanding of the evidence provided in Court by medical men. Much of this must depend on some knowledge of anatomy and physiology. A medical report that will be satisfactory to all interested parties cannot be written without using some academic jargon, and lawyers may well need an explanation of the phraseology that the medical witness uses. No apology is made, therefore, for an introduction that may seem unduly elementary to some readers but which may be useful, if only as a source of *aides-mémoire*, to others.

For anatomical descriptive purposes the human body should be regarded as standing erect with the palms of the hands facing forward (*see Figure 1.1*). Everything that can be seen in the mirror is then *anterior* while that which cannot be seen is *posterior*. These views are related to the *coronal* plane—the plane that

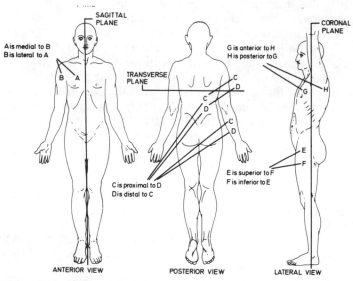

Figure 1.1 The planes of the body and some of the terms used for anatomical reference.

divides the body vertically through the shoulders. The vertical plane at right angles to this is the *sagittal* plane, and the sagittal plane that bisects the body into symmetrical left and right halves is the *midline*. If point A is on the same side of the body as point B and is nearer the midline, then A is *medial* to B and B is *lateral* to A. Thus, while the main torso has anterior, posterior and lateral aspects, the limbs have anterior, posterior, medial and lateral surfaces. The great toe is medial in man as in four-footed animals, but the human and primate thumb is on the lateral side of the hand.

Dividing the body horizontally results in the *transverse* section. From a section taken through the middle of the chest, one can move upwards towards the cephalic extremity and downwards to the caudal extremity. If one assumes that the limbs are extended to form an 'X', then if point C is nearer to the midchest transverse plane than is point D, it is *proximal* to D whereas D is *distal* to C. These terms can, however, be used functionally rather than anatomically; thus, while anatomically the small intestine lies distal to the transverse colon, the former is functionally a proximal portion of gut.

Strictly speaking, the body has also a *superior* surface which is seen from above and an *inferior* surface which is the soles of the feet. The terms 'superior' and 'inferior' are, however, far more important in regard to the surfaces of individual organs; all the above descriptions of the whole body are applicable to its component parts. Points on the body can also be described as superior or inferior to one another depending on whether they are nearer the head or the foot. The terms 'anterior' and 'posterior' can likewise be used relatively.

At its simplest, the body is divided into the head, the limbs and the torso. The interior of the head is the *cranial* cavity while the torso consists of the *thoracic* and *abdominal* cavities. The protection of these cavities differs markedly. The cranial cavity, which contains the brain, is surrounded by the rigid skull which, while giving a high degree of protection, is itself subject to shattering forces which can be propagated through its substance; once fully developed, the skull also inhibits expansion of its contents. The thoracic cavity houses the heart and the lungs. The governing functional principle is that of elasticity. The contents have considerable freedom of movement and the chest wall consists of a mobile combination of ribs and muscle which is only partially protective. The abdominal cavity lacks a bony structure, except where the massive lumbar spine protects it posteriorly, and its contents are therefore susceptible to injury both by penetrating and by blunt force. The major contents, which lie within a covering envelope, the *peritoneum*, include the stomach and greater part of the bowel, the liver and the spleen; these are loosely connected by ligaments and have considerable mobility. Those lying behind the peritoneum, including the pancreas and the kidneys, are more rigidly fixed but, in general, are better protected. The lower part of the abdominal cavitiy is bounded by the two pelvic bones and is known as the *pelvic* cavity which contains the urinary bladder and, in the female, the uterus and ovaries.

The ability of the various organs to move has much importance in relation to accidental injury. A mobile object can, to some extent, slide away from direct violence; the more fixed an organ is, the more susceptible it is to bruising and crushing. On the other hand, even the most mobile organ must be attached at some point to a relatively rigid structure; organs that can move are thus particularly susceptible to shearing forces and to indirect injury. The size of the organ will influence the likelihood of its being directly affected—the liver is a good example—while the extent of air/fluid/solid interfaces will partly determine the damage likely to result from internal vibration and other stresses. The *elasticity* of the organ is another major determinant in this type of trauma, while the condition of an individual organ at the time of stress may affect its response—a diseased spleen, for example, is more likely to rupture than is a normal organ.

The solid portions of the body are composed of myriads of *cells* held together by *ground substance*. The cells are organized so as to form either *epithelium* or *connective tissues*. Cancerous overgrowth of the former is known as *carcinoma* and, of the latter, as *sarcoma*. Epithelium either lines or cloaks the organs of the body. It is often specialized—for example, to secrete, as in the gut, or to waft particles (e.g. of dust); in the latter case, the epithelium is said to be *ciliated*. The skin is a most complex epithelium with many functions, perhaps the primary one of which is to retain the body fluids; thus, destruction of the skin by burning leads to a massive loss of fluid—the potentially lethal condition of *dehydration*. The *connective tissue* connects not only the various epithelia but also the major parts of the body—it includes fat, muscle, fibrous tissue including tendons and bones, the whole being permeated by a network of blood vessels. The connective tissues are of great importance in the healing of wounds. When the continuity of part of the body, for example the skin, is interrupted, a variable quantity of bleeding takes place; this is partly stemmed by contraction of the cut ends of the vessels and by the pressure exerted by the extravasated blood. Wandering tissue-repair cells then enter the bruise and the dead area is penetrated by new blood vessels which, in turn, provoke the appearance of young fibrous connective tissue cells. These vessels then age and become tough and bloodless, the result being a *scar*. The recognition of these stages is the basis of 'ageing' of wounds.

The blood itself is a specialized form of connective tissue which consists of cells and fluid; the latter is the *plasma* which carries soluble foodstuffs and electrolytes, waste products and messenger substances, or *hormones*, which provide the body's system of communication between organs. The blood cells are either *red* (erythrocytes) or *white* (leucocytes); the function of the former is the carriage of oxygen while the latter are, in general, concerned with the defence of the body against infection. Sarcomatous overgrowth of the white cells results in *leukaemia*. *Platelets*, concerned with blood coagulation, also circulate in the plasma.

All cells other than the erythrocytes consist of two main parts—the *nucleus* and the *cytoplasm*. The nucleus controls cell reproduction and contains 23 pairs of *chromosomes*, one of each pair being derived from a parent. Normal cell division and tissue growth results from *mitosis* in which each chromosome reproduces itself; the two new cells therefore contain the same chromosomes as did their progenitor. The exception lies in the sex cells, spermatozoa in the male or ova in the female, which divide by a process of *meiosis* and contain only 23 single chromosomes; the fusion of two sex cells thus results in a *zygote* with the normal nuclear configuration. The chromosomes are composed of a number of *genes* which are transmitted hereditarily and which determine the constitution of the body.

One pair of chromosomes dictates the sex of the subject. These sex chromosomes are designated X and Y. The presence of a Y chromosome in the pair indicates maleness.

In addition to describing the body on anatomical grounds, it is often useful to consider it systematically—that is, relating those parts which are functionally integrated irrespective of their position. These 'systems' are referred to frequently in medical reports and most are dealt with in greater detail in the opening chapter. In summary, the medical witness may refer to:

1. The *nervous* system, comprising the brain and spinal cord (central nervous system) and the peripheral nerves.
2. The *musculoskeletal* system, or the bones, tendons and muscles.
3. The *cardiovascular* system, consisting of the heart and blood vessels.
4. The *respiratory* system, running from the nose to the lungs and including the diaphragm and chest muscles.
5. The *gastrointestinal* system, which includes not only the gut from mouth to anus but also those organs whose function is to control the processing of food, i.e. the salivary glands, the liver and the pancreas.
6. The *genitourinary* system. Although quite distinct functionally, the genital and urinary systems are commonly combined on anatomical grounds. The genital system includes the ovaries, uterus, vagina and vulva in the female and the testes, ducts and penis in the male. The main components of the urinary system are the kidneys, the ureters, the bladder and the urethra, and the prostate gland in the male.
7. The *lymphoreticular* system, which is responsible for many functions particularly related to defence against infection. The main solid organs are the spleen, the thymus gland and the numerous lymph nodes including specialized nodes such as the tonsils.
8. The *endocrine system*, comprising those glands that control body function by secretion of hormones into the bloodstream. The most important from the forensic aspect are the pituitary, the adrenal and the thyroid glands.

All these systems are interlinked—all, for example, depend upon their component of the cardiovascular system and its contained blood, while the musculoskeletal system, in particular, cannot function in the absence of a nervous system. They form useful descriptive compartments in so far as the functional result of disease or injury within a system is immediately understandable.

Many medical terms are made up of the Latin names for the organ or tissue associated with a descriptive prefix or suffix. A selected list of these is given in Appendix A.

1

Some aspects of applied anatomy and physiology

The cardiovascular system

Animal life depends upon the supply of oxygen to the tissues. This is the function of two biological systems—the respiratory system which collects or harvests the oxygen and the cardiovascular system which distributes it for consumption. The two are closely interrelated, the common factor being the *erythrocytes* or red cells of the blood, of which there are about 5 million to the cubic millimetre of blood.

Red cells derive their colour from the pigment *haemoglobin*, a combination of iron and protein, the function of which is to accept oxygen in the lungs and to surrender it in the tissues. Maximum contact with the surroundings is achieved at both these points by passing the blood through vessels that are approximately the diameter of individual red cells—these vessels are known as *capillaries*. The extremely delicate nature of their walls allows controlled transference not only of gases but of water and salts or *electrolytes*; this system is most sensitive to oxygen deficiency and it is abnormal capillary permeability that is mainly responsible for the condition of *surgical shock*. This is an important concept—shock in medical terms is not a matter of mental distress; it is a profound biochemical disturbance which, triggered by capillary hypoxia (*see* page 353), leads to alterations in the distribution of body water and, particularly, of blood volume. Surgical shock is a condition of immense medico-legal importance as it occurs most commonly as a result of trauma; anything that reduces the peripheral blood pressure, particularly haemorrhage or fluid loss due to burning, can precipitate the condition which is self-perpetuating— low peripheral pressure means oxygen starvation which leads to capillary damage, local fluid loss and increasing failure of the blood pressure.

The blood pressure that is commonly described in medical reports is measured in the arteries; its maintenance is a function not only of peripheral resistance but also of the pumping action of the heart. The pressure is described in two phases—the *systolic* pressure, which is the maximum achieved as a result of the heart beat, and the *diastolic*, which is the residual pressure maintained while the heart is refilling; in general, it is the diastolic pressure that reflects most accurately the level of strain upon the system.

The *heart* consists of specialized muscle tissue, the *myocardium*, and is enclosed in a fibrous sac, the *pericardium*. Essentially it consists of two separate pumps (*see*

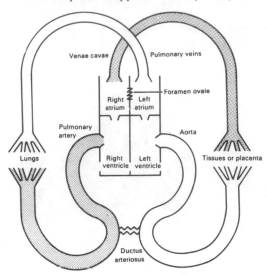

Figure 2.1 Diagrammatic illustration of the cardiovascular system. The fetal connections used to bypass
the lungs are shown as zigzags.

Figure 2.1), the left and right *ventricles*, which are fed with blood through
non-return valves from the left and right *atria*. The size and weight of the heart are
dictated largely by the condition of the ventricles which, in turn, depends mainly
upon the peripheral resistance to the flow of blood. A ventricle that is coping with
increased resistance will grow in bulk or *hypertrophy*; one that is failing to do so
will *dilate*. These observations are, therefore, of great importance in assessing
matters such as life expectancy in compensation cases. Blood passes from the
ventricles to the tissues through *arteries*. The main artery of the body is the *aorta*
which branches into vessels of descending calibre until the capillaries are reached.
The capillaries then coalesce into tributaries or *veins* which ultimately form two
main rivers—the *superior vena cava* coming from the upper part of the body and
the *inferior vena cava* from the lower—which return the blood from the *systemic
circulation* to the right atrium. All blood vessels have three coats—the *intima*, a
normally thin lining which is subject to the degenerative change of atheroma; the
media, a muscular coat; and the *adventitia* which is a loose covering responsible for
the supply of nutriments to the vessel itself and for its stability in the body. Since
the arteries are steadily decreasing in size, a considerable pressure must be
maintained within them to ensure adequate blood flow; the arteries therefore have
thick muscular walls. The situation in the veins, however, is that of a flowing river;
the walls are thin and the deoxygenated blood shows through them as dark purple
in colour.
    The blood returning in the venae cavae has shed much of its oxygen which must
be replenished. It passes into the right ventricle and thence to the *pulmonary artery*
which again divides until it forms capillaries within the lungs. These capillaries now
surround the smallest air pockets, the *alveoli*. The blood here accepts more oxygen
and returns via the *pulmonary veins* to the *left atrium* thus completing the
pulmonary circulation. The pulmonary capillaries are just as sensitive to changes in
blood volume and oxygen content as are those of the systemic circulation; fluid loss

from them results in *pulmonary oedema*, or water in the lungs, which, again, is self-perpetuating, in that displacement of the air in the alveoli by water simply decreases still further the supply of oxygen to the tissues.

The blood thus circulates in something of a figure-of-eight—that in the systemic arteries and pulmonary veins is oxygenated while that in the systemic veins and pulmonary arteries requires regenerating. Such a circulation will be useless for the fetus which has no access to atmospheric air. The lungs of the fetus *in utero* are, therefore, replaced by the *placenta*—a mass of capillaries derived from both the infant and the mother by means of which the former is supplied with oxygen as a 'tissue' of the latter; the pulmonary artery and veins are replaced functionally by the umbilical vessels. The fetal lungs must be bypassed and this is accomplished through two main mechanisms. First, the two atria are allowed to communicate through the *foramen ovale*. Some of the blood therefore passes from the right atrium to the left atrium rather than to the right ventricle and pulmonary artery. Secondly, a connection, the *ductus arteriosus*, is established between the aorta and the pulmonary artery by means of which the great majority of blood pumped from the right ventricle can be diverted to the aorta and, thence, to the placental circulation. The ductus usually closes a few days after birth and the foramen ovale some weeks later. These points are of major medico-legal importance as so much forensic pathology revolves round the fetal and neonatal period and, in particular, the post-mortem diagnosis of a 'separate existence'.

Damage to the heart or blood vessels results in haemorrhage, one of the most constant complications of trauma of all types. Its severity depends on three main factors. First, there is the size of the vessel. In this respect, the heart itself is the most important part of the system; apart from this, the larger the vessel damaged, the more dangerous is the injury to life. Second, the type of vessel is all-important—damage to an artery, subject to high internal pressure, will obviously be more dangerous than damage to a vein of comparable size. Third, there are the secondary effects, not only those resulting from oxygen deprivation in specific organs but also those due to occupation of space by extruded blood—thus, haemorrhage into the skull will have very different effects from the same amount of bleeding into the abdomen.

The *haemostatic* mechanism of the body—that is, its ability to control haemorrhage—rests first, on the properties of blood and, second, on the capacity of the vessels to contract, a matter of vascular health and size. The properties of the blood derive from two distinct sources—the *coagulation factors* and the *platelets*. The former, designated by Roman numerals, are protein substances circulating in the plasma that, when activated in the presence of calcium, take part in a complicated chain reaction. The result of this reaction is to form *thrombin* which then reacts with the circulating protein *fibrinogen* to form *fibrin* which is, in effect, the scaffolding of a clot. Deficiency of any factor can break the chain and cause one of what are collectively known as *bleeding diatheses*; for practical purposes, Factor II or prothrombin, Factor VIII, Factor IX and Factor I (fibrinogen) are the most important. Prothrombin is formed in the liver; severe liver disease will therefore predispose to a bleeding condition. Deficiency of Factor VIII results in the hereditary disease *haemophilia* (lack of Factor IX is responsible for haemophilia B or Christmas disease). The function of the platelets is twofold. In the first place, they release substances that activate the coagulation mechanism and, secondly, they aggregate to form 'plugs' at the site of injury to a vessel and thus consolidate the fibrin clot. Excessive bleeding is therefore likely if platelets are absent, as happens in disease or poisoning of the bone marrow, or if they are abnormal.

The medico-legal importance of bleeding diatheses lies in several fields. The response to injury will be abnormal—trivial wounds may result in severe haemorrhage or excessive bruising—and this will greatly affect their interpretation as to the time of infliction, the force used and the like. Secondly, the abnormal condition can be remitted by replacement of the deficient substance; it follows that failure to identify and neutralize the abnormal state before a surgical or dental operation might well be construed as negligent practice. Thirdly, the treatment of the excessive bleeding is expensive and wasteful; pugnacious haemophiliacs are doubly antisocial.

Blood coagulation and haemostasis occur normally only at the site of injury. The reverse of haemorrhage is the very dangerous condition of *intravascular coagulation* which occurs either locally in a diseased vessel or as a generalized condition resulting from severe surgical shock. A *thrombus* forms within the vessel; if this breaks off it becomes an *embolus*. The major significance of these abnormal states is discussed in Chapter 7.

Cardiovascular damage may be the result of indirect or direct trauma. The former is largely a matter of accidental injury and is described in Chapter 10. For present purposes, the most important causes of direct injury include stab wounds—when these are fatal, it is generally by virtue of penetrating the heart or a major vessel; incised wounds, when a major vessel presents under the surface as at the wrist or in the neck; and gunshot wounds, in which damage is likely from not only the bullet but also fragments of bone which act as secondary missiles.

Natural disease of the heart and vessels accounts for some 80 per cent of the sudden deaths reported to the Coroner or Procurator Fiscal. It represents perhaps the major preoccupation of a forensic pathologist and is discussed in detail in Chapter 7.

The blood

As has already been described (*see* page 3), the blood consists of two major fractions—the *cellular component* and the *plasma* in which the cells float. If the blood is clotted, the resulting altered fluid component is known as *serum*. Serum is technically easier to work with in certain laboratory examinations and it is common to speak loosely of 'serum substances'; but such substances circulate naturally in the plasma.

The plasma is responsible for transport of carbon dioxide and of the products of ingestion and of metabolism of fat, proteins and carbohydrates. It contains many of the mineral salts on which the biochemical balance of the body depends and also the hormones. The clotting factors, described above, are also present in the plasma which, normally, constitutes approximately 60 per cent of the blood volume; a relative fall in this proportion leads to a viscous blood and local tissue hypoxia due to stagnation.

The cells of the blood are divided into the red series (*erythrocytes*) and the white series (*leucocytes*); there is also a platelet component (*see above*). The oxygen transport function of the first has already been described. A relative lack of red cells constitutes *anaemia* which may result from haemorrhage or from an inability to form haemoglobin, usually because of a lack of its inorganic component, iron. There are other forms of functional anaemia which are important medico-legally. First, some poisonous substances convert the haemoglobin into forms that are less capable or incapable of accepting oxygen—the most important of these is carbon monoxide but there are other substances, particularly of an industrial nature, that achieve much the same end. Secondly, inherited abnormalities of the haemoglobin occur which are known as *haemoglobinopathies*; the best known of these is *sickle cell anaemia* but it is by no means the only member of the group[1]. The medico-legal significance of these diseases is not inconsiderable. First, sufferers from the conditions, which may be present in severe or mild form, are hypersensitive to low blood oxygen tensions arising from any cause; they are at some risk in air travel or in conditions of severe oxygen demand, a situation which might raise a valid defence when sudden death occurs during a struggle. Secondly, most of them show a strong ethnic distribution and are a hazard to the unwary surgeon or anaesthetist.

The *leucocytes* are basically of two types—the *polymorphonuclears* and the *mononuclears*. The former constitutes the body's tactical defence against acute infection; the latter are more akin to a strategic force which comes into action more slowly but whose influence persists for some time. The mononuclears are particularly responsible for the formation of *antibodies* and for the ability of the body to recognize a foreign intruder; an immediate reaction can thereby be set up should the intrusion be repeated. Certain poisons—and some drugs in excessive amounts—suppress the formation of the white cells and the subject is then left prey to infections that would be repelled easily in normal circumstances.

The blood cells are formed in the *bone marrow* which is found in the centre of virtually all the bones of the body; any poison or ionizing radiation that affects the bone marrow will affect the blood and its function. The bone marrow consists of cellular and fatty elements, the proportion of the latter increasing with age.

Effete blood cells must be removed and their important components preserved. This is mainly the function of the *spleen,* an organ which lies in the left upper abdomen covered by the lower ribs. It is one of those odd organs that are not essential to a normal life and its main medico-legal significance lies in the ease with which it is ruptured in vehicular accidents. Deliberate rupture of the spleen also had a vogue as a method of murder in malarial areas, the organ being particularly fragile in that disease.

The spleen and bone marrow are parts of the *lymphoreticular system* which is completed by the *lymphatic* system of the ducts and glands responsible not only for the immune response of the body but also for the circulation of the extracellular fluid which bathes all the cells of the body. The lymphatic and cardiovascular systems are united where the main lymph duct empties itself into the larger veins of the upper thorax. Cancer cells are readily disseminated in the lymph and set up secondary deposits (*metastases*) when they are filtered in the lymphatic glands.

The respiratory system

Without oxygen, there is no enzymatic activity and there is cellular death. The requirement is urgent—the urgency depending on the sophistication of the cells concerned. The body as a whole can survive without food for about 10 weeks; the cells of the brain will die if deprived of oxygen for some 10 minutes. The function of the respiratory system is to trap the oxygen which constitutes about one-fifth of the normal atmosphere, to transfer it to the haemoglobin of the blood and to remove

[1] Abnormalities may be structural—as in *sickle cell anaemia*— or qualitative—*thalassaemia*— resulting, for example, from the persistence of a fetal type of haemoglobin in the adult.

the product of combustion—carbon dioxide—which circulates dissolved in the blood plasma.

Air is passed to the lungs from the nose or mouth, through the *larynx* to the windpipe or *trachea*. The larynx is protected by three bones or cartilages—the *hyoid, thyroid* (Adam's Apple) and *cricoid*—which are of very great importance in the post-mortem diagnosis of strangulation (*see* Chapter 13). The trachea splits into a left and a right main *bronchus* which, in turn, divide into *lobar bronchi*—one to each major lobe of the lungs[2]. The bronchi split into *bronchioles* which end in the air sacs or *alveoli* which, as we have seen, are surrounded by the pulmonary capillaries. The lungs are contained in two layers of a fibrous envelope—the *pleura,* which has two main functions; first, a negative pressure between the two layers serves to maintain the lungs in a position of expansion and, secondly, the surfaces combine to reduce the friction which would otherwise exist between the lungs and the chest wall; the formation of pleural *adhesions* is a frequent result of pulmonary disease.

Air is drawn into the lungs as the muscles of respiration—the chest muscles and the diaphragm—create a negative pressure. As compared with the heart, which is innervated by the autonomic system only, the lungs are directed by both the autonomic and voluntary nervous systems (*see* page 13)—we normally do not consciously think about our respiration, but we are able to alter our breathing should we so wish. In the event of conflict, the autonomic innervation will succeed—it is impossible to die from holding one's breath and, ultimately, an irrespirable medium—whether water or poisonous gas—must be inhaled despite conscious resistance. Expiration requires no muscular effort and, in the event of respiratory failure, positive pressure breathing must be applied as when on a ventilator or in mouth-to-mouth resuscitation, or the whole chest must be subjected to artificial vacuum as in a respirator.

In essence, the process of respiration is one of equilibrating the tensions of the various gases in the air and body fluids. If the oxygen tension is high in the alveoli and low in the pulmonary capillary blood, the gas will pass into the plasma and form oxyhaemoglobin in the red cells; if the oxygen tension is high in the capillary peripheral blood and low in the tissue fluids, oxyhaemoglobin will dissociate and the oxygen will be made available to the tissues. Similar principles apply to dissolved carbon dioxide. Tissue respiration is comparable to an engine boiler—the fuel is oxygen which is used to burn the foodstuffs to produce energy; the resultant 'ash' represents carbon dioxide. The analogy is elaborated in *Figure 2.2* which also indicates the ways in which oxygen deficiency can occur.

The lungs are continually attacked by dust particles present in the air and, normally, the specialized lining of the air passages can cope with this hazard efficiently. In certain circumstances, these defence mechanisms may be destroyed and the lungs will then become diseased as a result of exposure to the environment. The most common precipitating causes are smoking and atmospheric pollution. Alternatively, the lungs may be exposed to unreasonable quantities of dust which may, of itself, be dangerous—most of these *pneumoconioses* or dust diseases are industrial in nature and are discussed in Chapter 15.

Injuries to the lungs are generally of obvious type. They may be penetrated by instruments, by foreign bodies—in particular, bullets—or by the ends of broken

---

[2] The right lung has three lobes, the left only two. The right lung is therefore slightly larger than the left which must make way for the heart which lies in the left thorax.

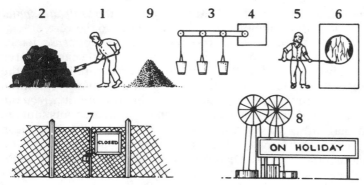

Figure 2.2 An illustrative concept of the respiratory system. A man (1) has to move coal (2) with a series of buckets (3) moved by an engine (4) to a stoker (5) who feeds the factory furnace (6) which represents the tissues of the body. Many things may interfere with the transport of the coal (2) which is supplied to the body in the form of *oxygen*:

   1. The man may get tired = respiratory paralysis.
   3. There may be insufficient buckets (red blood cells) = anaemia.
   4. The bucket transporter may break down = heart failure.
   5. The stoker may be ill = toxic hypoxia.
   7. The factory gates may be closed to coal trucks = mechanical asphyxia.
   8. There may be no coal = environmental anoxia.
   9. So much dust may accumulate that the man cannot reach the buckets
      = lung disease.
In the end
   6. The furnace goes out = death.
(After Lucas, B. G. (1956) In *Practical Forensic Medicine*. Ed. by F. E. Camps and W. B. Purchase, pp. 61. London; Hutchinson's Medical.)

ribs. Two consequences arise. First, the negative pressure in the pleural space may be broken and the lung collapses—not only does this lead to inefficient oxygenation of the blood but the immobile lung is a nidus for infection. Secondly, haemorrhage is inevitable and its severity depends on the size of the vessel involved. Blunt injury is commonly caused by crushing, as in vehicular accidents. Additionally, the large number of gas/fluid interfaces in the lungs renders them particularly sensitive to the passage of shock waves. Generalized pulmonary trauma is typical of falls from a height or of exposure to an explosive blast. The injuries consist of haemorrhage, laceration and destruction of the walls of the alveoli.

One of the most important medico-legal involvements of the lungs is that type of inflammation known as *hypostatic pneumonia* which is likely to follow enforced bed-rest after any injury. The lungs are inadequately expanded and oedema is common; the situation is ripe for the establishment of widespread infection. The less fit the subject, the more probable is the onset of pneumonia and the less likely is he or she to withstand the assault. The common fatal injuries in elderly persons are not those that are of immediately lethal severity; they are those that entail lengthy periods in bed.

The nervous system

Anatomically, the nervous system is divided into the *central nervous system* (CNS) and the *peripheral nervous system* which involves all those nerves that pass out from the CNS to the remainder of the body. The CNS consists of the *brain* and *spinal cord,* the latter being divided into a number of segments related to the vertebrae of the spinal column; a major efferent or *motor* root and an afferent or *sensory* root pass through the lateral aspects of each vertebra. The motor and sensory nerve pathways pass respectively downwards and upwards in the spinal cord between the brain and the nerve roots appropriate to the area of the body they supply. It follows that damage to the spinal cord will result in functional abnormality of a *regional* distribution, the region affected being that which is supplied by nerve roots situated below the point of damage; thus, severance of the cord at the neck will result in paralysis of all four limbs (*quadriplegia*) whereas severance in the thoracic region leads to paralysis of the legs (*paraplegia*). Division of a nerve root, on the other hand, will show itself in a segmented distribution—either anaesthetic or paralytic— whereas damage to a peripheral nerve will cause similar changes either in a group of muscles (or wide area of skin) or in an individual muscle depending on the size of the nerve affected. One further major difference in response to injury must be noted. While some regrowth and recovery of function is possible in the peripheral nerves (the degree depending to some extent on the surgeon's skill) there is no true regeneration in the CNS[3]; this applies not only to the nerve fibres (akin to electric flex down which the impulses travel) but also to the nerve cells—or batteries—from which derives the ultimate nervous function; a child is born with the maximum number of brain cells it will possess and the decreasing mental capacity of senility is to some extent a measure of how these degenerate during life.

In the event of damage to the spinal cord, some functions can be retained through the medium of spinal reflexes which operate without the control of the brain; after division of the cord some useful reflex actions such as the uncontrolled emptying of the bladder when it is full may be established.

It is convenient to regard the central nervous system as a core running from the head to the 'tail' with nerve fibres carrying information and commands in both directions. The spinal cord forms the lowermost part and, above this, lies the hindbrain consisting of the *medulla* and *pons* where many centres organizing the vital functions of the body—e.g. respiration—are situated; the pons is of very great medico-legal importance owing to the frequency with which it sustains fatal haemorrhage after head injury. There is then a narrow midbrain and, above this, the forebrain of which the central core is the *thalamus* and *hypothalamus* where, as a great simplification, the instinctive or animal processes are organized. Two major, bilaterally symmetrical, masses are connected to the centre core; these are the *cerebellum* which overlies and is part of the hindbrain and the *cerebrum* (covered by the *cerebral cortex*) which forms the major part of the forebrain. These masses are concerned with the more complicated functions of the body. The cerebellum essentially co-ordinates movements and posture. Anatomically, the cerebrum is divided into four lobes—the frontal concerned mainly with personality but also with the initiation of muscle movements, the parietal which is the area associated with sensation, the occipital concerned with vision and the temporal which is mainly associated with speech, hearing and equilibrium. Special areas within each lobe are related to special areas of the body, the important feature being that head injury can have reasonably predictable results[4]. The highly developed cerebral

---

[3] Clinical recovery of *functions* may appear when the effects of haemorrhage, oedema, etc., resolve.
[4] Within the head, cranial nerves are given off to supply the head and special senses and are analogous to the peripheral nerves of the spinal cord.

cortex acts in many ways as a controller of the instinctive thalamus. Thus, some drugs—and, in particular, alcohol—which appear to be stimulatory in nature are, in fact, depressants; the most highly developed part of the brain is most easily affected and this leads to diminished conscious control of activity.

This concept of conscious control extends also into the peripheral innervation where, in addition to the nerve supply already described, all the organs are subject to nervous control through the *autonomic system*. This consists of two functional moieties—*sympathetic* and *parasympathetic* systems; the vagus nerve forms a major component of the latter. The autonomic system is responsible for all those activities that are subconscious—for example, the beating of the heart, the production of sweat, movement of the bowel, etc. By and large, its two components are antagonistic; thus, it is the function of the sympathetic system to quicken the heart beat while impulses acting through the vagus nerve will slow it. This raises an important concept in forensic pathology—that of death due to cardiac inhibition resulting from vagal activity[5]. Basically, a sudden and, particularly, an unnatural stimulation of the sympathetic nerves will lead to reflex compensatory action of the vagus nerve; this, being equally severe and unnatural, may so slow the heart as to paralyse it completely. The mucous membranes contribute a potent source of such dangerous reflexes but pressure on special centres of sympathetic activity— especially the *carotid sinus* in the neck or the *solar plexus* in the abdomen—may lead to a similar result. No pathological proof of this sequence can be shown at autopsy but it is widely accepted as the physiological explanation of sudden deaths of this type.

The coverings of the brain and spinal cord are of great medico-legal importance. From without inwards, the brain is covered, first, by the skull and the cord by the component parts of the backbone. These rigid structures, designed to protect the delicate nervous structure from direct external violence, also have obvious disadvantages—there is no room for expansion or displacement of the contained organs and, if fractured, the broken bones themselves become potential lacerating instruments; skilled treatment of injury to the skull and spine is, therefore, a matter of urgency. Within its bony coverings, the CNS is surrounded by a tough membrane known as the *dura mater*. Large blood vessels flow between the bone and the dura; internally, numerous small veins drain into the *dural sinuses*. Head injury can therefore result in either *extradural* or *subdural* haemorrhage. The *arachnoid mater* is a thin membrane lying under the dura. A relatively wide space exists between this membrane and the *pia mater* which invests the brain closely and, in this subarachnoid space, are to be found *cerebrospinal fluid,* the main function of which is to give some leeway for expansion and to act as a water cushion, and also the main arteries as they pass from the neck to supply the brain substance; rupture of these vessels due to injury or natural disease results in *subarachnoid haemorrhage*. The thin pia mater invests the brain so closely that there is, effectively, no subpial space—any haemorrhage occurring in this area is of superficial *intracerebral* type. Deep intracerebral haemorrhage is often divisible into two types—petechial (or capillary), which is commonly associated with asphyxial states of all types, and massive, which may be traumatic in origin but is more likely to be due to natural disease. Intracranial haemorrhage is discussed in detail in Chapter 11.

---

[5] This is often loosely known as 'vagal inhibition'—an abbreviation of 'vagal inhibition of the heart action'. The shorter term is unfortunate as the physiological principle involved is the opposite of that implied.

A review of the nervous system is incomplete without consideration of the special senses but such a discussion is beyond the scope of this volume. It is obvious that the loss of a special sense is of particular civil medico-legal importance and that, of these senses, vision is not only the most important but is also, perhaps, the most vulnerable. In addition to penetrating wounds, partial or complete loss of vision due to trauma can result from damage to the outer covering (*corneal abrasion*), to infection due to the presence of foreign bodies, to intraocular haemorrhage and to *retinal* detachment; *sympathetic ophthalmia* is a particularly distressing situation in which the other eye may lose its function 'in sympathy' with one that is damaged. Internally, the *optic nerve* may be damaged in association with fractures of the skull and, finally, blindness may result from damage to the occipital lobe of the cerebral cortex where the centres for vision are located—falls on the back of the head are, therefore, important in regard to vision. The importance of the eyes as a *cause* of death due to accidents—particularly vehicular—requires no emphasis.

The gastrointestinal system

The function of the gastrointestinal system is to accept food, digest it, store it, circulate it to the tissues in a form that provides a ready source of energy and to excrete unused residues. The whole process is controlled by a complex system of enzymes (*see below*).

The *alimentary canal* starts at the mouth and leads into the straight *oesophagus* which traverses the length of the thorax. The oesophagus opens into the *stomach* which, in turn, empties into the *duodenum* or first part of the small intestine. The *jejunum* and *ileum* form the second and third parts of the small intestine which is about 6 m (20 ft) in length and closely coiled within the abdomen. The large intestine consists of the *caecum* and its attached *vermiform appendix;* the ascending, transverse, descending and sigmoid *colon;* and the *rectum* which opens to the exterior at the *anus*.

The *peritoneum* lines the abdominal cavity and invests the small and large intestines. The envelope of peritoneum that is attached to the posterior abdominal wall and from which the small intestine is suspended is known as the *mesentery* and the major blood vessels lie within this. Tissues that lie posteriorly in the abdomen behind the mesentery are said to be *retroperitoneal* in position.

Constituents of food absorbed from the bowel are passed to the *liver* where they are both processed and stored. The liver is the largest organ in the body and occupies the upper right quadrant in the abdomen. It has numerous functions including the metabolism of carbohydrates, fats and proteins; the storage of a readily available source of energy (glycogen); the processing of waste material derived from breakdown of body tissue; the preparation of many of the substances essential for blood clotting; and the formation of bile which is stored in the *gall bladder* and passed into the intestine where it assists in digestion. Failure to secrete bile or to excrete it into the bowel shows itself as *jaundice*.

Ferments from the *pancreas* are also essential to digestion; this organ lies in the posterior part of the abdomen and empties its secretion into the duodenum.

The forensic importance of the gastrointestinal system is very great. The majority of poisons that are administered homicidally must be given by mouth; it follows that the primary symptoms of poisoning are commonly gastric or intestinal in nature and the early diagnosis of this form of crime depends greatly on the skill of the family doctor (*see* Chapter 22). The liver itself is also very sensitive to poisonous substances many of which are industrial in nature; jaundice is, therefore, an important sign of poisoning at work. The function of the liver may also be greatly impaired by infection of the organ—when the condition of *hepatitis* is established. A proportion of these cases result from the 'hepatitis B virus' which is transmitted from the blood of infected persons; the significance of the condition in blood transfusion is discussed in Chapter 31[6].

The results of trauma to the bowel may be very serious. The contents of the bowel may be irritant—as in the stomach—or they may be heavily contaminated by bacteria—as in the large bowel. In either case, rupture of the viscus will result in severe damage to the abdominal cavity and death may follow due to shock (*see* page 353); stab wounds and gunshot wounds of the abdomen thus require urgent surgical treatment. The hollow organs are also sensitive to explosive blast, particularly if this is transmitted through water. The bowel itself is surprisingly resistant to blunt, non-penetrating trauma, but both the intestine and its mesentery can be ruptured when massive force is applied from outside over a limited area; the single lap-belt type of restraint used in some motor cars and light aircraft is a modern means of transmitting such forces during a crash.

The sheer bulk of the liver increases its susceptibility to penetrating injury but it is at its most vulnerable in crushing accidents or in conditions that set up severe vibrations in the body, such as falls from a height.

The pancreas, on the other hand, is well protected and is only occasionally injured. The organ is, however, prone to damage by disease in alcoholics and degenerative changes are found when cold injury occurs in the undernourished.

The urinary system

When considering the respiratory system, the body was compared to a furnace; following the same analogy, a mechanism for waste disposal or removal of the ashes is essential if the organism is not to be poisoned. Gaseous products of combustion are eliminated in the breath but soluble waste products circulating in the plasma of the blood are excreted in the urine, which is prepared and voided through the urinary system (*see Figure 2.3*).

This consists of a pair of *kidneys*, placed posteriorly in the abdomen with their upper portions covered by the lower ribs, from which pass a pair of tubes, the *ureters*. Each ureter drains into the *bladder*, a muscular reservoir whose outflow is protected by sphincters. Urine which is stored in the bladder is passed to the outside of the body through a single pipe—the *urethra*. The urethra in the female is short; in the male it is long and assumes a serpentine shape as it passes through the *prostate* gland and the *penis*.

The kidneys play a major part in the regulation of the body's biochemical status and have two further roles in the maintenance of health. First, as indicated above, there is the elimination of waste products. The primary mechanism of clearance is pressure filtration through a vast network of blood capillaries. Secondly, it follows that any disease of the kidneys will have a profound general effect on the

---

[6] It used also to be transmitted during mass immunization procedures but, nowadays, the reuse of unsterilized needles for this purpose would be unacceptable.

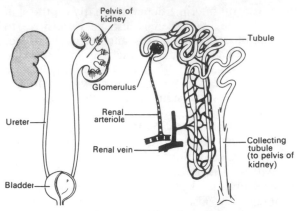

Figure 2.3 The anatomy of the urinary system. (*a*) Macroscopic structure. (*b*) Microscopic appearance of a nephron. Note that the blood supplies the tubule after it has passed through the glomerulus.

cardiovascular system; the most common adverse result is a raised blood pressure—the condition of *hypertension*. Disturbance of the blood pressure may, indeed, be the cause of death from a primary disease that started in the kidney tissues.

The excretory function with which this section is most concerned is based on the individual excretory units, the *nephrons,* each of which consists of a *glomerulus* and a system of *tubules*. A glomerulus, of which there are approximately 2 million, is essentially a skein of blood capillaries enclosed in a capsule. The wall of the capillary acts as a semipermeable membrane—semipermeable because it will allow the passage of water and small dissolved particles but will retain particles of large molecular size, especially proteins. Filtration pressure, aided perhaps by diffusion, results in the appearance with the capsular space of what is effectively protein-free blood plasma. This contains not only waste products but also materials that are of value or even essential to the body, notably glucose and sodium; moreover, the body cannot lose all its water. Some sort of selective concentration is needed.

This is the role of the tubules which, from the functional aspect, can be divided into proximal and distal portions. The glucose, sodium and much of the essential water are reabsorbed in the former while complex reactions designed to regulate the degree of acidity of the blood take place in the latter. The distal tubules run into collecting tubules which act as tributaries to the ureters. The importance of clearly distinguishing between the glomeruli and the tubules is that the function of the latter is active and requires the use of much energy. They are, therefore, very dependent on an effective blood supply and, since the vessels to the tubules have already supplied the needs of the glomeruli, conditions at tubular level are ripe for the development of an 'energy crisis'; any condition that interferes with the free delivery of oxygen to the tissues will affect the renal tubules with particular severity.

Abnormal conditions that damage the glomeruli differ markedly from those affecting the tubules and, while the former have comparatively little medico-legal significance other than in respect of treatment, they illustrate some important principles of pathology that have widespread implications and which might well be considered at this point.

Immunity

The body has a remarkable capacity to recognize strange materials within its substance and, save in exceptional circumstances, will defend itself against invasion. The defence mechanism is referred to as an *immune reaction* and the foreign substance that precipitates it is known as an *antigen*. The immune reaction may be of two types: 1, humoral—this involves the formation of circulating antibodies which react specifically with antigens and can generally be demonstrated to do so in the laboratory; 2, cellular—in which the body musters forces of migrant cells which will actively attack and either destroy or eliminate the intruder.

A major result of antigenic challenge is to stimulate the body's powers of recollection. Thus, the first intrusion causes comparatively gradual recognition followed by reaction. The pattern of the foreign substance is remembered, the templates of antibody production are retained and a second attack can be met by the immediate mobilization of reserves. Repeated stimuli result in increasing immunity. Normally, this system is entirely to the body's advantage—it forms the basis, for example, of vaccination against various infectious diseases. Occasionally, however, the body may fail to distinguish between self and non-self, with disastrous consequences; this occurs in two basic ways. The first mechanism is incompletely understood but, possibly because of abnormal position rather than abnormal constitution, the body reacts against its own tissues without any stimulus from outside. This constitutes *auto-immune disease* and need not be considered further. As to the second form, it must be appreciated that antigens are molecular in nature and that any organized biological particle contains a number of antigens; individual antigens may, therefore, be common to substances of dissimilar nature. Once having recognized an antigen, the body will react to it similarly irrespective of mode of presentation. As an analogy, the body might remember being attacked by a villain armed with a willow bough; it will react violently and defensively to a subsequent friendly offer of a cricket bat.

Such a direct error of identification may occasionally result in severe disease of the glomeruli. Additionally, however, *immune complexes* are formed when a foreign antigen stimulates and combines with an antibody. These immune complexes—often associated with the *streptococcus* which causes sore throats—may become deposited on the glomerular capillary walls and establish a secondary reaction. The subsequent damage to the capillary walls and the efforts of the glomeruli to remove the deposited material result in *glomerulonephritis*, a diffuse condition in which all the glomeruli are equally at risk. Fortunately, in most cases the glomeruli return to normal and clinical recovery is the rule. Occasionally, however, the disease progresses and, after a variable time, the kidneys cease to function. Medico-legally, the importance is that treatment then depends on replacement by machine or transplant and this important subject is discussed later.

Frequently, in the less acute cases, the functional integrity of the glomerular filtration membrane is compromised and, as a result, the body protein is lost steadily into the urine—the condition known as the nephrotic syndrome. Few of the causes of this condition have forensic interest but it may be associated with certain medical treatments, particularly by drugs containing heavy metals.

Acute renal failure[7]

In contrast with conditions affecting the glomeruli, extraglomerular disease of the

[7] The condition is often referred to as 'renal tubular necrosis'. Recent research, however, indicates that this may be a misnomer.

nephrons is a common complication of unnatural disease and is of special medico-legal interest.

Shock as defined medically is discussed on page 353. Essentially it results in inadequate oxygenation of the tissues. The condition may arise from blood loss which, in turn, may be due either to bleeding or to destruction of the blood (haemolysis) within the body. Haemolysis may result from inherent enzyme deficiency diseases, autoimmune diseases, infection of the blood cells as in malaria or, occasionally, from the inadvertent precipitation of an immune reaction, the most obvious example of which is a mismatched blood transfusion. Oxygen lack may be induced during anaesthesia (see Chapter 31). Reduction of the plasma component of the blood may follow burning, severe surgical trauma or unusual conditions such as crushing of the muscles or subatmospheric decompression.

Acute renal failure may accompany any of these conditions. The medico-legal significance of this condition is twofold—first, nearly all the basic causes are unnatural and, secondly, the condition is in many cases recoverable provided that some mechanism can be substituted for the kidneys during a period of recuperation. This substitution treatment is known as haemodialysis, or 'the artificial kidney', in which the blood is diverted to a man-made membrane simulating the glomerulus. Passage of dissolved substances from the blood across this membrane can be controlled by altering their concentration in the 'bath' fluid which takes the place of the filtrate in the glomerular capsule—in effect an 'osmotic gradient' can be established for any constituent of the plasma.

Sometimes, the kidneys fail to recuperate (treatment is notoriously difficult when the condition has been precipitated by burning) and haemodialysis carries hazards of its own including the increasing possibility of blood transfusion reactions and cross-infection between staff and patients—especially by the agent responsible for infective hepatitis. Generally, however, treatment is successful after a finite number of sessions.

By contrast, dialysis used for the treatment of glomerular death must be continued throughout life. This process involves sustained and regular occupation of machines which are unlikely ever to be available in numbers adequate for the needs. It is also expensive in bed space and nursing manpower so that the tendency is to encourage home dialysis treatment despite the attendant difficulties associated with asepsis and like problems. Decisions as to treatment must involve socio-economic considerations and the treatment of chronic renal failure is a good example of the modern doctor's inability to treat many of his patients on purely medical criteria; much must nowadays be a compromise with external factors. Habits and opinions change but, at the time of writing, many physicians would regard haemodialysis for irrecoverable kidney failure as an ideal treatment only while awaiting transplantation (see Chapter 12).

Both the glomeruli and the tubules may be involved in inflammation resulting from infection ascending from the bladder; this important subject is referred to later in this section.

Injury to the urinary system

The kidneys lie posteriorly in the body and are comparatively well protected by large muscle masses; they also lie in a good shock-absorbing bed of fatty tissue. Laceration by indirect trauma is, therefore, comparatively rare and the kidneys are not often torn in fatal accidents that inflict severe damage to other solid organs such as the liver and spleen. None the less, damage to the kidneys is surprisingly frequent in non-fatal automobile accidents—a situation probably associated with the great vascularity of the organs and consequent severe bleeding as a result of compression.

The kidneys are also prone to injury during violent attack. They are common targets in assaults by kicking—in which case very severe internal injury may be present in the absence of obvious external damage—and they may be involved in knifings. It is fortunate that the body can function perfectly well with only one normal kidney.

The ureters are well protected from external injury but, as they pass into the pelvis, they come close to the female generative organs; they are therefore at risk when the latter are subjected to surgical operation. The error of tying the ureters during gynaecological operations is well known and may occasionally be very difficult to avoid in the presence of widespread chronic inflammation.

The bladder in both male and female is closely associated with the bones of the pelvis. Fracture of the pelvis—which results from a variety of accidents, such as those associated with transportation, falls from a height, crushing, etc.—is commonly accompanied by rupture of the bladder or of the urethra. Both these injuries are treatable by surgery but often the condition of the casualty dictates a delay in operation. The possibility is then raised of ascending infection of the urinary tract with consequent involvement of the kidneys as discussed below.

Bladder disorders of medico-legal importance

The bladder itself is under control of the autonomic nervous system and the muscle is generally in a state of relaxation; distension results in reflex contraction and expulsion of urine. Autonomic urination is prevented by additional control of the external sphincter through the voluntary nervous system.

Since the nerve supply to the bladder sphincter originates in the lower part of the spinal cord, any injuries of the cord are likely to upset the capacity to control the act of micturition—the organ will revert to automatic action. Apart from the social inconvenience, the stage is then set for ascending infection of the urinary tract and it is not uncommon for the life of a paraplegic to terminate years after the spinal injury as a result of inflammatory destruction of the kidneys.

The different shape of the urethra in the male and female has a profound effect on the establishment of infection in the bladder. Thus, in the female, it is not difficult for organisms on the skin of the external genitalia to pass in retrograde fashion to the bladder, while the inherent laxity of the perineum predisposes to prolapse and inefficient emptying of the viscus. Inflammation of that organ (*cystitis*) is, therefore, common in women. The male urethra, by contrast, can protect the bladder from external invasion relatively well but the prostate gland is subject to enlargement of either a benign or cancerous nature. Obstruction to the flow of urine due to prostatism is a common accompaniment of later middle age; the resultant 'back pressure' may have serious effects on the kidneys themselves while the stagnation of urine induced is, as in the female, conducive to the establishment of infection; the process may be accelerated by the need to pass catheters into the distended organ.

Stagnation of urine leads to its prolonged contact with the inner wall of the bladder. Injurious substances that are excreted in the urine might be expected, therefore, to strike selectively at the bladder and this is indeed the case. Some hydrocarbons are active in the production of epithelial cancer (carcinoma) which may arise as a result of occupation (*see* Chapter 22).

Infection of the kidney

It is convenient to complete this section by returning to the kidneys themselves with a comment on inflammation due to infection. In the end, infection of the kidney probably results in as much glomerular destruction as does primary glomerular disease and, in contrast to the latter, inflammatory disease has considerable direct medico-legal significance. Thus, anything that facilitates the introduction of, or encourages the growth of, organisms within the bladder—including injury, surgery or simple instrumentation—may ultimately lead to severe disability or even to death.

The reproductive system

The male reproductive system consists of the twin *testes* which usually descend into the *scrotum* just before birth. The organs are formed of coiled tubules in which the *spermatozoa* mature. A spermatozoon consists of a head (approximately 4 μm in length), a neck and a tail which is some 50 μm long. When stained, the head shows a typical dark nucleus at its base, an appearance that is quite characteristic even when the tail is lost. Some 400–500 million spermatozoa are shed with a normal ejaculation. The bulk of the seminal fluid is derived from the *epididymis,* one of which lies close to each testis; together they drain into the *vas deferens.* The vas deferens on each side opens into the *urethra* at the base of the bladder. Other small glands contribute to the total seminal ejaculate.

The female reproductive organs consist first of two *ovaries* which lie on each side of the pelvis. Each ovary has a finite store of *ova* which is greatly in excess of the requirements for the maturation each month—between the onset of menstruation and the menopause—of, normally, a single egg. The ovaries on each side are connected to the *uterus* by the *Fallopian tubes* down which the ova pass. There is a potential space between the ovary and the receptor end of the tube; occasionally, ova are fertilized and yet do not reach the uterus, in which case the dangerous condition of *ectopic pregnancy* is established. The outlet of the uterus is a tightly closed canal surrounded by the *cervix* which juts into the *vagina.* The vagina opens through the *vulva.* In the virgin state, the vaginal opening is protected by the *hymen,* a sheet of fibrous tissue with, usually, a small opening which will permit the passage of normal secretions. The size of the hymenal opening varies—it may be large originally or it may be dilated by tampons or masturbation. In general, however, the size is such that the first penetration by the penis results in laceration which is usually posterior in position; the distinction between the virginal hymen and one showing old or recent rupture is of obvious importance in accusations of rape. The vulva consists, internally, of paired *labia minora* which join anteriorly and posteriorly as commissures. The posterior commisure is known as the *fourchette;* this again is likely to be damaged during forceful intercourse and during childbirth. The *labia majora* lie outermost; they are joined in front at the *mons veneris* but posteriorly dissolve into the tissues of the perineum.

Spermatozoa injected into the vagina make their way into the uterus or tubes where they may meet a mature ovum; the ovum is fertilized by penetration by the spermatozoon. An unfertilized ovum will die in some 2 days but the fertilized ovum implants itself on the uterine wall and begins to divide. After some 3 months' development, a *placenta* forms which is attached to the developing fetus by the *umbilical* cord. The fetus is surrounded by a fibrous sac known as the *amnion* and floats in the *amniotic fluid*.

The birth process is started by contractions of the uterus and dilatation of the cervix, usually with rupture of the amnion. If the placenta becomes detached, the fetus will die and be expelled as a foreign body; it will be similarly rejected should the fetus itself die. Unnatural dilatation of the cervical canal will, of itself, cause the uterus to contract. Any of these situations can be simulated in order to procure abortion (*see* Chapter 19).

The endocrine system

The body contains a number of glands that discharge 'hormones' into the bloodstream. These hormones have specific actions on various parts of the body; overproduction or failure of the 'endocrine' glands can, therefore, result in disease or dysfunction of the target organs.

There are seven different glands secreting some 30 hormones which are commonly likened to an orchestra. The 'conductor' of the orchestra is the *pituitary* gland which lies in the base of the skull. The pituitary stimulates activity in many of the other glands but is itself sensitive to circulating hormones; once sufficient hormones are present in the blood, this servomechanism inhibits further stimulation. In addition to its supervisory function over the other glands, the pituitary itself controls growth, the secretion of urine and the contraction of the uterus during childbirth. Damage to the pituitary gland is, therefore, a very serious matter; it is a common result of fracture of the base of the skull and the gland may be damaged by the effects of haemorrhage after complicated childbirth.

The remainder of the endocrine glands, while vital to health, are of little medico-legal significance, but, as the names will certainly appear in autopsy reports, a brief description is given.

The *thyroid* gland lies in the neck and is responsible for mental and physical growth in childhood and for the general rate of metabolism in the adult body— deficiency of thyroid hormone leads to cold and apathy, excess results in production of heat and hyperexcitability. The position of the thyroid renders it susceptible to bruising which may be of considerable evidential value in strangulation.

The *parathyroid* glands are small and closely associated anatomically with the thyroid. They control the distribution of calcium, as between the bones and the body as a whole.

The *adrenal* glands lie against the kidneys and are of immense importance to the body. Their central parts secrete *adrenalin* which affects the tone of the blood vessels and also the heart rate; its action is similar to that of the sympathetic nervous system. Adrenalin is secreted in response to sudden stress and, in effect, brings the body to a fighting trim in response to alarm. When given therapeutically, it has profound effects on the blood pressure and blood distribution; these must be considered in relation to death associated with surgical operations. The outer parts of the adrenal glands control the salt and water balance of the body, exert an effect on the metabolism of carbohydrates, influence the sex glands and are very much concerned with the response of the body to infection or other conditions resulting in inflammation. Large doses of adrenal hormones are used to suppress the immune response that underlies the rejection of transplanted organs (*see* Chapter 12).

The *pancreas* secretes the hormone *insulin*, absence of which causes the disease *diabetes* in which the storage of carbohydrate is inhibited and the blood contains large amounts of sugar. The converse situation, *hypoglycaemia*, results from an excess of insulin. This is a rare natural condition but is an obvious hazard of the treatment of diabetes; hypoglycaemia can be fatal and insulin has been used as a refined method of homicide. Hypoglycaemia may occur spontaneously in sensitive persons independently of insulin secretion; the syndrome closely simulates alcoholism and was a not uncommonly successful defence to motoring charges prior to the enactment of the Road Safety Act 1967.

The *testes* and the *ovaries* secrete hormones which, in the former, are concerned with the secondary sex characteristics and physique of maleness and, in the latter, with the control of menstruation and pregnancy. Perhaps their main medico-legal connotation is in the use of sex hormones in competitive sport (*see* Chapter 16).

The musculoskeletal system

This system consists of the bony skeleton (*see Figure 2.4*) to which the muscle masses are attached often through the medium of tendons. These muscles, which can be activated at will, are known as *voluntary* muscles (or *striated* muscles, because of their appearance under the microscope). Many organs—for example, the bladder or bowel—are equipped with muscle that is not under conscious control and is therefore known as *involuntary* or, from its microscopic appearance, *smooth* muscle; such muscle is, however, an integral part of the system with which it is associated. Where bones articulate with one another in joints, the surfaces are covered with cartilage; cartilage is also formed at bony junctions when some mobility is needed—the prime example being the junctions betweeen the breast bone and the ribs.

The *skull* is divided simply into the vault, which covers the brain, and the base on which the brain rests—on each side the base forms the anterior, middle and posterior *fossae* or cavities in which are accommodated the lobes of the brain (*see Figure 2.5*). The skull rests on the spine which is formed of a number of individual vertebrae; the uppermost is known as the *atlas* bone. The atlas and six small vertebrae form the *cervical* spine or neck; below this are 12 *thoracic* vertebrae with which the ribs articulate posteriorly; five large vertebrae lying in the small of the back form the *lumbar* spine and below this are the fused vertebrae of the *sacrum* which makes up the rear wall of the pelvic cavity; the tail of the primates is represented by the small *coccyx*. The sacrum joins the two *pelvic* bones posteriorly; anteriorly the pelves are united by a cartilaginous band known as the *symphysis pubis* which is often split in severe accidents.

The front of the chest is protected by the solid breast bone or *sternum* which is, again, a common casualty of accidental trauma. The shoulder girdle is formed by the *scapulae* or shoulder blades posteriorly and the *clavicles* or collar bones anteriorly. The *humerus* articulates with these to form the shoulder joint and, at the elbow, forms a joint with the two bones of the forearm—the *ulna* and the

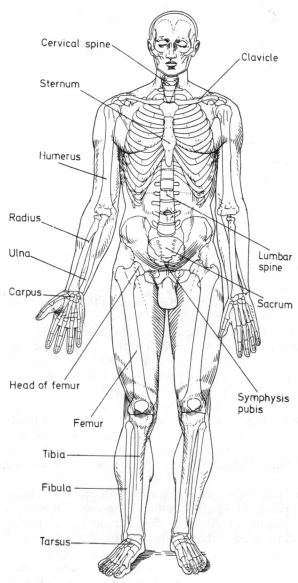

Cervical spine

Clavicle

Sternum

Humerus

Radius

Ulna

Carpus

Lumbar
spine

Sacrum

Head of femur

Symphysis
pubis

Femur

Tibia

Fibula

Tarsus

Figure 2.4 The major relationships of the human skeleton. (From an
original diagram by Professor G. J. Romanes.)

radius which is on the thumb side. The bones of the wrist are collectively known as
the *carpus,* those of the hand as the *metacarpals* and those of the fingers the
phalanges; the knuckles may, therefore, be either metacarpophalangeal or
interphalangeal joints.

The thigh bone or *femur* has its large circular head embedded in the *acetabulum*
of the pelvis. The hips must be wide in order to accommodate the massive leg
muscles and the first part of the femur—known as the neck—must therefore adopt
a relatively horizontal position before joining the main thigh bone at an obtuse

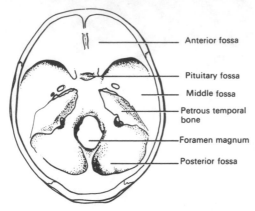

Anterior fossa

Pituitary fossa

Middle fossa

Petrous temporal
bone

Foramen magnum

Posterior fossa

Figure 2.5 The inner surface of the base of the skull.
The frontal lobes rest in the anterior fossae, the
temporal lobes in the middle fossae and the
cerebellum lies in the posterior fossae. The spinal
cord passes through the foramen magnum.

angle which approximates, as will be seen later, to a right angle in the female. The
neck of the femur is therefore a mechanically weak point and is of great forensic
importance owing to the ease with which it can be accidentally broken in elderly
women whose bones are becoming brittle; the condition then requires either
prolonged bed-rest or the surgical insertion of a pin before the broken ends will
reunite—conditions are ripe for death from hypostatic pneumonia or from
pulmonary embolism (*see* pages 11 and 71)[8]. The femur articulates at the knee
joints with the large *tibia*, which lies medially in the lower leg, and with the slender
fibula which lies laterally. Unlike the bones of the forearm, the bones of the lower
leg cannot cross over—the foot cannot be pronated or supinated as can the hand.
The bones of the ankle are known as the *tarsus* and contain two particularly large
individual bones—the *talus* and the *calcaneus*. The foot contains the *metatarsals*
and the toes the *phalanges*.

The voluntary muscles are rarely described individually in post-mortem reports
and need not be detailed at this point. Paralysis of individual muscles may be of
great importance in relation to claims for compensation but, in those circumstances, far more information will be needed than could be provided in a book of
this size.

The importance of fractures in virtually all aspects of forensic medicine is clear.
Apart from their frequency in violence, they are demonstrable and readily
presentable by means of X-rays (*see* Chapter 27), they can be 'dated' and many are
of specific type; fractures are therefore discussed in regard to special situations
throughout this book.

Otherwise, the major forensic significance of the skeletal system lies in its
relationship to the identification of an unknown body.

The bones of the body consist of calcium salts deposited in an organized fashion
in a protein medium. Calcification and the laying down of bone in soft connective

[8] The application of the modern operation of total hip replacement to increasingly elderly patients has
greatly modified the outcome of such an injury.

tissue begin in *centres of ossification* which are demonstrable visually and by X-ray at different times in individual bones. Although there is considerable biological variation, ossification centres are generally established in a regular order and with reasonable constancy so that their assessment can give a fair guide to the age of a fetus or young infant—it is only in these age groups that such early development is progressing.

Centres of ossification in the long bones are generally multiple and at least triple—one centre appearing in the shaft or *diaphysis* and one at each end or *epiphysis*. These must fuse in order to form adult bone and, again, this process is one of some regularity which extends throughout childhood and adolescence.

The individual bones of the skull unite in older age. This feature is, however, extremely variable.

The skeleton also gives considerable evidence as to sex. The bones of the female are, in general, less robust than are those of the male and the ridges formed where muscles and tendons are attached are less massive. Certain bones give particular indications of sex and, amongst these, the pelvis is pre-eminent, being designed to allow the passage of the fetus in the female. Other bones—notably the thigh bone and the skull—show particular sex differences, but the appearances are not always easy to interpret; the advice of a skilled anatomist will be found very valuable in all aspects of the identification of skeletal remains.

This is particularly true when estimating stature in life from the findings in one or two bones. The number of formulae which have been devised for this purpose testifies to the difficulties involved—whichever figures are used, allowance must be made for drying of the bone, for the age of the subject and for race.

The application of the principles outlined above is further described in Chapter 3.

Biochemistry of the body*

The cell is the basic building block of the body; the human body may consist of up to 5×10^{12} cells. To remain alive, each cell must manufacture energy from a series of chemical reactions that take place within the cytoplasm and are controlled by its nucleus. The sum total of these diverse chemical reactions taking place within a cell is known as cell metabolism and biochemistry defines and describes the nature of metabolism. The fuel for the metabolic process comes from ingested food, which consists of proteins, carbohydrates and fats; these are themselves composed of varying combinations of molecules of carbon, hydrogen and oxygen, with lesser amounts of nitrogen, phosphorus and sulphur. Energy is obtained and stored during the process of breaking down these compounds to carbon dioxide and water. This process requires a constant supply of oxygen (aerobic metabolism) although an alternative pathway (anaerobic metabolism) provides lesser amounts of energy for a limited time where oxygen is lacking. The energy thus provided has two main purposes—the maintenance of equilibrium and the manufacture of new material.

The metabolic processes are conducted in a fluid medium which is an aqueous solution containing chemicals that exist as electrically charged particles known as *electrolytes* or *ions*. The most important chemicals, in addition to hydrogen and

* This section on biochemistry is by T. J. Anderson, MB, PhD, MRCPath.

oxygen, are sodium, potassium, chloride, calcium, phosphate, sulphate and bicarbonate. However, there is a difference in chemical composition between the fluid which is intracellular and that which is extracellular. To function properly, cells must sustain a difference across the membrane of the cell surface such that the fluid inside is more concentrated than that on the outside. This is effected principally by the constant pumping out of water and sodium, with a resultant perpetual requirement for energy. It is also necessary to ensure an environment within and around the cells that is neither acidic nor alkaline but is neutral as valued in units of pH[9].

The second use for energy is in the acceleration of the chemical reactions of a constructive nature. The cell is in a constant state of turnover and not only must it keep manufacturing new components to replace those lost or broken down, but it may also have a specific function to store and release compounds. Many and complex components are utilized in the formation of the ultrastructure of the cell, for there are numerous membrane-bound organelles—such as *mitochondria* and *lysosomes*—in its cytoplasm. These membranes are composed of proteins, sugars and fats that are assembled together in as yet poorly-understood ways. The most important, and also the simplest, components, which are in fact often attached to these membranes, are *enzymes*. Enzymes are proteins having the property to accelerate chemical reactions and each cell must manufacture enzymes to accelerate the chemical pathways not only essential to maintain life but also for which it is particularly specialized (or differentiated). Regulation of the specific qualities and quantity of such enzymes is determined by information contained in the genes of the chromosomes. Errors in this information may occur, resulting in faults in or absence of particular enzymes, and these errors may be transmitted to succeeding generations via the chromosomes of the sex cells. Diseases due to such enzyme abnormalities are termed *inborn errors of metabolism*.

It is important to realize that interference in enzyme functions within cells is directly responsible for the lethal effects of ingestion or inhalation of many poisons such as cyanide, arsenic and mercury. In the case of cyanide the enzymes of the mitochondria are inactivated with subsequent blockage of oxygen transfer for metabolic processes.

Other factors that influence the activity of enzymes are temperature, pH and, perhaps most importantly, the presence of specific substances in trace amounts. This last group are termed 'essential *co-factors*' and may be simple chemicals such as magnesium or zinc, or may be more complex molecules known as *vitamins*. The vitamins, which are designated alphabetically, are either fat soluble (A, D, E and K) or water soluble (B, C) and are essential constituents of the diet.

While it is convenient to consider the biochemistry of the body at a cellular level, it is important to appreciate that an equilibrium must be maintained within and between the body fluid compartments, defined as intracellular, extracellular and vascular. For example, the concentration in the blood of glucose and calcium must be carefully monitored to remain within upper and lower limits. The endocrine system is principally responsible for controlling this balance, and achieves it by the elaboration of specific *hormones* in the cells of this system. These hormones are secreted into the blood to be carried to distant tissues where they affect the functions of specific 'target' cells. The release of these hormones is in turn

---

[9] pH is a logarithmic notation of hydrogen ion concentration in a solution, with 7 representing neutrality. Acid solutions have a pH less than 7, and alkaline solutions have a pH greater than 7.

regulated by the level of the target-cell product in the vascular compartment. This 'feedback' control exists to maintain normal biochemical values. The function of individual hormones has been described above (page 21).

Another factor in the maintenance of biochemical equilibrium is the requirement to replace the water and electrolyte loss that occurs continuously (and often insensibly) in urine, faeces and perspiration. Situations in which this replacement assumes critical significance arise in the surgical patient who requires intravenous fluid therapy because of inability to receive or retain any food or fluid by mouth over a sustained period. Provision of this balance is further complicated by the change in general body metabolism that takes place in response to trauma, of which surgical intervention represents a more planned form. A distinct alteration in the nature of metabolic processes, to become destructive (catabolic) as opposed to constructive (anabolic), results in loss of important nutriments, electrolytes and water. These changes are hormonally induced and constitute a reaction to stress—the so-called preparation for fight or flight. The observed decrease in body temperature in the period after trauma provides a further index of the profound alteration in body metabolism.

2

Comparative medico-legal systems

All countries have developed methods of primary inquiry into sudden or unnatural death. The major systems from which these derive can be described in the simplest way as the English, or Coroner, System and the (European) Continental System. The further distribution of these throughout the world largely follows the pattern of early colonial expansion. The Scottish Procurator Fiscal has absorbed points from both these systems; it is therefore convenient to leave discussion of his office until the others have been described.

The Coroner

The office of Coroner in England and Wales developed from the twelfth century, at which time the Coroner was largely responsible for supervising the material interests of the Crown in criminal cases. As these could well be affected by the status of the dead person and the precise conditions surrounding the death, the Coroner's office became intimately concerned with the overall investigation of suspicious deaths; the identity of the deceased was always fundamental, the Coroner had to view the body[1]—at the locus if possible—and inquests were held with juries. The financial connotations of sudden death gradually relaxed, or were diverted to other offices, and the position of the Coroner declined until it was revived in the Middle Ages. At that time, the Coroner's attention was specifically directed to the establishment or exclusion of criminality, a principle that persisted until the nineteenth century and that still motivates the Procurator Fiscal's office in Scotland.

It was not until 1860 that Coroners could fairly claim that they were free to act independently of outside influences, and the election of Coroners was abolished in 1888. The major legislation establishing the present system was the Coroners Act 1887 which stated (s. 3(1)):

> Where a Coroner is informed that the dead body of a person is lying within his jurisdiction, and there is reasonable cause to suspect that such person has died either a violent or an unnatural death, or has died a sudden death of which the cause is unknown, or has died in prison, or in such place or under such

[1] A duty only abolished under the Coroners Act 1980.

28

circumstances as to require an inquest in pursuance of any Act, the Coroner, whether the cause of death arose in his jurisdiction or not, shall, as soon as practicable, issue his warrant for summoning not less than 12 nor more than 23 good and lawful men to appear before him at a specified time and place, there to inquire as jurors touching the death of such person as aforesaid.

This compulsion to hold an inquiry with a jury was greatly modified by the Coroners (Amendment) Act 1926, which enabled a Coroner to look into certain types of death without recourse to open inquest. The 1926 Act also laid particular stress on the Coroner's function in establishing the causes of sudden natural death and reduced his responsibility for the investigation of homicide. This process has continued, still further restriction being imposed by the Criminal Law Act 1977, s.56. Similarly, the basic regulations governing the functions and *modus operandi* of the Coroner have been restated in the Coroners Rules 1984[2]. Amongst other restrictions, neither the Coroner nor his jury may now make recommendations designed to prevent a recurrence of the conditions leading to the inquest (r.36 (2))[3].

A Coroner is appointed under the Local Government Act 1972. He must be medically or legally qualified and be of at least 5 years standing in his profession; he is independent of the Government and is solely responsible for his actions—only the High Court can give him instructions. Many of the more controversial aspects of his office have been gradually whittled away although the requirement to hold his inquiries in public remains.

A general duty rests on 'any person about the deceased' to inform the Coroner of circumstances that indicate the need for an inquiry. Otherwise, there is no statutory obligation on a doctor to report a death directly to the Coroner although, in practice, he commonly does so when he judges it necessary[4]. The duty by regulation to do so is vested primarily in the Registrar of Deaths[5]. In brief, the circumstances in which he must refuse to register a death without reference to the Coroner include:

1. When no medical certificate of death is available because there was no doctor in attendance during the last illness.
2. When the certifying doctor states he has neither seen the body after death nor attended the deceased within 14 days prior to death.
3. If the cause of death is in doubt.
4. All deaths that were unnatural, were due to or associated with accident, violence or neglect, were due to any form of poisoning, which includes alcohol, or that were in any way suspicious.
5. Deaths occurring during an operation or before recovery from the effects of an anaesthetic.
6. Deaths associated with industrial disease or poisoning.

The only other statutory duty to report directly to the Coroner is imposed on Governors of Prisons, Borstals, Detention Centres and other similar institutions.

---

[2] S.I. 1984/552.
[3] But the Coroner may still report a matter of concern to an appropriate authority at any time during or after his inquiries (Coroners Rules 1984, rule 43).
[4] The Medical Protection Society has drawn up a list of circumstances in which the doctor concerned is advised to inform the Coroner as soon as possible; this is reproduced in Appendix B.
[5] Registration of Births, Deaths and Marriages Regulations 1968, Regulation 51 (S.I. 1968/2049).

On being informed of a case that he considers to be within his jurisdiction, the Coroner has certain options open to him. He can decide that no further action is called for; in this case, he notifies the Registrar to accept the certificate of death granted by the medical practitioner. He can order a post-mortem dissection and, if he decides as a result of this that no further investigation is required, he himself may certify the cause of death as indicated by the autopsy; this Coroner's certificate invalidates any previous medical certificate as to the cause of death. In any other circumstances, he may hold an inquest and he must do so when death was due to any unnatural event. As a result of the Criminal Law Act 1977, s.56 (2), an inquest must be held with a jury only when it is suspected that death:

1. Occurred in a prison or in such circumstances as to require an inquest under any Act other than the Coroners Act 1887.
2. Was due to an accident, poisoning or disease that must be notified to any Government department or an Inspector approved under s.19 of the Health and Safety at Work etc. Act 1974.
3. Occurred in circumstances, the continuance of or possible recurrence of which is likely to be prejudicial to the public.
4. Occurred when the deceased was in police custody, or resulted from an injury caused by a police officer in the purported execution of his duty[6a].

Condition 3 is obviously open to interpretation, but it would seem that the governing principle is that the case should be put before a jury if a recurrence could be prevented or safeguarded against as a result of action taken by some authority[6]. The 1977 Act does not preclude the Coroner from summoning a jury in the case of a road-traffic accident if he thinks it necessary, but he is very greatly restricted in a case of murder, manslaughter, infanticide, causing death by reckless driving or suicide in which there may have been abettment. In these cases, the Coroner must accede to a request from the chief officer of police to adjourn his inquest; the Coroner need not resume the inquest after the relevant criminal proceedings but, if he does so, the finding of his inquest must not be inconsistent with the outcome of those proceedings. No Coroner's verdict may be framed in such a way as suggests criminal or civil liability on the part of a named person and, in the event of evidence of unlawful killing coming to light during the inquest, the case must be adjourned and the Director of Public Prosecutions must be given the necessary details.

A list of conclusions open to the Coroner's inquest is given in Appendix C. Subsequently, the Coroner provides the registrar with a certificate after inquest which includes the circumstantial as well as the medical causes of death. Statements signed by both the witness and the Coroner are known as depositions and can be used in subsequent legal proceedings, provided that they were taken in the presence of the person who is accused at any later criminal trial.

The Committee on Death Certification and Coroners headed by Judge Brodrick have made it abundantly clear that, in their judgment, it is the accurate certification of the cause of death that has become the most important function of the Coroner: 'Today (1971) the role of the Coroner as an investigator of crimes against the person has become a relatively insignificant one'[7]. This view has been underpinned by the recent legislation. In practice, while very nearly a quarter of all deaths occurring in England and Wales are dealt with by the Coroners Service, natural disease accounts for at least 80 per cent of the cases currently examined by Coroners' pathologists. For the Northern Ireland coroner's system see page 38.

[6] R. v. H.M. Coroner for Hammersmith, ex parte B. Peach (No. 1) [1980] 2 W.L.R. 496.
[6a] Administration of Justice Act 1982, s.62.
[7] Report of the Committee on Death Certification and Coroners (1971). Cmnd. 4810, p.130. London; HMSO.

The system in Europe[8]

It is impossible to generalize about the comparable systems in Continental Europe, because the procedures for investigating sudden and unexpected death vary not only from country to country but also within national boundaries.

A legal code based on Roman Law operates in many States, and as a result the medico-legal system is almost expressly designed to obviate the need for post-mortem dissection. In general, deaths that are due to violence or that cannot be certified are reported to the police, who are often represented by a lawyer—the *procureur, magistratura*, etc. A selected doctor—comparable with the British police surgeon—is called upon to make an external examination, the purpose of which is to exclude the possibility of criminality; further action is improbable once this has been achieved.

If the case is a serious one, the responsible Judge—e.g. *juge d'instruction*, examining magistrate—appoints a qualified specialist in forensic medicine to make a further external examination, and as a result of this an internal autopsy may be authorized. The widespread establishment on the Continent of Medico-legal Institutes very often results in the provision of opinions that are backed by several individuals of high repute. The magistrate or his equivalent is normally responsible for certification of the cause of death in those cases falling within his disposal; in criminal cases this function is assumed by the higher court.

Interesting systems have developed in Scandinavia. There is no uniformity but the principles are based on direct co-operation between the police and specialized forensic pathologists (with the interposition of a public health officer in Denmark), the performance of autopsies by two doctors, reporting to the Court rather than to the prosecution or defence and the authority of a higher forensic medical body. One side effect is that forensic pathologists very rarely go to Court to give evidence, and if they do they are there as advisers to the Court rather than as witnesses for one or other side. The system has been perfected in Denmark, where medico-legal reports can be referred to the Medico-Legal Council at the request of the Court or of either side. The medical intricacies are then thrashed out by experts in private and the opinion of the Council is binding.

The Medical Examiner

The medico-legal system of many of the United States rests on the office of Medical Examiner. This has much in common with the European system, with the major difference that the investigation of sudden and suspicious deaths is the responsibility of a medical rather than a legal organization. Thus, a single medical man inspects the locus of death, decides the need for internal autopsy and, in many instances, performs the post-mortem dissection himself. Only when his inquiries are complete and these indicate the possibility of criminality does he notify the District Attorney of his findings although, in the meantime, a close liaison has been maintained with the police.

His powers of investigation are wide but his jurisdiction is very limited; two courses are open to him—he can either issue a death certificate and dispose of the case or refer the case to the prosecutor.

[8] An excellent extended review has been undertaken by Knight, B. (1977). Medico-legal systems in Europe. *Forensic Science*, **10**, 3–86.

The Procurator Fiscal

The office of the Procurator Fiscal in Scotland was not known until about the time of the Reformation other than in the Ecclesiastical Courts. The public Prosecutor, a concept clearly imported from France, first appeared in the Burghs in the middle of the sixteenth century and the practice of appointing such officials spread rapidly. The office was formally recognized as one of service to the Crown in 1746 and about a century later became financially independent of fines collected. Modern Procurators Fiscal are appointed by the Lord Advocate. Their function is to receive reports from the police of all crimes committed in their districts—and to direct the police in their task[9]; additionally, the Fiscal prepares the Crown case in criminal trials committed to the High Court and conducts the prosecution in the Sheriff Court. It follows that the Procurator Fiscal must be a lawyer and is very unlikely to be also medically qualified. For the purposes of this chapter, the main responsibility of the Fiscal is to investigate any sudden, violent, suspicious or accidental deaths or any other death that is reported to him. A list of reportable deaths is given in Appendix D[10]. Although some of the items on this list are clearly associated with public health or with the possibility of civil negligence, it remains true that the basic medico-legal function of the Fiscal is to exclude criminality; it is no part of his duty to establish the precise cause of death.

As in England and Wales, the statutory responsibility to report appropriate deaths to the Fiscal rests with the Registrar but, by common usage, most of his preliminary information stems from the police, medical practitioners or the next-of-kin, the last two often working through the medium of the first. The Fiscal will then call for a report from the 'sudden deaths' officer (a member of the police force) and from the Police Surgeon who will have examined the body externally; these reports will include information about the medical history of the dead person. If the Fiscal decides that no further inquiry is needed, he will invite the Police Surgeon to grant a death certificate; the system clearly operates very much more smoothly when there is a close working relationship between the Fiscal and his medical adviser.

Should the Fiscal decide, or should he accept the advice of the Police Surgeon, that a post-mortem dissection is required, he will seek the authority of the Sheriff giving one of the following reasons for so doing:

1. That his inquiries cannot be completed unless the cause of death is fully established.
2. That there are circumstances of suspicion.
3. That there are allegations of criminal conduct.
4. That death was associated with anaesthesia in connection with a surgical operation and the fact that all precautions were taken must be established.

The dissection is carried out by two doctors whenever the circumstances give grounds for suspicion or suggest the possibility that criminal proceedings may follow; it is only necessary for one pathologist to give evidence in Court[11]. After the autopsy, the Fiscal's pathologist may issue a death certificate.

All the Fiscal's inquiries are conducted in private. In the event that further

---

[9] Smith v. H.M.Adv. 1952 J.C.66 at pp.71–2.
[10] Registration of Births, Deaths and Marriages (Scotland) Act 1965, s.28.
[11] Criminal Justice (Scotland) Act 1980, s.26(7).

proceedings are likely he has the power to precognosce material witnesses. Precognition implies the private interrogation of witnesses which will amplify their preliminary statements and which will form the basis of the Fiscal's final report to Crown Counsel in whom is vested the ultimate decision as to what proceedings, if any, are to follow upon a death. In passing, it is worth observing that not every death reported to a Fiscal requires to be reported by him to Crown Counsel. Sudden deaths that, in the opinion of the Fiscal, are free from suspicion and certain other difficulties may be cleared by him upon his own responsibility; a list of those conditions that must be reported by him to Crown Counsel is given in Appendix E. Precognitions are informal and the evidence is not usually taken on oath, although it may be. The defence have a right to precognosce witnesses but they may have to call upon a witness to take the statement which he is under a duty to give to them. They can cite an unwilling witness to attend Court at a trial even though he or she failed to attend for precognition.

Outwith criminal proceedings—in which, it will be noted, privacy is maintained until the hearing in the definitive court[12]—the Fiscal's inquiries can be made public by way of the Fatal Accidents and Sudden Deaths Inquiry (Scotland) Act 1976.

Under s.1(1), the Procurator Fiscal for the district with which a death is most closely associated must apply to the Sheriff for the holding of a Public Inquiry under the Act when:

(a) (i) it appears that the death has resulted from an accident occurring in Scotland while the person who has died, being an employee, was in the course of his employment or, being an employer or self-employed, was engaged in his occupation as such; or
   (ii) the person who has died was, at the time of his death, in legal custody; or
(b) It appears to the Lord Advocate to be expedient in the public interest that an Inquiry under this Act should be held into the circumstances of the death on the ground that it was sudden, suspicious or unexplained, or has occurred in circumstances such as to give rise to serious public concern.

Public Inquiries are mandatory in respect of deaths detailed in s.1(1)(a) but it is entirely within the discretion of the Lord Advocate whether a Public Inquiry is held under paragraph (b); serious public concern might, for example, attend cases of alleged negligence in hospital, accidents involving public transport, etc. Any person with an interest may make representations to the Lord Advocate that an Inquiry should be held. Such representations will be considered but the Lord Advocate's decision is final. The Sheriff sits without a jury but an expert assessor may be appointed at the request of any properly interested party. No witness can be compelled to answer any question indicating that he is guilty of any crime or offence. The Sheriff determines as to when and where the accident and the death(s) took place, their cause or causes, the reasonable precautions that might have prevented the accident, any defects in the system of working that contributed to the accident and any other relevant facts. The determination of the Sheriff is not admissible in evidence in any judicial proceedings, of whatever nature, arising out of the accidental death. The Act applies to fatal accidents resulting from North Sea operations.

---

[12] This used to contrast with the procedure in England where much publicity arose as a result of the preliminary Magistrates' hearing. The situation has approached more closely to that applying in Scotland since the passing of the Criminal Justice Act 1967.

Systems in some parts of the Commonwealth

Australia*

In common with the majority of Commonwealth countries, Australia retains the Coroner as the primary medico-legal authority. However, the autonomy of the States and Territories is such that, while practices are very similar, there is no absolute uniformity[13]. Medico-legal autopsies are performed at varying rates which extend from the unusually high proportion of 30 per 10 000 population in the Northern Territory, through the fairly steady range of 12–15 which holds in Victoria, New South Wales, Australian Capital Territory, Queensland, Western Australia and Tasmania, to 10 per 10 000 population current in South Australia. The comparable rates in the United Kingdom are 25 in England and Wales and 5 per 10 000 population in Scotland.

In general, all stipendiary magistrates are Coroners *ex officio* for the whole of their respective State or Territory. The Governor or appropriate Minister of a State or Territory may appoint other persons to be Coroners or Deputy Coroners. Deputy Coroners often have limited jurisdiction or powers; Justices of the Peace may act as Coroners in remote areas and are then often restricted to ordering post-mortem examinations.

As in England and Wales, the Coroner's autopsy is considered part of the ordinary process of certifying the medical cause of death; death is certified on the basis of autopsy as being due to natural causes in approximately 70–80 per cent of Coroners' cases. A minimum of 70 per cent of cases reported to the Coroner are examined by internal dissection.

The Coroners' powers to dispense with Inquest are varied. Such a course is open in most States and Territories. Except for those deaths where it is provided by Statute that an inquest must be held, Coroners generally exercise their discretion in first directing post-mortem examinations without ordering an inquest and subsequently dispensing with an inquest if they think fit; in Queensland, the Coroner can only recommend to the Justice Department that an inquest is unnecessary if it would serve no useful purpose.

A Coroner almost invariably sits without a jury unless he is requested to do so by relatives or if it is a requirement of some other State or Territory Act that he does so. For example, in Western Australia, the Coroner must sit with a jury of three in the event of death being due to an accident in a factory or mine. There are no provisions for Coroners' Juries in Queensland, South Australia and the Territories.

In Victoria and the Australian Capital Territory, a Coroner may commit a person charged with murder, manslaughter, wilful fire and other similar indictable offences to stand trial before a Court of competent jurisdiction. In the other States of Australia, such committals may be carried out by a Coroner only when evidence taken at his Inquiry leads him to believe that such a crime has been committed. The Coroner will also adjourn his Inquiry until after the conclusion of the criminal proceedings if he is informed that such a charge is pending.

New Zealand†

Primary medico-legal responsibility rests with the Coroner, whose function is similar to

---

* Based on information kindly supplied by Dr J. I. Tonge, Dr V. Plueckhahn and Dr J. Hilton.

† From Cairns, F. J. (1974). Concerning forensic services in Australia and New Zealand. Presented at *The 26th Annual Meeting, New Zealand Society of Pathologists*, Auckland.

[13] The relevant statutes include: New South Wales—Coroners Act 1980; Victoria—Coroners Act 1958; Tasmania—Coroners Act 1978; South Australia—Coroners Act 1975; Western Australia—Coroners Acts 1920–1960; Northern Territory—Coroners Ordinance 1974–75; Queensland—The Coroners Act 1958–78; Australian Capital Territory—Coroners Ordinance 1956.

that of his English counterpart—that is, to decide who died, when and where and from what cause. He has no authority to commit for trial. The relevant statute is the Coroners Act 1951. The Justice Department has recommended that all autopsies for the Coroner should be carried out by specialist pathologists; while usually acceding to this, the Coroner may choose his own pathologist—an option that is generally subject to agreement with the police authority in cases of suspected homicide.

The proportion of autopsies performed on cases referred to the Coroner is similar to the high figure found in England. Public inquests can be dispensed with but the opportunity to do so is generally taken only when death has been shown by autopsy to be from natural causes. The situation in New Zealand therefore approximates very closely to current English practice—there is a firm commitment to establishing the precise cause of sudden death.

Canada*

The Federal Government of Canada has no overriding authority over the medico-legal system, which is established on a Provincial basis.

The Coroners' system operates in Ontario (The Coroners Act 1972) where there are a full-time Provincial Coroner and a Deputy Provincial Coroner who act in a supervisory capacity. Under them are Regional Coroners and each city and district has one or more Coroners; there are 380 Coroners in Ontario, all of whom are appointed. Medical qualification is a prerequisite for the position. The Coroner visits the scene of death and carries out a full investigation of all cases notified; as a result, an autopsy is requested in some 20 per cent of these. Inquests are, in some cases, mandatory—e.g. when death occurred in custody or was due to a mining or railway accident; otherwise, an Inquest may be ordered by the Coroner investigating the case or by the Chief Coroner. Inquests are heard by a jury and the bases for their being called are generally similar to those described under the Scottish Fatal Accident Act; the Coroner is generally motivated by a concern for public safety. The jury cannot make any finding of legal responsibility.

Alberta, by contrast, has created a Medical Examiners' system. The Chief Medical Examiner is based in Calgary and the Deputy Chief Examiner in Edmonton. Each Pathologist/Medical Examiner has a staff of part-time medically qualified assistants who function somewhat similarly to Coroners. Post-mortem dissections are carried out either by or on behalf of the Chief Medical Examiners in major hospitals. Inquiries are held into selected cases before a Provincial Judge. Somewhat similar systems operate in Manitoba and in Nova Scotia.

British Columbia and Saskatchewan still use lay Coroners who are assisted by trained investigators. There seems a probability that these Provinces will shortly alter their medico-legal systems to correspond to those operating either in Ontario or in Alberta.

The system in Quebec is rather less precise but is based on a form of coronial hierarchy served by a Government Medico-Legal Institute to which many of the more serious cases are directed. Understandably, there is an influence from the system that operates in Continental Europe.

* Based on information kindly supplied by Dr J. A. J. Ferris and Dr Margaret Milton.

The Far East*

Malaysia, Singapore and Hong Kong retain the Coroners' system but this has adapted pragmatically to prevailing circumstances.

The Coroners' system in Singapore can be taken as an example of practice in conditions of exceptionally high-density population. The Coroner is legally qualified and, as in England, his duty is to decide who died, when, where and from what cause. He has comparable status to a Magistrate and has power to commit for trial. All sudden, unexpected, unnatural, accidental, violent and cause-unknown deaths are reportable to the Coroner; in Singapore some 2200 cases are reported annually. The autopsy rate is 75 per cent giving a medico-legal autopsy rate of 7·5 per 10 000 population. The Coroner can dispense with a post-mortem examination if the cause of death is known to be natural, and in such cases, certification by a doctor is required; post-mortem examination will also often be waived in cases of suicide and in certain accidents of a domestic nature where the circumstances are clear. The Coroner can dispense with an inquest when death is due to natural causes, but in all other cases a Public Inquiry must be held unless the case is proceeding to the Criminal Court. In these circumstances there is a reversal of the usual findings in forensic practice—70 per cent of the autopsied cases disclose death to be due to unnatural causes with only 30 per cent due to natural disease. Although there are various religious and customary objections to post-mortem examination, the Coroner's ruling is final and binding.

Malaysia is, by contrast, a predominantly rural country. The primary medico-legal system operates less precisely, and in general the decision as to post-mortem examination rests with the investigating police officers; dissections are not carried out on cadavers of persons of the Muslim faith.

Sri Lanka and India†

The medico-legal system of the Indian subcontinent largely reflects the contents of the original Indian penal code, compiled by Lord Macaulay. The first recorded list of Coroners was published in 1844; the Sri Lankan penal code dates from 1883.

The investigation of sudden death in Sri Lanka centres around an Inquirer (known in the principal towns as a Coroner) who is appointed by the Minister for Justice; Inquirers appointed for the main towns are usually qualified either in law or in medicine. The Inquirer is assisted by the police and, when necessary, by a medical officer. The law requires that anyone who knows of a sudden, unnatural or suspicious death must report it to a police officer; a magistrate must be informed if a person dies in custody or in a mental or leprosy hospital.

The Inquirer may call upon a qualified medical officer (not necessarily a Judicial Medical Officer) to perform an autopsy and may summon witnesses to give evidence upon oath. The Coroner's Court is public but there is no jury. The Inquirer's report is forwarded to a Magistrate or, in case of homicide, to the Director of Public Prosecutions.

In India, the Coroners' system operates only in Bombay; the Coroners' Courts function with a jury. Elsewhere, the inquiry into an accidental or unnatural death is conducted by a senior police officer in the presence of two respected citizens of the area who subsequently sign the report. The report, known as Panchnama,

* Based on information kindly supplied by Professor Chao Tzee Cheng.
† Based on information kindly provided by Professor N. Kodagoda.

embodies the significant findings at the scene, the external appearances of the body and the apparent cause of death. An autopsy by a medical officer is requested in cases of doubt or suspicion. Deaths in prison or while in police custody are subject to a Magisterial Inquiry (Coroner's Inquiry in Bombay).

In both Sri Lanka and India, the Medical Officer—who, outside the large towns, usually undertakes medico-legal duties as part of a more general commitment— may also be called upon to report to the police on non-fatal injuries sustained. He thus combines the roles of Coroner's pathologist and police surgeon, the system being very similar to that obtaining in Scotland.

An analysis of the various systems

Although the reader will have formed his own opinions, it is not out of place to present a brief review of the advantages and disadvantages of the systems described. Before doing so, a cause of some confusion must be removed. Much unfounded suspicion of the Coroners' system is based on the nature of this office in the United States. In practice, the office of Coroner in the USA has little more than nominal similarity with that in the English system, the Coroner in the United States being generally elected or a political appointee. He is often unqualified either medically or legally and there is considerable basis for distrust of the system; but this is no reason for extrapolating that the English Coroner would be better replaced by a Medical Examiner.

Perhaps the most frequently raised valid criticism of the system in England and Wales relates to the publicity given to many cases which are of no public concern. The increasing use of the dispensation given in the 1926 Act has done much to dispel this objection but, nevertheless, there are instances—of which suicides are the most prominent—in which much unnecessary distress must be given to relatives. Privacy, on the other hand, is dependent on the qualities of those acting within its protective ramparts; all the other systems described will be effective only if there is public confidence in the officials concerned—perhaps this is most evident in the case of the Medical Examiner. At the same time, these systems have an inbuilt protective mechanism in that, unlike the Coroner who is solely responsible for his actions, all other comparable officials are subject to an immediate higher authority. The system whereby two doctors must attest to the autopsy findings in serious cases, which exists in Scotland, the USA (under the Medical Examiner system) and in many European countries, undoubtedly enhances the quality of the medical evidence, and nullifies many of the arguments in favour of publicity.

The true function of the primary medico-legal system is currently receiving much attention[14]. The undoubted trend towards the role of adjusting the records of the Registrar, which is evident in England, leads to a very high autopsy rate with a potential limitation in standards. The rigid interpretation of the Fiscal's function to exclude criminality would, on the other hand, lead to undue constriction of the pathological service and, in practice, a wider spectrum of sudden death is examined by dissection; even after selection by external examination, natural disease accounts for some 55 per cent of deaths in which a Fiscal's autopsy is performed— from about 5 per cent of the total deaths in Scotland.

At present however, it seems that neither system ideally meets its function of eradicating conditions that operate against the public interest. The power of the Coroner's Court in this respect is now almost nominal. There is greater scope in

[14] See for example, Mason, J. K. (1983) Coroners from across the border. *Medicine, Science and the Law*, **23**, 271.

Scotland under the 1976 Act but this avenue of life-saving propaganda is used surprisingly seldom. For example, some 800 road deaths occur annually in Scotland, yet such deaths are rarely the subject of a Public Inquiry.

I do not agree with the Brodrick Committee in its attempts to overwhelm the Coroners' service still further with diagnostic autopsies, many of which would, if undertaken, be more beneficially routed through academic departments of morbid anatomy. The Fiscals' service strikes a good balance between available resources and value to the public, although support to community health might be still further improved by greater use of the Public Inquiry.

It is difficult to complete this section without drawing attention to the great attractions of Scandinavian practice, particularly as regards the presentation of expert medical evidence in the higher courts. The acceptance of a wholly objective assessment by a superior medical authority eliminates the sometimes unhappy suggestion of partisanship on the part of witnesses; of perhaps greater importance, it ensures that expert evidence is treated as a whole, and unwitting omissions which may compromise justice are avoided[15].

Northern Ireland*

Northern Ireland has a Coroner's system but it differs from that in England in a few important respects. The coroners operate under the Coroner's Act (Northern Ireland) 1959 and the Rules made thereunder. Coroners are appointed by the Lord Chancellor in England and they have to be practising solicitors; the coroner for Greater Belfast is full-time but the other six coroners are part-time. The cases coming within their jurisdiction are clearly stated in s.7 of the Act:

> Every medical practitioner, registrar of deaths or funeral undertaker and every occupier of a house or mobile dwelling and every person in charge of any institution or premises in which a deceased person was residing, who has reason to believe that the deceased person died, either directly or indirectly, as a result of violence or misadventure or by unfair means, or as a result of negligence or misconduct or malpractice on the part of others, or from any cause other than natural illness or disease for which he had been seen and treated by a registered medical practitioner within twenty-eight days prior to his death, or in such circumstances as may require investigation (including death as the result of the administration of an anaesthetic), shall immediately notify the coroner within whose district the body of such deceased person is of the facts and circumstances relating to the death.

This section also places a duty on a number of people, including doctors, to report these deaths to the coroner and the doctor's duty in this regard is reinforced by the legislation governing death certification which requires a doctor to complete a death certificate *only* when he has seen and treated the deceased for the fatal illness within 28 days of death, knows the cause of death and knows it to be entirely natural. In all other circumstances the coroner must be informed and no death certificate must be issued.

The coroner's functions are similar to those of his English counterpart. Section 8 of the Act provides for the involvement of the local police in the investigation of the circumstances of the death. A police officer carrying out this duty is thus acting as a coroner's officer. Also, the Government provides a full-time forensic pathology service with four forensically-trained pathologists to assist the coroners in these investigations. About 1400 coroner's autopsies are carried out annually. This service and its counterpart dealing with forensic science are provided to coroners without charge.

[15] Blom-Cooper, L. (1981). A miscarriage of justice—English style. *Medico-Legal Journal*, **49**, 98. *See also* the opinion delivered by Emslie, L.J.-G. in Preece v. H.M. Adv. [1981] Crim. L.R. 783.
    * A note kindly contributed by Professor T. K. Marshall.

3

Identification of the dead and of remains

The problem of identification of the dead arises in two ways which require rather different methods of solution. First, there is the identification of the single unknown body. The most difficult situation is provided by the body that is discovered in some place unrelated to habitation—the classic example being the body discovered in a wood or a shallow grave. Such subjects may well have died by criminal means and are commonly decomposed. It is likely that no immediate clues to identity will be available and the problem will therefore be one of deductive identification—fitting a name to a body. If, on the other hand, a body is discovered in a house, there is, at least, a possibility that it is a cadaver of a person associated with that house and, in the initial stages, the identification team can work from that premise. The problem is then the much simpler one of fitting a body to a name; only when the probable names have been excluded does one have to revert to the random situation.

The second type of identification problem relates to conditions resulting from a major disaster. Even here, the subject is not quite homogeneous—the identification of a large number of victims of a flood is likely to be more difficult than in the case of a train accident which, in turn, may well be more complex than is the air disaster, in which an accurate list of those presumed killed is usually available. In all such cases, crime is the exception and—other than in aircraft accidents, when extensive mutiltation and burning is likely—the bodies will probably be found in a reasonably preserved condition; at least some clues as to likely identity will be to hand and, in particular, circumstantial evidence in the form of clothing, documents, jewellery and the like may well be available. Identification in the mass is a matter of fitting a number of bodies to a number of names known with varying certainty.

These categories will certainly overlap but, for descriptive purposes, it is convenient to discuss primary characteristics, comparative methods and circum-stantial means of identification and to relate these to the random body, to the single body of likely identity and to the mass disaster.

The purposes of identification

Excluding such philosophical concepts as the right of every free-born person to an identity after death, which has been implied from the United Nations Declaration of Human Rights, identification of a dead body is needed, in the first place, in the field of criminal investigation; the chances of apprehending a criminal are greatly increased once the identity of the victim has been established. Secondly, many important procedures in the civil field—e.g. grant of probate, resolving of partnerships and the general administration of estates—depend upon accurate identification; failure in this respect may result in a delay of up to 7 years before death can be presumed. In disasters of an explosive nature, the process of identification might well have to be limited to establishing the total number of deaths—this may be the only way in which the standard period required for presumptions of death may be acceptably shortened. Thirdly, there are purely social reasons for assigning a correct name to a dead body—many people have an understandable affection for the remains of their next-of-kin and certain religions have strict and conflicting rules as to the disposal of the dead. Finally, accurate identification of the fatal casualties and correlation of their injuries with their environment in transportation accidents—particularly those involving airlines— may greatly assist the accident investigation authorities, either in relation to the cause of the accident or as to the prevention of fatal injury in the future.

Identification of the single unknown body

Proof that the remains are human

Surprising as it may seem, mistakes as to the human or animal origin of skeletonized remains are not uncommon at first assessment. At least one murder investigation has been mounted because a bear's paw was mistaken for a human hand, and bones are often referred to forensic departments suspected as being the remains of human infants but which are, in fact, derived from middens. Such errors are, however, generally corrected rapidly: in case of doubt, the opinion of a specialist anatomist should always be sought and be backed, if necessary, by a veterinary or zoological appraisal.

A more difficult situation arises when only soft tissues or unidentifiable bones are available; it may then be necessary to invoke immunological evidence. All tissues of animal species, including humans, contain antigens (*see* page 17) which are more or less specific to that species[1]. Artificial antibodies may be prepared to these antigens which can thereby be identified in the laboratory. The commonest method is to precipitate the antigen/antibody complex and, for this reason, the test is often referred to as a 'precipitin test', the details of which are not needed here. A similar technique is used in the preliminary study of blood and other biological stains (*see* Chapter 18).

Determination of sex

It may be difficult to establish the sex of a body by cursory superficial examination even in the absence of severe burning or putrefaction. In a case investigated by the author, 2 hours was allowed for the examination of 114 coffins primarily to establish the total number of dead; despite the observations of three pathologists, it was found that, while the total number was correct when compared with the manifest, the division of males and females was still not accurate. Unisex fashions

---

[1] There may be some cross-reaction between closely related species but this is of little practical importance in human forensic medicine.

in hairstyle and clothing contribute to the difficulty and problems may arise from congenital deformities of the genitalia. Such difficulties are, however, unlikely to be serious in single bodies other than in those that are severely damaged.

Early putrefaction and burning short of combustion may actually accentuate secondary sexual characteristics—particularly the size of the breasts. On the other hand, severe burning, putrefaction and the ravages of animals may destroy the genital region. The sex can then generally be determined by the finding of either a uterus in the female or a prostate gland in the male; these organs are among those most resistant to putrefaction in the body. In the event of complete skeletonization, the sex of the dead person can be derived, with varying degrees of certainty, from a study of the total skeleton or from individual bones. Many bones show *comparative* differences between male and female but the pelvis very often provides definitive indications of sex (*see Figure 3.1*).

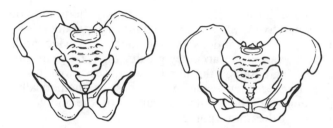

Figure 3.1 The pelvic bones of the male (left) and the female (right).

There are many sophisticated measurements that can be made to this end but, for present purposes, only a general summary is needed—the female pelvis is wider and squatter, with a far straighter sacrum, than is found in the male; the dorsal surface of the pubic bone also becomes pitted during childbirth. An accuracy of 95 per cent or more is claimed for the determination of sex from the pelvis. The wide hips of the female dictate a more acute angle between the neck and shaft of the femur than is needed in the male in order to bring the knees together; the thigh bone is perhaps the most valuable of the long bones that may be available for sexing—provided the ethnic origin is known, an accuracy of some 80 per cent can be obtained. Sex differences are also notable in the skull which is one of the bony specimens most frequently presented to forensic departments. The features that are sought include the round orbits and more vertical forehead of the female; the greater surface area of the mastoid process in the male; and the prominent supraorbital or eyebrow ridges that are a feature of masculinity.

Determination of age

In the presence of putrefaction or burning, a superficial examination can result in gross error as to the age of a cadaver; objective parameters are needed. The condition of any remaining organs may provide these but again, the skeleton can give very useful clues. The significant findings in the bones depend to a large extent on the age group; it is convenient to consider the fetus and neonate, the adolescent, and the adult as separate categories.

The fetus and neonate

Objective evidence of age at this stage is to be obtained from the development of the bones and, in particular, from the presence of certain centres of ossification; these have been described on page 25 and a representative list is given in Appendix F. The most important centres are those that distinguish the legally viable (28-week pregnancy) and the full-term fetus (*see* Chapter 19 for details). Although it is simple to demonstrate these centres at autopsy, the most objective, and permanent, record is obtained by the routine radiological examination of unidentified fetuses. Anomalous appearances occur in individual centres but, at this stage of development, the *overall* picture can produce an accuracy of ±1 month.

In childhood and adolescence

Up to the age of 20, the most useful information on age is given by the joining of the epiphyses to their shafts (Appendix G). Although such unions generally follow in a definite chronological order, the variations in individuals are wide and, certainly when using a single observation, an accuracy greater than ±2 years can rarely be claimed. The accuracy increases as the number of observations made increases and numerous attempts have been made to sum these mathematically, allowance being made for 'weighting' the relative accuracy of the individual observations. Such problems are for the anthropologists.

Adult life

After the age of 20, the ageing of an unknown body becomes progressively more difficult. The sutures of the skull close in adult life but, apart from the interfrontal suture, union does not commence until approximately the age of 35 and, even then, the findings are subject to wide variation. It is extremely doubtful if it is possible to age the skeletal remains of an adult to closer than within one decade.

Other gradual changes associated with use, such as the angle of the jaw bone, occur as part of the natural process of ageing; the presence of disease states either in remaining soft tissues or in the bones may give general indications of age but only within very wide limits.

Ageing from the teeth

In the experience of nearly all observers, the most valuable indication of age from infancy to adulthood can be obtained from the teeth and it is in this field that the greatest advances have been made. The subject is discussed in detail in the section on forensic odontology (Chapter 29).

Determination of stature

The determination of the stature in life from post-mortem remains is fraught with difficulty. Even if the whole cadaver is available, a direct measurement has its own inaccuracy as the body in life measures some 2.5 cm (1 in) less than the body when dead. There is also the complication of age. After the age of 30, the natural processes of senile degeneration are said to result in an average decrease in stature of something of the order of 0.6 mm (¹⁄₄₀ in) per year.

It follows that mathematical formulae designed to assess the *in-vivo* stature from limited remains must be treated with reserve. Moreover, the exact height of an individual during life is available only rarely—far more likely, only a subjective assessment or, at best, a fairly rough measurement will be forthcoming.

The bones of the lower limb provide the best evidence, and the more bones that are examined, the narrower will be the range within which is put the final estimate of living height. Taking everything into consideration it is doubtful whether an accuracy of greater than within 2.5 cm can ever be achieved by studying individual bones and this may represent considerable overconfidence; the interested reader is referred to specialized monographs[2]. Simple calculations are probably best used in practice. A useful rule of thumb is that the humerus (arm bone) is 20 per cent, the femur (thigh bone) 27 per cent and the tibia (lower leg bone) 22 per cent of the subject's height in life. The spine, if available, is some 35 per cent and the distance between the outstretched fingertips approximates to the total height.

The use of comparative methods

The problem of allotting a body to a probable name is very much simpler because information concerning many characteristics individual to the presumed person is likely to be available. The matter is then one of comparing these with the findings in the cadaver. It is not necessary to discuss here such obvious characteristics as colour of hair or eyes, save to point out that these may alter considerably *post mortem*. The forensic medical practitioner will, however, be much concerned with the provision of medical information in relation to identity.

Medical information

Recognizable disease states, evidence of past surgical procedures, deformities and tattoos can be included under this general heading.

The value of the past medical history depends on the nature of the information. Thus, a history of cardiac pain in a missing person is relatively useless as damage to the heart muscle is discovered at post-mortem examination in a very high proportion of persons beyond middle age. A history of gall bladder disease might, on the other hand, be much more significant. A combination of evidence—e.g. severe arthritis of the spine together with disease of the thyroid gland—will provide far greater probability of identification than would be suggested from the sum of the diseases present in the population as single entities.

Similar considerations apply to surgical procedures. A history of removal of the appendix is unhelpful; partial removal of the female genitalia is less common but would certainly be insufficient evidence by itself on which to base an identification. Each case requires individual assessment as to significance and, again, a combination of surgical procedures may provide virtually incontrovertible evidence of identification. The presence of surgical prostheses—particularly if X-ray or other in-life records are available for comparison—may provide evidence that would satisfy even the most sceptical. Old fractures, which can also be compared by X-ray, can be very useful.

[2] Of which the classic is Krogman, W. M. (1962). *The Human Skeleton in Forensic Medicine;* Springfield, Ill; Thomas.

Deformities may also be common or rare. They may be congenital—that is, present from birth—or acquired. Very often, they provide little more than confirmatory evidence of identification made on other grounds.

Tattoos present some interesting problems in identification. First, it has been pointed out that many tattoos are of standardized pattern and the presence, say, of a heart pierced by an arrow cannot be regarded as proof of identification. Secondly, the investigator must be wary of descriptions of tattoos; what may be a clear illustration to one party may be quite differently interpreted by another. It is, however, fair to say that so long as an adequate description of tattoos in life is available—particularly in the form of photographs—they may provide excellent evidence of identification. It is of practical importance that, although tattoos may be superficially obscured by the carbonization of burning, scrubbing of the area may reveal an easily identifiable pattern in the deeper tissues.

Personal identification

Two methods of positive, personal identification are outstanding—fingerprinting and dental comparison.

The science of dactylography or fingerprinting is one for the expert and is outside the province of this book. Indeed, for present purposes, fingerprints have a limited use in identification since permanent records[3] are available in the United Kingdom only for criminals and merchant seamen. The main value of fingerprints in the identification of a body from the general population depends on the ability to compare the prints from the cadaver with those on the personal possessions of the supposed person. The more personal the possessions, the more certain becomes the identification. The preservation of heel or sole prints in those who are at risk of sudden death with mutilation—e.g. airline crews—is probably of more practical value, and less emotive, than is the taking of fingerprints, as the feet are commonly preserved from burning by boots or shoes.

The importance of dental identification is becoming increasingly recognized, particularly as dental records are available for a very high proportion of a population served by a National Health Service. The methods involved in and the limitation of dental identification are discussed in Chapter 29. It is enough to say here that the method is wholly dependent on the quality of record-keeping by practitioners and that the certainty of identification increases in almost geometrical progression with the number of positive correlations present; ultimately, a comparison of ante- and post-mortem charts may be as personalized a method of identification as is a fingerprint. A comparison of X-rays taken before and after death may provide incontrovertible evidence of identification. *Table 3.1* indicates some relative merits and demerits of dactylography and odontology in identification.

Identification in a major disaster

The identification of a large number of casualties presents problems that are mainly organizational and that are, in other respects, dictated by the nature of the disaster. It may be that the subjects are well preserved but that there is little knowledge of their origin, as may occur in a rail accident; they may be relatively unclothed and severely carbonized, as in a hotel fire. The aircraft accident is, perhaps, the least

[3] Fingerprints taken in the course of a criminal investigation must be destroyed if there is no conviction (Police and Criminal Evidence Act 1984, s.64).

TABLE 3.1 Some advantages and disadvantages of dactylography and odontology as methods of identification (*see also* Chapter 29)

TEETH	FINGERPRINTS
Fire resistant	Destroyed by fire
Durable	Subject to putrefaction
Records readily available	Limited recording
'Compatible inconsistencies' due to incomplete charting	Unchanging
No acknowledged criteria of proof	Well-established criteria
Useless without records	Possible value of personal possessions in absence of records
Comparative dental X-rays are as personalized as are comparative fingerprints	

uncommon form of mass disaster and, by virtue of its unforeseeable and varied location, is certainly likely to present the most urgent difficulties in identification. The aircraft accident can be taken as a model for mass disaster investigation so long as it is appreciated that there are certain unique features involved. Great differences are likely even within the category of aircraft accident—thus, one accident may present as a problem of disintegration while another may approximate to a mass cremation.

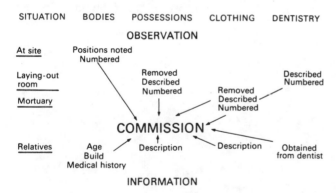

Figure 3.2 Diagrammatic representation of the identification commission established for a major disaster. Sources of observations and information are shown. The importance of numbering the bodies—and of maintaining a single set of numbers—is emphasized.

The secret of accurate, rapid identification of mass casualties lies in the organization. The essential is to establish a 'commission of identification' which, on the one hand, is receiving information about missing persons and, on the other, is being advised of observations on the dead bodies from various sources. The scheme is illustrated in *Figure 3.2*. Standardized documentation that can be completed easily is essential; the disaster victim identification form introduced by the International Criminal Police Organization has been criticized on many counts, and alternative forms, which have been recommended by the International Civil

Aviation Organisation, are used by the Accident Investigation Branch of the United Kingdom Department of Trade[4]. Whatever forms are used, the process of identification is essentially one of sorting through numerous 'information' files and attempting to 'marry' these to 'observation' files.

The main difference between identification in the mass and identification of the single unknown body lies in the enforced use in the former of much circumstantial evidence. Thus, a large amount of preliminary or 'primary' identification is done on the basis of documents carried, recognizable jewellery and clothing; jewellery, being fire resistant, is especially valuable in this context.

The use of such evidence requires much care—it is, for example, essential to ensure that possessions attributed to a given body in the furore of cadaver retrieval were, in fact, incontrovertibly associated with that body. Vagaries such as exchange of tickets and the widespread use of chain-store clothing must be accepted as potential hazards and it is important that any circumstantial evidence should be confirmed by an alternative method, preferably one involving 'personal' identification. Of these, dental evidence is of outstanding importance; medical evidence, particularly if it is of an unusual nature, has a significant part to play.

Visual identification, the standard 'personal' method of many police forces, is highly suspect in the context of a mass disaster. Not only may recognizable peculiarities be erased or mimicked but the observers are often under such emotional stress that they are particularly prone to unwitting error. It is generally far better to present next-of-kin with a maximum of three bodies, ideally already identified by other means, when subjecting them to the ordeal or recognition. In practice, the enforcement of visual identification would be inhumane in the majority of aircraft disasters.

[4] The use of these forms has been well described by Stevens, P. J. (1973), in *Modern Trends in Forensic Medicine—3*. Ed. by A. K. Mant; London; Butterworths.

4

Post-mortem changes and the timing of death

For present purposes, death is defined as the irreversible failure of the cardio-vascular system. Functioning heart and blood vessels are essential for the transport of oxygen, without which the body tissues must die; on the other hand, the heart may continue to beat and nourish the tissues despite the presence of irrecoverable damage to the central nervous system—the judicial hangings of the past were examples of such action. For these reasons, the cardiovascular system provides the most useful index of true life or death; the concept of 'brain-stem death' arises only in relation to artificial survival and is considered in Chapter 12.

The main practical function of the doctor called to the locus of an unexplained death is to decide whether death has taken place; other considerations must take second place. This decision may be difficult in the event of grossly diminished cardiac output—as may occur in hypothermia or in drug-induced central depression of the vital functions. But some form of heart activity, even if demonstrable only by special techniques, is always present when death is apparent rather than real.

The changes that occur after death can be deduced from the functions of the cardiovascular system. The cessation of oxygen transfer results in cellular death. Those components of the cell that are most sensitive to hypoxia—the enzyme systems—will be first affected. After a variable period of residual activity, energy production ceases and the body cools. Blood which has been circulating is now stagnant and settles under the influence of gravity. There is a final attempt at metabolism in an environment increasingly deprived of oxygen and waste products accumulate where they are formed; the ground substance of the body degenerates and the individual cells lose cohesiveness. In the absence of an effective bloodstream, the body is defenceless, and bacteria, whether derived from within or without the corpse, are left to multiply at the expense of the tissues—the process of putrefaction is set in train and may be augmented by the flesh-eating larvae of various flies. The process of skeletonization may be hastened by carnivorous animals and, ultimately, the skeleton itself may crumble to chalky dust. These changes can be used to estimate the time of death.

The timing of death

The first 24 hours

It is only within the first 12–18 hours that any reasonable accuracy can be expected as to the time of death. Even then, it is important that the basic inaccuracies inherent in any biological phenomenon are appreciated.

The estimate of the time elapsed during the first 12 hours after death is based mainly upon the body temperature. Theoretically, this temperature falls according to a sigmoid curve; numerous attempts have been made to liken the body to an experimental cylinder to which the laws of physics can be applied without reservation. However, no matter how many variables are introduced into a mathematical calculation, accuracy cannot be guaranteed in a practical situation.

Factors that must influence the rate of cooling include:

1. The body *temperature* at the time of death. Conditions that tend to raise the temperature at the time of death—for example, infection or cerebral haemor-rhage—will result in an artificially short estimate of the post-mortem interval based on temperature recordings; hypothermic and algid states will produce the opposite effect.
2. *Clothing*. The rate of fall in body temperature of a reasonably clothed body is approximately two-thirds that of a naked one.
3. *Body insulation*. A fat body is better insulated against heat loss compared with a lean one, while those with a large surface area in relation to the body weight will cool faster than will those of more massive physique; thus children and the aged will always cool faster than will well-nourished adults;
4. *Convection currents*. A body will cool faster in the presence of moving air than does one in a closed environment. The effect may be considerable.
5. The *environmental temperature* is a variable that will always affect the rate of cooling, but the time taken for the body to reach either a high or a low ambient temperature is the same because the rate of fall will be correspondingly slow or fast.

The practical difficulties in using temperature as a measure of the time elapsed since death are illustrated in *Figure 4.1*. While it might be possible to compute a formula that would accommodate the measurable variables, no such formula could take into account variations whose extent is unknown—e.g. the effects of moving the body before measuring the temperature, changes in environmental tempera-ture and the action of draughts. It is better that a relatively simple approach be adopted and its limitations freely admitted. A method is described by Knight[1] in which the temperature at death is assumed to be 37 °C and the difference between this figure and that recorded by a rectal thermometer is the degree of cooling observed. The degree of cooling is then multiplied by 1, 1¼, 1½, 1¾ or 2, according to an air temperature of 0 °, 5 °, 10 °, 15 ° or 20 °C respectively; the resultant figure is taken as the time in hours elapsed since death. In my experience, the rigid application of this method tends to exaggerate the length of the post-mortem interval. It is simpler, though more subjective, to accept an average fall in temperature of 1 °C per hour. The resultant 'time' is then modified by personal assessment of the conditions at the *locus* of death. In practice, it is surprising how the variables may cancel each other out—a person in a cold room will wear more clothes which may themselves mitigate the effects of draughts, etc. It is abundantly clear that the practical results are a long way from the accuracy of detective fiction

[1] Knight, B. (1982). *Legal Aspects of Medical Practice*. 3rd edn., p. 119. Edinburgh; Churchill Livingstone. Knight now questions the validity of this formula (personal communication).

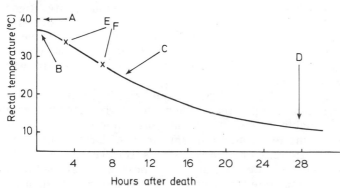

Figure 4.1 The uncertainties in the post-mortem body temperature. A = The deceased's temperature in life; B = The isothermic stage, greatly dependent upon the body's insulation; C = The rate of fall which is influenced by the environmental conditions; D = The room temperature. In the event, two readings taken at E and F and extrapolated to 37 °C will give as accurate a result as is likely to be obtained.

and can achieve no more than a 'bracket of probability' representing ± 1 hour of the actual time of death—and the more remote that time is, the more optimistic does such an evaluation become. Greater confidence is gained if it is possible to make repeated readings at the scene, particularly if the body has been dead for less than 10 hours—it is then possible to extrapolate backwards using the straightest part of the temperature curve. It is everywhere agreed that temperature measurement loses all meaning once the temperature of the body has decreased by 85 per cent of its original difference from that of the environment.

These considerations apply to bodies found on land. As expected, cooling of the body is more rapid in cold water although, here again, much will depend on the quantity and the flow of the medium.

1–3 days

As the enzymatic processes of the body fail, so too does the elimination of waste products. The tissues of the body become altered in consistency and the most prominent representation of this is the phenomenon of *rigor mortis*. Biochemically, this is associated with a massive increase in the lactic acid content of muscle; clinically, the resultant stiffening and shortening of the muscle fibres presents as a fixation of the joints which can be broken down only by force.

Rigor results from reduction of the chemical constituent of the muscles known as adenosine triphosphate. The stiffening of the muscles commences when the level of this substance is reduced to 85 per cent of the normal but the process is not demonstrable clinically until some time has passed. All muscle fibres are affected but stiffening will be demonstrable earliest in those bundles of smallest mass; joints supplied by very large muscle groups will be affected the slowest.

In theory, therefore, one would expect the muscles of the face to be the first to demonstrate rigor. The larger muscles would then become involved, the arms appearing stiff before the knees and hips. In practice however, this order is not always maintained. The condition is apparent some 5–7 hours after death and is usually established throughout the body in 8–12 hours. The muscles remain in rigor until the processes of degeneration and putrefaction cause secondary laxity. Rigor has been observed to disappear clinically in much the same anatomical order as it became established but, again, the process is variable. The body is generally free of rigor some 36 hours after death, but it is by no means uncommon for the condition to persist for 4 days. Relating the degree of rigidity to the body temperature will help to indicate the phase of the rigor 'cycle'.

Theoretically, the degree of distribution of rigor should give a useful indication of the time elapsed since death but, in practice, a phenomenon that depends upon biological processes is inevitably capricious in its presentation. Its onset is accelerated in conditions leading to an ante-mortem excess of lactic acid in the tissues including, in particular, exercise or a pyrexial illness. It will come on slowly, if at all, in persons whose muscle is degenerate, as in those who have suffered wasting illnesses. Children demonstrate the phenomenon far less readily than do adults and it is to some extent dependent upon the ambient temperature, being accelerated in the summer months and retarded in the winter. Probably, the best that can be hoped for from a consideration of rigor mortis is a 'time of death' at the centre of a bracket of probability extending over some 6–12 hours—and this only over a very limited total period.

Certain conditions simulate rigor mortis but are easily distinguished. The most common of these is cold stiffening; a body that has been placed in the refrigerator is virtually beyond assessment as to rigor. At the other end of the scale, intense heat will result in shrinkage and stiffening of the muscles; but the effects of the heat will be readily seen on the skin. Cadaveric spasm deserves a mention. This is a contraction of the muscles which is probably mediated by the central nervous system when death occurs in conditions of high emotional tension; it is instantaneous and permanent until putrefaction occurs. The most common manifestation is seen in the hands which may be found grasping some object, particularly one that gives some hope of support. Cadaveric spasm may occasionally involve the hand which has held a firearm used suicidally. The medico-legal importance of this is that, while the absence of spasm is of no significance, cadaveric spasm cannot be simulated after death in an attempt to disguise a homicide. It should be stressed that this phenomenon is uncommon.

Attempts have been made to improve the timing of death during this difficult period by investigating other biochemical changes that occur in the body after death. For obvious reasons, the parameters must be simple to measure and resistant to putrefaction; effort has therefore been primarily concentrated on the changes in the distribution of inorganic salts found in those fluids that classically remain sterile after death—in particular the cerebrospinal fluid and the vitreous humour of the eye. The level of, say, potassium alters with time after death and does so very nearly in mathematical progression in a single individual. The variations between individuals are, however, so wide as to eliminate any real hope of improvement in the accuracy of the timing of death by the routine use of such laboratory investigations.

Beyond the 3rd day—putrefaction

The process of putrefaction begins with death but only becomes manifest after a few days. Again, many variables have to be considered, particularly the condition of the body before death, the temperature and humidity of the environment and the relative sterility of the area. Thus, the bodies of persons who have died while suffering an acute infection or of those subjected to open injury will decompose faster than the norm; particularly rapid changes occur in dead bodies that are allowed to lie in bed under activated electric blankets.

Generally, there is discoloration of the abdominal skin in 2–3 days and swelling of the tissues, with the formation of blisters, towards the end of the first week. Gross disfiguration is present in some 3 weeks. Partial liquefaction is commonly evident in the body at the end of a month. It will be seen that an estimate of the time of death in a putrefied body can generally be given only in terms of weeks.

Putrefaction of the body is normally delayed in water unless this is heavily contaminated by sewage. In ordinary circumstances, an immersed body will tend to float after a week to 10 days but this will be greatly modified by clothing and water temperature; in deep cold water a body may not surface for some 3 weeks or, indeed, may never do so. There is a similar retardation of putrefaction in coffins in which bursting of the body, an almost invariable accompaniment of putrefaction in the open, is an uncommon finding.

Some features of putrefaction are of forensic importance. Muscular and, particularly, fibrous tissues are resistant and certain organs—for example, the uterus and the prostate gland—may be recognizable for a considerable time; this is of obvious importance in identification. Vascular walls tend to resist decomposition and evidence of coronary insufficiency can often be discovered when the general appearances would suggest that a search would be unlikely to be rewarding; this will be particularly so if calcification has occurred.

The combination of destruction of the blood and formation of gas may lead to the issue of bloody fluid from the orifices. The appearances may closely simulate those of ante-mortem haemorrhage and must be interpreted with caution.

Finally, there is the problem of the body that appears to have resisted decomposition to an unusual degree. This may happen as a natural phenomenon in the closed environment of the coffin. Nevertheless, it has been stated that the finding of such a cadaver should raise the suspicion of poisoning by metallic compounds; this association between preservation and poisoning may, however, be little more than folklore.

Two well-known modifications to the normal process of putrefaction require mention. The first of these is mummification where, in the presence of drying conditions and the absence of bacterial contamination, the tissues may become desiccated rather than putrefied. Ultimately, the mummified tissues may be reduced to powder but, in the meantime, the general format of the body may be remarkably preserved. The bodies of infants tend to mummify very readily.

Secondly, there is the formation of adipocere which results in the transformation of the normal fluid fats of the body to solid compounds. This variant of putrefaction may occur in any tissue containing fat if associated with moist conditions; it is therefore prevalent in bodies recovered from the water and in bodies exhumed from coffins. Adipocere adheres to the bone, the result being that, even after the skin has disintegrated, the body may retain recognizable characteristics of importance in identification; injuries to soft tissues may also be preserved. The presence of adipocere almost invariably means that the body has been dead for some weeks if not months.

Skeletonization

Ultimately all the soft tissues of the body will decompose, the tendons and other highly fibrous tissues being most resistant.

The time for complete skeletonization is extremely variable and depends not only on the natural processes of decomposition but also upon predators from the insect and animal worlds—and from fungi and other moulds. The author has seen two bodies reduced to skeletons within their clothing in a light aircraft which remained undiscovered for 2 months in an English summer; it is doubtful if such rapid skeletonization would occur in winter.

Although the time can be much shorter, it is probably fair to estimate a skeleton with which are associated remnants of fibrous tissue as having been dead for approximately 1 year, but from this point estimates of the intervals since death can be assessed in brackets only of years or even decades. The environment is all-important—bones many hundreds of years old have been discovered well preserved, particularly in dry caves. Numerous scientific techniques, including some of great sophistication—such as the analysis of radioactive carbon—have been introduced for the dating of skeletons but are beyond the scope of this book.

Hypostasis

As the stagnant blood pools under the influence of gravity, its presence becomes apparent on the skin and contrasts vividly with the exsanguinated portions. Similar changes occur in the internal organs where it is important that they are not confused with ante-mortem haemorrhage, for example in the lungs.

Hypostasis, or lividity, can often be seen within 1–2 hours after death and is generally fully established in 6–12 hours. At this point, although fluid blood itself may be displaced, there is sufficient staining of the tissue to maintain some evidence of hypostasis irrespective of the subsequent position of the body. Sustained pressure prevents pooling of the blood and it is common to find that generalized lividity of the back is notably absent from the buttocks and shoulder blades which take the main weight of the recumbent body.

Hypostasis is of relatively little value as a method of timing the interval since death although—taken in conjunction with other signs—it has some use in this respect during the first 6 hours. Its distribution is, however, a fundamental observation in establishing the position of the body after death and, particularly, whether it has been changed. In the event that the body has been moved, the examining doctor may discover either a dual distribution of lividity or a distribution that is incompatible with the locus as presented to him. Either finding must raise the possibility of outside interference.

There are two conditions that require differentiation from hypostasis. The first of these, bruising, is a relatively simple decision. Apart from the fact that bruises are commonly localized, they are, by definition, the result of bleeding into the tissues as opposed to stagnation of blood in the vessels. A rather more difficult situation arises in the distinction between hypostasis and the congestion of an asphyxial death; this has considerable practical significance. Thus, a baby dying in the prone position will show a facial distribution of lividity with pallor over the pressure points—the centre of the forehead, the tip of the nose, the chin and cheek bones. The contrast between this appearance and that of congestion of the face resulting from an asphyxial death may be difficult to appreciate.

The colour of the lividity also provides evidence as to the mode of death. No great reliance can be placed on the 'blueness' as all deaths are, ultimately, anoxic in type. A lividity of bright red colour, however, indicates the presence of fully oxygenated blood which is typical of death in the cold or of exposure to cold after death. Cyanide poisoning gives a rather similar result. Perhaps the most well-known example of this type of observation is the diagnosis of poisoning by carbon monoxide. The cherry-pink colour is usually obvious when sought in a good light.

Post-mortem artefacts

Artefacts resulting from efforts at resuscitation are not uncommon. Heat, be it in the form of direct application or resulting from electrical stimulation, is the most common form encountered. It is perfectly possible to produce burns in a dead body, but these can be differentiated by the absence of so-called vital reactions—that is, the defensive reactions of the living body to injury. The most immediate vital reaction to a burn is dilatation of the surrounding capillaries which shows as an area of redness diffusing into the normal skin colour. Blisters formed before death contain more protein than do those arising *post mortem*. Infiltration of the area by white blood cells is evident microscopically in a few hours and, later, there is repair by connective tissue cells (*fibroblasts*). None of these signs will be present in a burn inflicted after death.

A very common series of artefacts result from attempted resuscitation by external cardiac massage. The breastbone is almost invariably bruised if not dislocated and fractures of the ribs are often caused. The difficulty in distinguishing such injuries from those inflicted during life on purely pathological grounds rests on the self-evident fact that *efficient* cardiac massage simulates a functioning circulation. Any bruise or fracture caused by this means will therefore closely resemble ante-mortem injury (*see also* page 106).

Severe post-mortem injuries may be inflicted by carnivorous animals or crabs on land and by fish or shellfish in water—the last may bare exposed parts to the bone in a matter of days. Injuries inflicted by rats may closely mimic those of suicidal origin; again, it is the absence of vital reaction and an awareness of the possibilities that simplify the interpretation.

Infestation and accelerated destruction of decomposing tissue by larvae of dipterous flies and of beetles is so common as to deserve special mention. It has forensic significance in that entomology has been used on numerous occasions in an attempt to assess the time interval since death. Thus, the insects present can be correlated with their known preferred feeding habits while the age of the larvae and the number of generations can give further information. The assessment is more complicated than would appear theoretically and is certainly a matter for the expert who should, ideally, collect his own specimens in the post-mortem room and at the locus.

Finally, traumatic injuries inflicted on the dead body must be mentioned. A body lying on a roadway may be damaged by vehicles whose drivers are genuinely ignorant of having done so. Post-mortem injuries are outstandingly associated with bodies in the sea where buffeting on rocks by the waves, contact with ships' propellers, grappling in fish nets and the like may result in a confused picture. The important practical point is that the possibility of such sources of injury must be considered in relation to the locus of death.

5

Legal disposal of the dead

With one minor exception[1], it has been illegal since 1836 in England and Wales to dispose of a body unless the death has been registered. There is a wider relaxation of the general rule in Scotland which was designed to take into account the difficulties of communication that used to exist in parts of the country but, in the event of burial before registration, the person in charge of the cemetery must notify the Registrar of the occurrence. The current legislation relating to disposal of the dead in Great Britain is contained in the Birth and Deaths Registration Act 1953, as amended, and in the Registration of Births, Deaths and Marriages (Scotland) Act 1965. In either case, legal disposal begins with medical certification.

Medical certification of the cause of death

Although the general layout of the certificate conforms in each case to the international system of certification of the cause of death, there are some important differences of practice in England and Wales and in Scotland.

In England and Wales, there is a statutory duty laid upon the doctor who attended the deceased during the terminal illness to issue a medical certificate of the cause of death. This obligation does not cease simply because the case is one reportable to the Coroner. If this is so, the correct procedure is for the doctor to issue the certificate, personally report the case to the Coroner and initial the box printed on the reverse of the certificate to indicate that he has done so. The practice of reporting the death to the Coroner and taking no further action is commonly adopted but has no foundation in law; conversely, there is no absolute obligation on the doctor to inform the Coroner—to pre-empt the Registrar in this duty is only a way of saving valuable time.

The English medical certificate requires the certifying doctor to state the date on which he last saw the deceased alive and, in common with the Scottish certificate, to indicate whether or not the body was seen after death and, if so, by whom. The

---

[1] A Registrar in England and Wales may issue a certificate for disposal before registering the death if he has received written notice of the death from a qualified informant and has received a medical certificate of the cause of death—provided the death was not one that should have been reported to the Coroner.

certifying doctor does not have to view the body after death,[2] but in the absence of such precaution, the Registrar must refer the case to the Coroner if the remainder of the certificate indicates that the doctor had not seen his patient during the last 14 days of the patient's life. The doctor in England and Wales further certifies that he was in medical attendance during the deceased's last illness; if no one can so certify—a situation that often obtains in holiday periods—there can be no medical certificate and, *ipso facto,* the case is referred to the Coroner.

A 'Notice to Informant' is attached to the English certificate and the doctor is required to furnish this forthwith. The medical certificate may be sent without delay to the Registrar but, since the death cannot be registered in its absence, it is often handed to the informant together with the notice.

The most important respect in which the Scottish process of medical certification varies from that in England is that, in Scotland, there is no requirement upon the certifying doctor to have been in attendance during the last illness. Under Section 24 of the 1965 Act, it is proper for any doctor who is able to complete the certificate 'to the best of his knowledge and belief' to do so. While this has the great merit of removing a large number of manifestly natural deaths from the intricacies of the medico-legal system, it carries some disadvantages; many doctors are unwilling to certify a cause of death of which they are not quite certain while, on the other hand, the Procurator Fiscal has no wish to accept the English Coroner's responsibilities as to the accuracy of the mortality statistics. There is, therefore, a tendency for certificates to be couched in such terms as 'death from natural causes, probably——', which is regarded as a generally satisfactory compromise. There is nothing in the certificate relating to the last time the deceased was seen alive; it follows that there is no obligation on the Registrar to refer a case to the Fiscal for reasons similar to the English '14-day rule'.

There is no space on the Scottish certificate for indicating that the Fiscal has been informed of the death; this is done in the great majority of cases by the doctor himself on a relatively informal basis—once the case has been referred, the certification of the cause of death is generally taken over by the Police Surgeon. Nor is there a 'Notice to Informant'. The certificate as to the cause of death must be transmitted either to a qualified informant or to the Registrar within seven days.

The informant

Persons qualified and liable to act as informants in England and Wales include a relation of the deceased present at the death, in attendance during the last illness or residing in the subdistrict where death occurred; a person present at the death; the 'occupier' of the house or any inmate of the house if either knew of the happening of the death; or a person causing the disposal of the body. If death occurred outside a house, informants may include any relative of the deceased having knowledge of the necessary particulars; any person present at the death; any person who found the body, who is in charge of the body or who is causing the disposal of the body.

In Scotland, the duty to give information of particulars of death devolves, in

---

[2] But he would be well advised to do so. There are many recorded instances of bodies being discovered alive in the mortuary (e.g. *Medicine, Science and the Law* (1981), **21**, 228).

succession, upon any relative of the deceased; any person present at the death; the deceased's executor; the occupier of the premises where the death took place; or any other person having knowledge of the details to be registered. If the deceased's home is unknown, any person finding the body, including the police involved in the investigation, has a duty to inform the Registrar but all such deaths are then reportable to the Fiscal.

Registration

The importance of registration of a death is often inadequately emphasized. The Registrar must be informed even in the unusual situation of a body being buried without registration; cremation without registration is not permitted (*see* below). In the event that the Coroner adjourns his inquest at the request of the Director of Public Prosecutions, he must now send a certificate to the Registrar giving such particulars as are required for registration 'so far as they have been ascertained' (Criminal Law Act 1977, Sch. 10, para 20(4)). The distressing delay in registration imposed by criminal proceedings is thus now very much reduced and brings English practice into line with that existing in Scotland.

Otherwise, registration can be completed only when the full details required by the Acts of 1953 and 1965 are supplied, and the process thus provides an essential back-up service in the detection of secret homicide.

Informants must attend personally at the Registry and provide the necessary information within 5 days of the death in England and within 8 days in Scotland; the Registrar will then issue a certificate for disposal after registration. If the death has been the subject of medico-legal inquiry, the appropriate authority informs the Registrar of the details and provides a disposal order.

Burial

Almost incredibly, there is no general statute that requires any individual to dispose of a body and there is nothing that says that a body must be buried or cremated. There is, however, an obligation at common law 'in the nature of a public duty' that rests on persons in possession of a dead body to dispose of it in a manner suitable to the estate[3]. Similarly, there is a common law right to be buried in one's parish churchyard. The local authority must take the responsibility when no other arrangements have been made[4] but, otherwise, only the general health laws govern the method of disposal; thus, the burial or cremation of a body may be ordered by a magistrate should its retention above ground be considered a danger to health[5]. The provision of burial grounds is now the responsibility of Burial Authorities[6], but, surprisingly, national laws restricting the position of cemeteries have been repealed; such matters are now subject only to by-law regulation. Burial outside England requires the authority of the Coroner[7]; the Procurator Fiscal must

[3] Rees v Hughes [1946] 1 K.B. 517.
[4] National Assistance Act 1948, s. 50, as amended.
[5] Public Health Act 1936, s. 162; Public Health (Scotland) Act 1897, s. 69; London Government Act 1963, s. 40.
[6] Local Government Act 1972, s. 214.
[7] Removal of Bodies Regulations 1954 (S.I. 1954/448).

authorize the removal of a body 'firth of Scotland' if the death has been subject to his inquiries—otherwise, the body is simply accompanied by a Certificate of Registry of Death in Scotland.

After burial or cremation, a notification that the body has been disposed of must be delivered to the Registrar within 4 days of the event. Failing such advice within 14 days, the Registrar must, after inquiry, report the matter to the appropriate Community Physician (or Specialist in Community Medicine).

Exhumation

Exhumation is an unpleasant procedure, particularly if the body has been buried only recently, and one that engenders considerable emotion. Although the practice is, as a result, very strictly controlled, there are occasions when the re-examination of a body already buried may be of overriding importance either to the State, as in the case of suspected criminality, to insurance companies or to individuals when civil actions for damages are contemplated or when identification is disputed. A Coroner in England and Wales may authorize exhumation of a person buried within his jurisdiction either for the purpose of holding an inquest, or of discharging any other of his relevant functions. He may also do so in connection with criminal proceedings relating to the death of the body exhumed, or to the death of another person that is related to the circumstances surrounding the death of the person to be exhumed[8]. In all other cases, permission must be sought from the Home Secretary[9]. Something of the order of two medico-legal exhumations are carried out annually in England and Wales; even before the widening of the powers enjoyed by the Coroner, only a minority of these were carried out under licence from the Home Secretary.

In Scotland, the person requiring the exhumation, whether it be the Procurator Fiscal or a member of the public, petitions the Sheriff to that effect. The Sheriff must notify the next-of-kin of the deceased, who are given the opportunity to make objections at a hearing. If the petition is granted, the Sheriff will issue a warrant for exhumation.

Presumptive identification is made by the superintendent of the graveyard consulting his records and by the undertaker's recognition of the coffin and of the internal wrappings. Whenever possible, relatives should be asked to confirm the name on the identifying plaque.

Many exhumations authorized for the purpose of establishing the precise cause of death are concerned with suspected poisoning. It is then incumbent upon the pathologist in charge of the operation to obtain a full series of control specimens which can be analysed for the poison along with the tissues from the body. These include earth from above, around and below the coffin, the wood of and fluid from inside the coffin, and portions of the burial robes. It is also advisable to collect further control specimens of soil from a distant area of the cemetery. Parallel analyses will provide valuable evidence as to the possibility of any poison having entered the body from outside after burial rather than having been ingested before death.

There is considerable onus on the pathologist to make a particularly thorough

[8] Coroners Act 1980, s. 4.
[9] Burial Act 1857, s. 25. An ecclesiastical faculty is also needed whenever a body is removed from consecrated ground, but a licence is not required when the sole purpose is to remove the body from one piece of consecrated ground to another. Local authorities have special powers of removal and reinterment (e.g. Town and Country Planning Act 1971, s. 128.).

examination of exhumed bodies—they certainly constitute cases that justify a full-body X-ray survey as a routine; so far as is known, no request for a second exhumation has ever been granted.

Cremation

As a reflection of its finality, cremation as a method of disposal of the dead is carefully regulated[10]. Cremation is the ultimate method of concealing a crime; on the other hand, it has certain advantages over burial as a legal method of disposal of the dead. Moreover the modern operation of the Coroners' (and Fiscals') system has greatly reduced the opportunity for the concealment of homicide. Any regulations must therefore be so designed as to permit without undue hindrance a process that is in the public interest and yet, at the same time, safeguard that interest in respect of criminality. The Cremation Act 1902 and the regulations made thereunder in 1930, 1935, 1952 and 1965 constitute the law in both England and Wales and in Scotland, although the regulations are currently subject to governmental review. The process of cremation can be described conveniently in relation to the Forms that must be completed before it can be allowed:

Form A. This constitutes an application for cremation which sets out, *inter alia,* the relationship of the applicant to the deceased, the wishes of the next-of-kin, the details of the death, an affirmation to the effect that there is no reason to suspect foul play or the need for further examination of the body and a statement by those who have been in medical charge of the deceased. The application must be countersigned by a householder who knows the applicant.

Form B. This is the certificate of the medical attendant who has 18 questions to answer relating to the mode and cause of death, the scope of his attendance on the deceased, operative treatment and nursing care in the recent past. The doctor must certify that he has no reason to suppose that further inquiry is needed and he must also affirm that he is not related to nor has he a pecuniary interest in the death of the deceased.

Despite its comprehensiveness, Form B does not replace the medical certificate as to cause of death; the latter is essential for the registration of the death whereas Form B is related only to the process of cremation.

Form C. This is a confirmatory medical certificate which must be completed by a practitioner of at least 5 years standing who has no family or professional relationship with the practitioner signing Form B. He must state whether he has seen the body and whether he has made a careful external examination. There is no statutory requirement for him to have done so but the Regulations clearly indicate the need; a negative answer would certainly result in the rejection of the certificate. There is provision for stating whether or not he has performed a post-mortem dissection[11]. There are five questions relating to his having questioned various categories of person as to the circumstances of the death;

[10] In contrast to the surprisingly lax attitude to burial, the Cremation Regulations 1930 prohibit the burning of human remains in any place other than a recognized crematorium.

[11] The fact that a post-mortem examination has been made on a person dying in hospital may, in some circumstances, obviate the need for Form C (Cremation (Amendment) Regulations 1985 (S.I. 1985/153) (S.I. 1985/820 (s.73))).

there must be a positive reply to at least one of these. Finally, the certifying doctor must affirm that he is satisfied as to the cause of death.
Form F. This form is completed by the Medical Referee (a medical officer nominated by the Crematorium and appointed by the Home Secretary or Secretary of State). The signature confirms that the Referee is satisfied that the regulations have been complied with, that the cause of death has been established and that no further examination is required; cremation of the remains is authorized.

The Cremation Act gives very wide powers to the Referee. He can complete Form C himself; he can withhold Form F without giving reasons and can make any inquiries he thinks fit; he can report the case to the Coroner or Procurator Fiscal; he can also invite a pathologist to perform a post-mortem examination or make such an examination himself. In the last circumstance, the person performing the autopsy completes *Form D,* which will then replace Form C and will also override Form B. In the event that the case has been reported to the Coroner or Procurator Fiscal, the certificate of those officials, *Form E,* replaces Forms B and C and clears the case for the Medical Referee. Form E may be issued before the conclusion of the medico-legal inquiries but, in England and Wales, it does not state the cause of death; it does not replace either the Coroner's death certificate or Certificate after Inquest. The version of Form E provided by the Procurator Fiscal does indicate the cause of death but, notwithstanding, a normal certificate must be provided by his medical adviser.

It is re-emphasized that the discretionary powers under which a body can be buried without certification as to the cause of death and prior to registration of the death do not apply to cremation. Surprisingly, a body that has been buried for not less than a year may be cremated without further documentation or authorization; the situation is subject only to the requirements for exhumation.

The Anatomy Act 1984

This Act governs the retention of a body for the purposes of use in an Anatomy School. The Human Tissue Act 1961 extends the scope of, but does not replace, the Anatomy Act; the 1961 Act raises issues of far more general application and is discussed in detail in Chapter 12.

In general, the disposal of a body through the dissecting room is subject to the dissection being conducted only by a licensed person in a licensed establishment. The person in lawful possession of the body can give permission for the examination unless the deceased is known to have objected or the spouse or a relative objects; in this instance, the 'person in lawful possession' means the hospital authority or the management of a similar institution in which the death occurs[12]. The body cannot be possessed without a valid certificate of the cause of death and it must not be dissected unless the death has been registered. No new regulations have yet been promulgated and, currently, the receipt of the body must be acknowledged within 24 hours by supplying the local Inspector of Anatomy with details as to the source of the body and

[12] R. v. Feist [1858] Dears & Bell 590. The situation is clarified in s.4(9) of the Act (*see* Chapter 12 for further discussion).

of the date and place of death, the sex and, if known, the name of the deceased; the certificate of cause of death is attached to these details. The body must be disposed of within 3 years by interment in a proper cemetery or by cremation and the Inspector must be so informed[13]. In the event of cremation, a special *Form H* must be completed.

One medico-legal distinction between the Anatomy Acts and Section 1(1) of the Human Tissue Act is that, whereas the former is specially designed for the provision of teaching material to medical schools, dissections under the latter must be carried out by registered medical practitioners. The power of veto of a spouse or relative which existed even when the deceased had bequeathed his body has now been withdrawn[14].

The disposal of stillbirths

A stillbirth is defined as a child that issued from the mother after the 28th week of pregnancy and that did not at any time after being expelled from its mother breathe or show any sign of life.

The pathological distinction between stillbirth and perinatal death is discussed in Chapter 19. We are concerned here only with the regulations surrounding the actual disposal of the body; these are governed in England and Wales by the Births and Deaths Registration Act 1953 (s. 11) and in Scotland by the Registration of Births, Deaths and Marriages (Scotland) Act 1965 (s. 21). The process is essentially similar under both statutes.

The body of a stillbirth cannot be disposed of without a valid medical certificate of stillbirth which, throughout Great Britain, can be completed by virtue of the certifier either having been present at the birth or having examined the body following information as to its birth. The certificate may be signed by a registered medical practitioner or by a certified midwife. In the event of the Registrar being in any doubt as to whether the child was born alive, the case must be reported to the Coroner or to the Procurator Fiscal; in practice, many cases are reported direct when the certifier thinks it necessary. There is provision under both jurisdictions for a declaration by the informant that the child was stillborn when, for some reason, there is no professional person available to provide a certificate.

A stillbirth is, technically, a birth rather than a death. The informant therefore has 42 days in England and 21 days in Scotland to register the event. Stillbirths do not come within the compass of the Human Tissue Act and, in the present state of the law, must be buried or cremated. Disposal is contingent upon the issue of a Certificate for Disposal or of the appropriate Coroner's Certificate. Specially adapted Forms A and F are used in the event of cremation. There is no requirement for the superintendent of the place of disposal to notify the Registrar of disposal of a stillbirth—as there is in the ordinary case of death—unless the body has been buried without a certificate of registration. It scarcely needs mention that, if a child has survived birth for even a fleeting time, certificates both of birth and death are required—the normal medical certificate as to cause of death is then used.

[13] The limit of three years is not negotiable (s.4(8)).
[14] The 1984 Act generally brings conditions for anatomical dissection closer to those of the Human Tissue Act 1961.

The disposal of fetuses

There is no law as to the disposal of a fetus that is expelled from the mother dead before the 28th week of pregnancy. There is no requirement for registration and the method of disposal must simply comply with current standards of proper public behaviour and with the various Public Health Acts. Fetuses of this type are not subject to the restrictions of the Human Tissue Act and may be retained for scientific purposes, but there are serious ethical problems. The Advisory Group[15] have proposed that fetuses weighing less than 300 g are previable and may be suitable for research purposes. The same group, in attempting to distinguish between the viable and non-viable, has proposed that the dividing line should be at 20 weeks' gestation when the fetus is obtained as a result of hysterotomy. The problem is bound up with the working of the Abortion Act 1967 but the areas of legal doubt have not been clarified particularly as to the rights of parents to have a fetus properly buried.

Disposal of bodies returned from outside the United Kingdom[16]

Although the procedure is not quite uniform—any differences depending upon the actual country in which death has occurred—it follows generally similar principles.

The death is certified acording to the regulations of the country in which it occurred and, usually, the death certificate is accompanied by further certificates as to freedom from infection and to embalming. The papers are notarized by the Consul who may also add his own certificate.

In the event of burial in the United Kingdom, all the documents are referred to the Registrar of the area where the body is to be interred. Since the death has already been registered abroad, the Registrar will then issue a Certificate of Non-liability to Register which, in effect, takes the place of the usual Disposal Certificate. Notification of disposal is still required within 96 hours of the event. No Certificate of Non-liability is required in Scotland where burial is controlled by the appropriate cemetery authority. If the next-of-kin wish for a cremation, an application must be made on Form A which is sent, with all the relevant documents, to the Home Office or the Secretary of State whence a licence to cremate is provided.

It is now clear that the Coroner for the district in which the body lies must hold an Inquest if the circumstances of the death indicate a need, despite the fact that both the death and the cause of death occurred abroad[17].

---

[15] Department of Health and Social Security (1972). *Use of Fetuses and Fetal Material for Research.* London; HMSO.

[16] Based on information kindly provided by Messrs. J. H. Kenyon Ltd.

[17] R. v. West Yorkshire Coroner, *ex parte* Smith [1982] 3 W.L.R. 920 CA.

6

The spread of communicable disease: some aspects of public health

Epidemiology is the study of the determinants and mode of distribution of disease. All natural disease is to some extent subject to outside influences but communicable disease is that type that can most obviously be controlled by legislation[1]. Community health is therefore a part of the general spectrum of forensic medicine, and virtually all the early university chairs in Forensic Medicine combined Medical Jurisprudence with Public Health; at the present time, certain categories of death reportable to the Fiscal (Appendix D) are there by virtue of their importance to the health of the community. Actions for tort or delict may well be based on transference of preventable disease, an aspect of forensic medicine that has come to greater prominence with the availability of cheap, world-wide travel facilities. Some understanding of the spread of communicable disease should be available to the lawyer concerned with medical aspects of the law; it is the purpose of this chapter to present this in outline.

Organisms responsible for infectious disease

Organisms capable of causing human disease vary greatly in habit and in size. Ascending from the smallest, the groups that are of greatest concern include the following.

The Viruses

The characteristic of these minute organisms is that they are incapable of a free existence and must live as true parasites within living tissue. As a corollary, viruses can be grown in the laboratory only in cultures of live tissues. Examples of virus disease include smallpox and measles[2].

The Bacteria

These unicellular organisms of great simplicity are omnipresent. Those that cause disease are described as *pathogenic* and those that produce a purulent reaction are

---

[1] Examples of attempted legal control of non-communicable diseases include that of disease associated with cigarette smoking, through regulations as to packaging and advertising.
[2] Slightly different viruses, known as *Rickettsiae*, cause typhus fever.

pyogenic. Bacteria come in various shapes—the round *cocci* which, *inter alia*, cause sore throats, boils and pneumonia; the *bacilli*, which include the organisms responsible for typhoid fever and tuberculosis; the curved *vibrios*, which are responsible for cholera; and the coiled *spirochaetes*, which cause several diseases additional to syphilis. The *anaerobic bacteria* form a group that is of special importance in forensic medicine; they will grow only in the relative absence of oxygen and proliferate particularly well in wounds, causing tetanus and gas gangrene. Bacteria that are not pathogenic in their normal habitat may produce disease when displaced in the body so-called *opportunistic infection*.

The Protozoa

These are more sophisticated unicellular organisms which cause many diseases of world-wide economic importance including malaria, sleeping sickness and the bowel disease amoebic dysentery.

The Fungi

These are branching organisms of simple type which are increasing in importance as they may flourish in severely ill patients, particularly those on antibacterial treatment.

The Helminths or Worms

These take many forms and vary from those that are scarcely visible to the naked eye to others that are several metres long. They are often of considerable medico-legal importance due to their close association with food and its preparation. Many have no more than a nuisance value but others—for example, one tapeworm of dogs which causes hydatid disease in man—are potentially dangerous to life; the pork tapeworm may cause an intractable form of epilepsy.

The spread of communicable disease (*see Figure 6.1*)

If a disease is to spread, the responsible organism must be passed from person to person. The simplest way in which this can be done is by *direct contact*, in which case the organism must be either on the skin or in secretions that are passed directly from person to person. The most obvious examples of such contact diseases are those that are sexually transmitted and the infectious skin diseases.

Otherwise, human-to-human transfer of disease depends upon excretion of organisms and this can take several routes—particularly via the sputum, the urine and the faeces. Sputum does not mean necessarily the tangible mass of phlegm seem in sufferers from bronchitis but rather the invisible spray known as *droplets* that is spread each time a person coughs; in so far as this can be directly inhaled by others, droplet infection is a matter of *proximity contact* and is fostered by conditions of overcrowding with inadequate ventilation. Urine is a vehicle for surprisingly few communicable diseases—typhoid fever is of the most immediate concern but, on a world-wide basis, the condition of schistosomiasis, due to a worm, is a far more important source of morbidity. Contrastingly, the faeces may

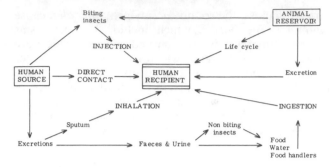

Figure 6.1 Schematic representation of the spread of disease due to microbiological organisms.

contain large numbers of pathogenic organisms—not only those associated with the many infectious bowel diseases but also those that become pathogenic when displaced—for example, when contaminating wounds.

When an excretion is passed it may remain on the hands and any organisms can then be transferred to the utensils or food of others—the role of the food handler in the transmission of disease is therefore of great importance. Alternatively, the excretion may be passed into the water supply—either localized, as into a well, or generalized, as into a stream or river; sporadic disease in the locality, or explosive epidemic disease involving a whole distant community may then arise. The major contribution of the public authorities to the health of the people probably depends upon the provision of an efficient system of sewage disposal. Otherwise, the excretions may dry and become incorporated in dust; control of those pathogenic organisms that are resistant to desiccation is a major problem within institutions—it is the standard route of cross-infection of patients in hospital. Finally, infected excretions may be transferred to foodstuffs by insects, of which the house-fly is the most important.

In many communicable diseases, the responsible organism is not excreted but remains in the blood. Transfer from case to case must then depend upon blood-sucking insects[3]—the importance of *insect-borne disease* is vast in the world as a whole but slight in temperate climates. Pandemics of arthropod-borne disease, among which are included yellow fever, typhus, plague, malaria and sleeping sickness, have changed the course of history, and it is only an efficient public health system that prevents their recurrence or limits their effects. Certain arthropod-borne diseases are essentially human in distribution—louse-borne typhus fever, which is associated with overcrowding in conditions of poor personal hygiene, is the outstanding example. Others, however, depend upon an animal reservoir—the most historic example being the rat as a source of bubonic plague. Human diseases that are animal dependent are known as *zoonoses*. Zoonoses may also persist by means of a direct association between man and animals. Some are industrial in nature—for example, the infective jaundice of sewer workers or hydatid worm disease of sheep farmers—but the most urgent contact zoonosis is undoubtedly

---

[3] Used in a colloquial sense. Ticks and mites which also transmit disease are not, zoologically speaking, insects; a better general term is 'arthropod-borne disease'.

rabies—a disease particularly apposite to the theme of this chapter because its control in Great Britain rests almost entirely on legislation[4].

The control of communicable disease

The general methods for control of infectious disease are clear from the foregoing paragraphs. First, one can attempt to eliminate—or, in human instances, isolate—the source of infection; secondly, knowing the mode of spread, an effort can be made to break the chain at some vital point; thirdly, one can use artificial means to promote immunity in the population.

Statutory powers to achieve these ends are contained in the many Acts and regulations pertaining to public health; the main United Kingdom legislation is contained in the Public Health Acts 1936 and 1961 and the Public Health (Scotland) Acts 1897–1945. Many of the powers are wide and far beyond the ambit of the individual—they include adequate supervision of housing, the control of sewage, drainage and water supplies, the whole range of inspection and control of foodstuffs, the control of imported biological goods likely to be infected such as animal bones or skins and the quarantining of animals. The law as it affects individuals is now consolidated in the Public Health (Control of Disease) Act 1984.

Much current attention is focused on what are described as exotic diseases—that is, diseases that are imported from abroad. They may be of little or no public concern—if a visitor becomes ill with malaria it will not be communicable in Britain because the insect carrier, the anopheles mosquito, has been so reduced in number as to be ineffective; this, in turn, is the result of efficient public health measures[5]. Exotic diseases may be of relatively severe consequence—a person with typhoid fever, for instance, could infect a number of contacts before discovery; at the other end of the scale, they could be catastrophic—a classic example would be the importation of yellow fever into an area where the mosquito vector was present in sufficient numbers to start an epidemic. Even in parts of Britain it would be a matter of very great concern if a human or animal case of plague were introduced into an area where rats and fleas abounded[6]. The control of exotic disease is largely a matter of port health control; while the control of shipping has been practised successfully for very many years, the problems are accentuated by the widespread use of air travel—aircraft can transport infected insects, persons incubating disease will reach their destination before becoming overtly ill and there is a rare possibility of infecting a high proportion of the passengers through one ill-prepared meal obtained *en route*. Special regulations[7] are applied to aircraft and, in those parts of the world at special risk, control is exercised on an international basis[8]. Other contact zoonoses are controlled either by prohibition of imported animals or compulsory quarantining—measures that are available only to an island State.

[4] Animal Health Act 1981.

[5] Most exotic diseases are specifically treatable and diagnosable in the laboratory. It would now be considered negligent to fail to take the necessary steps to make a diagnosis despite the infrequency of the disease; extensive damages have, in fact, been awarded for such mistakes (*see British Medical Journal* (1975), **iv**, 474).

[6] All ships must be in possession of either a Deratting Certificate or a Deratting Exemption Certificate; certificates are valid for 6 months (International Health Regulations (1969), Art. 54).

[7] Public Health (Aircraft) Regulations 1979 (S.I. 1979/1434); Public Health (Aircraft) (Scotland) Amendment Regulations 1974 (S.I. 1974/1017).

[8] The International Health Regulations (1969, amended 1973), drawn up by the World Health Organization, cover cholera, plague, smallpox and yellow fever.

These major concerns are of little interest in the present context. Of greater immediate importance is the fact that certain control measures impinge upon the rights of the individual and also on the doctor/patient relationship.

Notification of infectious disease

As indicated above, human infectious disease can be effectively controlled by isolation of infective cases; moreover, the original source of a disease can often be traced through a knowledge of those thereby infected. Both these public health control measures depend primarily upon notification of cases.

A number of diseases are statutorily notifiable[9] to the local Community Physician (or Specialist in Community Medicine) by the practitioner in charge of the case (Appendix H). The general list of some 29 diseases is not exhaustive as the Area Health Authority or Board has the power to add to the printed list when local conditions indicate the need or desirability[10]. There can, therefore, be no question of a binding confidentiality between doctor and patient in this respect (see Chapter 30); this statutory type of breach of confidence illustrates two important points of principle in medical ethics—first, the 'need to know' quality of the person to whom confidential information is disclosed and, secondly, the precedent that is thus established of the overriding importance of the public need when it is in conflict with that of the individual.

But statutory powers go deeper than this. It is an offence for a person knowing he has an infectious disease to expose himself to others or to carry on with his occupation. In the absence of consent, a Justice or a Sheriff may order a healthy person from a building in which he is considered at risk, he can make a hospital order and he can require a person to be detained in hospital if housing conditions are unlikely to be satisfactory upon discharge; clearly, however, such an order may be difficult to enforce. Perhaps the quickest preventive measure lies in the authority to order a medical examination of a person thought to be suffering from or to be the carrier of a notifiable disease[11], if it is considered to be in the interest of the person himself, his family or the public in general. Control of the carrier state is most important. In this condition, a person feels perfectly well, yet is excreting pathogenic organisms—the state may be a hangover from an overt attack of the disease but, equally commonly, the carrier will never have been aware of being infected. He may therefore resent compulsory medical treatment, but the devastation that could be caused by a typhoid carrier who persistently polluted a water supply or who was engaged in food handling of any sort needs no emphasis. Carrier states are notoriously difficult to treat and, in the event of failure, the Local Health Authorities are empowered to arrange a person's occupation so that he will be a minimal danger to the public[12].

Immunization

There can be no doubt as to the efficacy of mass immunization as a method of controlling infectious disease. At the same time, no immunity procedure is entirely

---

[9] Under the Public Health (Infectious Diseases) Regulations 1968 (S.I. 1968/1366) as amended.

[10] National Health Service (Scotland) Act 1972, s.53; Public Health (Control of Disease) Act 1984, s.16.

[11] Public Health (Control of Disease) Act 1984, ss.35, 36.

[12] Public Health (Control of Disease) Act 1984, s.20. See also Food Act 1984, s.28.

without risk; controversy centres on the right balance being struck between, on the one hand, the effectiveness and the risk of vaccination against a particular disease and, on the other, the chance of contracting that disease and its short- and long-term effects both on the individual and on the public. A good illustration is provided by smallpox. This very severe disease could have wreaked havoc if introduced into Britain and, consequently, preventive vaccination was at one time compulsory; the procedure had, however, a recognizable mortality and morbidity of its own. By the middle of this century, other control measures had become so effective that the risks of vaccination were considered to outweigh the dangers of contracting the disease and compulsion was abandoned in 1971; there has been no increase in the indigenous disease as a result. Nevertheless, a voluntary immunization programme is still an essential part of the control of many infectious diseases; within the United Kingdom, immunization is recommended as a routine against diphtheria, tetanus, whooping cough, poliomyelitis, measles, tuberculosis and German measles[13].

Immunization is of two types—active and passive. In the former, the body is presented with either an attenuated (made-safe) live strain of the wild pathogenic organism or with a killed form. This vaccine acts as an antigen which stimulates the formation of antibodies, which are then ready to repel the antigen when it presents in its natural disease-provoking form; antibody production can be boosted by repeated doses of the vaccine and is, therefore, long lasting. In passive immunity, the body is supplied with preformed antibodies; the action is short and is designed only to combat the actual or supposed entry of a dangerous organism before it can take hold in the body.

Active immunization—that type of inoculation or vaccination given in childhood or before travelling to an infected area—has a number of hazards, many of which are now only theoretical. The recipient may have a completely unforeseeable idiosyncracy to the injection and may sustain a severe allergic shock. More commonly, the organisms in the vaccine may reactivate an abnormal condition present in the recipient—classic examples are skin eczema after vaccination against smallpox and convulsions after whooping-cough immunization. The vaccine may cause a modified form of the disease it is intended to prevent—some children, for instance, suffer what is apparently a mild attack of measles following inoculation. In the case of live virus vaccines, the growth may not be pure—yellow fever vaccines that are grown on eggs may contain viruses that have been infecting the eggs themselves. This is of little consequence since it is virtually eliminated in modern manufacture. Of far greater importance is the possibility that antibodies may be provoked not only to the desired antigen, but also to the medium in which it is prepared. Thus, the original form of anti-rabies vaccine is grown in nervous tissue; when it is used, there is a possibility that anti-nervous tissue antibody will be formed in the recipient with disastrous results within his own brain[14]. A major danger, however, lies in the potential effects on pregnancy. This is a hazard almost specific to those vaccines composed of living viruses; these may cause abortion or, more seriously, may damage the growing fetus if given within the first 3 months of intrauterine life. This last possibility is particularly evident in immunization against

<hr>

[13] Standing Medical Advisory Committee for the Central Health Services Council (1972). *Immunization against Infectious Diseases*. London; Department of Health and Social Security.

[14] Research has now developed methods for preparing the vaccine in duck embryos or in human diploid cells.

German measles, a fairly predictable chance in that the only purpose in immunizing is to prevent a true attack of the disease during childbearing. The likelihood of damage to the fetus is such that a guarantee of contraception for at least 60 days is required of a woman before she can be immunized against German measles.

Formidable though this list may seem, the risks of immunization must be contrasted with the dangers of inadequate control of the relevant diseases; looked at in this way, the hazards as a whole are very slight[15]. Nevertheless, complications do occur and raise difficulties when public policy is involved; the Vaccine Damage Payments Act 1979 represents a pragmatic solution to the problems. Under this very limited statute, a lump sum is payable to a young person who can be shown to have been severely disabled as a result of vaccination carried out as part of the public health campaign. The same sum is payable when the damage was inflicted before birth. This legislation does not exclude the application of the wider social security provisions for disabled persons, nor does it inhibit an action for damages in the event of medical negligence (*see* Chapter 30). Such negligence would be shown only if the doctor had failed to follow accepted practice—for example, it might be suggested as being negligent to immunize against whooping cough a child who was known to suffer from convulsions, or to continue with a course of vaccination when the first dose had precipitated a convulsion. Even so, the balancing of the risks of contracting the disease against the risks of its prevention is a matter of clinical judgment; negligence would be difficult to prove in the majority of cases[16].

Persons travelling abroad present a special problem. There are two types of active immunization involved—those procedures undertaken for the obvious benefit of the individual, of which immunization against poliomyelitis and typhoid fever are good examples, and those that are required by the Health Authorities of the countries to be visited before entry is permitted. The former category poses little difficulty. If a woman is pregnant or has an infant child and wishes to travel to an area in which an immune state would be desirable but, at the same time, involves an injection that might present an above-average risk to her fetus or child, she should be warned of the dangers both of immunization and of travel while non-immune and should be given appropriate advice including that of postponing her travel. The choice is then up to the patient within the terms of 'informed consent' as discussed in Chapter 30. Travel to countries that insist on certain vaccinations poses difficulty if it is necessary during high-risk periods. In certain circumstances, such as travel from an area known to be free of a particular disease, a certificate giving a valid reason for non-vaccination may be acceptable; in other cases, for example, in travel from an area where yellow fever exists to one where it could be introduced, a period of quarantine on arrival may have to be accepted. The problem is, however, of less practical importance than might be supposed; a real risk for the fetus probably exists only in the case of smallpox vaccination and this is no longer required for travellers.

The dangers of passive immunization are of a different type but are very real. Antibodies are produced in the blood of animals. Therefore, when an antibody is injected, foreign antigens derived from the animal are also introduced and an

---

[15] Although, clearly, the balance need not necessarily be the same. Diphtheria immunization is, for example, virtually without risk while the disease is extremely dangerous; vaccination against cholera is again without risk but its protective value is very slight; smallpox vaccination has a hazard, although slight, but the chance of contracting the disease is now negligible on a world-wide basis.

[16] An action in tort might also lie in the Congenital Disabilities (Civil Liability) Act 1976.

immune reaction of varying severity may be established. This is of wide forensic importance due to the frequency with which anti-tetanus antibodies need to be given after wounds of all sorts. In many cases it might be at least arguable that the dangers of passive immunization were greater than the likelihood of contracting tetanus; but in the event of misjudgment it would be difficult to defend an accusation of negligence in the light of previous decisions[17]. Such dilemmas should, in practice, become very much rarer if the official policy of active immunization against tetanus in childhood is widely followed—the correct procedure in a wounded person who has been previously immunized is to boost the active immunity with a fresh dose of antigen; this carries no risk of an untoward species reaction.

[17] For example, Coles v. Reading and District Hospital Management Committee and Another, (1963) 107 S.J. 115. See also the case discussed in Taylor, J. L. (1970), *The Doctor and the Law*, p. 113; London; Pitman. (There were additional features in both cases.)

7

Sudden natural death

The mechanism of sudden natural death

Some 80 per cent of the cases coming to autopsy at the hands of the English Coroner's pathologist are found to have died from natural causes. Even in Scotland, where a high proportion of such deaths are certified without dissection, many medico-legal post-mortem examinations fail to disclose anything unnatural. The proportions differ very much from city to city and, particularly, as between city and rural areas; in Edinburgh, in 1978, a diagnosis of death due to natural disease was made in 47 per cent of the Fiscal's cases that were examined internally. These cases therefore form an essential part of forensic medicine, both in their own right and also because it is impossible to appreciate properly the medico-legal interactions between trauma—particularly that due to accidents—and incapacitating disease without a knowledge of the mechanisms underlying the latter.

For present purposes, 'sudden death' is defined as unexpected death following so rapidly from the onset of symptoms that the cause of death could not be certified with confidence by a medical practitioner unfamiliar with the patient—the type of death that is likely to disguise a 'secret homicide'. Sudden death of this sort is almost entirely a matter of disease of the cardiovascular system and will be discussed as such, first in the immediacy of death and, secondly, as to the age of those affected.

In order of increasing suddenness, death may be due to haemorrhage from vessels, to peripheral blockage of vessels or to inhibition of the heart's action (*see Figure 7.1*).

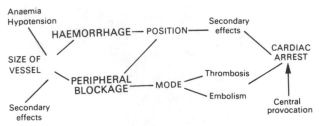

Figure 7.1 Factors involved in sudden death related to the cardiovascular system.

The mode of death due to *haemorrhage* depends on two factors—on the size of the vessel that bleeds and, when internal, on the ability of the cavity involved to accommodate the blood shed and of the contained organs to continue to function normally. The effects of bleeding from a small vessel should be less than from a larger one but, given the same size of small vessels in the cranial cavity and in the abdomen, the effect in the latter may be slight while, in the former, it may be lethal because of the concurrent effects on brain function.

The effect of *blockage of a peripheral vessel* is determined by the nature of the part deprived of blood, by the size of the vessel blocked and by the method of occlusion. The primary effect on an organ or area is to deprive it of oxygen; the secondary effect on the body as a whole depends on the function of that organ. Thus, a man can well survive a portion of his spleen being deprived of blood, but closure of a vessel supplying the respiratory centre in the brain will cause immediate death. The effect of the size of vessel is obvious—one might be able to withstand the sudden elimination of a lobule of lung, but sudden obstruction of a main pulmonary artery would be almost inevitably fatal. Three main processes lead to blockage of an artery. The slowest in effect is restriction of the lumen due to thickening of the wall. This process is one for which the body is often able to compensate by the development of new vessels—known as a collateral circulation. An urgent need for extra oxygen in the organ supplied by the vessel or a very rapid exacerbation of the restrictive thickening may result in sudden incompetence; the subject is discussed later in the context of coronary disease. A faster method of preventing blood flow is provided by local *thrombosis*, that is, abnormal clotting of the blood within a vessel[1]. Generalized intravascular coagulation occurs in surgical shock and in other conditions but the common presentation considered here is that of a single clot forming round a localized area of damage to the vessel lining. Clots of this type may arise in arteries or in veins. In addition to the dangers inherent in obstructing what may be a vitally important vessel, such as a cerebral or coronary artery, conditions are set up for the third and most rapid form of blockage which is known as *embolism*. In this condition, fragments of preformed clot break off. If this occurs in an artery, the particles are forced into vessels of decreasing size until they lodge and cause a sudden deprivation of blood to the parts beyond, the process being known as *infarction*—death of a particularly sudden type will occur if a cerebral vessel is embolized. If the clot that disintegrates is located in a vein, it passes to the right side of the heart where, if large enough, it will occlude the main pulmonary artery but, if smaller, will pass into the lung until it can go no further; this is the condition of pulmonary embolism which is such a common cause of death in persons whose blood tends to clot in the leg veins as a result of enforced immobilization in bed[2].

Inhibition of the heart action may result from any of these processes. The heart itself may perforate, in which case the blood held within the pericardial sac inhibits the normal heart action mechanically—this condition is known as *cardiac tamponade*. There can be blockage of the coronary vessels, which supply the heart muscle, either by thickening of the walls, by thrombosis or by embolism. The

[1] The important word is 'abnormal'. Thrombosis is a 'normal' part of the process of limiting haemorrhage from a vessel whose wall is broken (*see* Chapter 1).

[2] Strictly speaking, this type of embolism should be referred to as thrombotic embolism. Embolism by itself is a generic term for the process whereby vessels are blocked by particles of any sort. Thus we have conditions such as fat embolism, air embolism or embolism due to particles injected into veins, etc., but the origins in each instance are quite distinct.

feature distinguishing such occlusions from those occurring in peripheral vessels of comparable size is that sudden deprivation of oxygen in even a small area of heart tissue which is vital to its rhythmic function inhibits its action; the contractions become ineffective, the condition of *ventricular fibrillation* is set up and the tissues throughout the body are immediately deprived of oxygen. Additionally, any disease of the heart muscle—whether it be inflammatory, toxic or simply due to excessive loads imposed—may, at a particular moment, become just sufficiently severe to stop the heart beat and to cause sudden death. Finally, inhibition of the heart through abnormal stimulation of its regulatory nerves must be mentioned; the concept of vagal inhibition of the heart, which was introduced on page 13, is referred to at many points in this text.

These various processes are likely to present at different times in life; the underlying causes of sudden death must be related to age if their forensic significance is to be appreciated.

In infancy and early childhood

Death in this age group is discussed in detail in Chapter 20. Many sudden infant deaths are associated with congenital cardiovascular malformations; the presence of these will have been known previously and death will not be unexpected—they are therefore beyond the definition of sudden death that is adopted here. This age group, in which the important group of so-called 'cot deaths' occurs, provides the exception to the rule that sudden unexpected death is almost entirely associated with the cardiovascular system. Although it has been suggested that some 'cot deaths' may be due to primary disease of the heart, this is plainly not the common cause. A proportion of these baffling cases may be due to fulminating viral infection and, certainly, many sudden deaths in early childhood do result unequivocally from infection—either of the brain (meningitis), the lungs (pneumonia) or the bowel (enteritis). Such disease states can progress very quickly, and it is seldom that allegations of negligence on the part of the doctor—which are not uncommon in the emotional atmosphere surrounding the death of a child—can be shown to have any substance.

In the young adult

Bleeding in the form of subarachnoid haemorrhage is the most important process under this heading; since subarachnoid haemorrhage is also a frequent result of injury, the cases are of particular medico-legal significance.

The common form of naturally occurring subarachnoid haemorrhage is of congenital origin. As a result of malformation of the muscle wall, balloon-like swellings, known as *berry aneurysms*, form in the cerebral arteries at the base of the brain, most commonly at one of the comparatively abrupt, geometric junctions in the area. The wall of the aneurysm is thin and is liable to rupture. The resulting pressure effect of the extruded blood is particularly concentrated on the vital centres of the brain and can cause sudden unexpected death. Often, it is the death rather than the symptoms that is sudden—a fairly slow leak of blood may cause a headache for several hours but such premonitory signs are often overlooked.

The distinction between natural disease and injury as a cause of subarachnoid haemorrhage is not always a simple matter. Trauma may rupture even normal cerebral vessels; although there is some difference of opinion among various researchers as to the true cause-and-effect relationship, it is logical to suppose that abnormally weak arteries could be damaged by abnormally slight force. Similarly, while most berry aneurysms rupture in the absence of a permanently raised blood pressure, it would be hard to deny the probability that a transient rise in pressure could predispose to 'blow-out'. The contribution of an altercation to such a death may therefore be doubly difficult to interpret[3]. Aneurysms may be so small as to be invisible and, occasionally, it may be impossible to demonstrate a specific bleeding point; failure to do so must, however, raise a suspicion of an unnatural cause of haemorrhage (*see* Chapter 11).

The inclusion of the condition in a section devoted to the young adult does not imply that it does not also occur in older age groups; it most certainly does, and modern studies draw attention to the increasing average age at which spontaneous subarachnoid bleeding occurs. The incidence in older persons is increased by rupture occurring in cerebral vessels damaged by the degenerative disease of atheroma. Death is surprisingly often associated with straining on the lavatory pan.

Intracerebral haemorrhage is rare in young persons. When it occurs, it is likely to be due to bleeding into a tumour of the brain which, in turn, may be derived from a primary tumour of the genital system. Haemorrhage into tumours is a more common cause of death in elderly persons, secondary deposits from the stomach and lung being the most common findings.

Acute haemorrhagic deaths in young women may result from bleeding due to growth of the fetus in an abnormal position—the so-called *ectopic gestation* which results from the ovum 'losing its way' or being 'held up' in its passage to the cavity of the uterus. Such catastrophes have been largely eliminated by modern antenatal care, but it is still probably true that, from the medico-legal point of view, sudden death in a young woman should be suspected of being associated with pregnancy until proved otherwise.

Apart from such relatively obvious causes, the diagnosis of natural sudden death in young persons may present considerable difficulty. In some instances, the deaths appear to be due to one of a group of primary diseases of the heart muscle collectively known as cardiomyopathies. Occasionally, a toxic origin may be shown for such diseases—alcoholic cardiomyopathy is a good example; more often there is an abnormality of growth, one side of the heart being greatly enlarged. This condition is known as *asymmetric hypertrophic cardiomyopathy*; one possible mechanism of death is that an enlarged left ventricle occludes the outlets into the great vessels but, alternatively, the increasing bulk of muscle may outstrip the available capacity of the coronary arteries, a concept that is discussed further below. On other occasions, 'inflammation' of the heart muscle, so-called *myocarditis*, has been invoked as a cause of obscure deaths. The condition may be due to true infection, usually of viral type, to an allergic reaction or to disorders of the endocrine system—e.g. overactivity of the thyroid gland. All of these conditions can be diagnosed only by a microscopic examination and are characterized by collections of white blood cells in the muscle of the heart. While such a finding may satisfy some observers, others are sceptical of their true significance; the distinction between findings that are causative of death and those that are purely incidental is discussed in Chapter 10.

[3] There is a strong tendency not to prosecute such cases in the English Courts. A very useful review of this difficult subject is by Knight, B. (1979), Trauma and ruptured cerebral aneurysm, *British Medical Journal*, i, 1430.

The mention of scepticism draws attention to 'status lymphaticus' as a cause of sudden death in young persons. This diagnosis, based on the finding of an enlarged thymus gland, often with associated enlargement of the lymph nodes, is an example of a conclusion forced by the absence of recognized fatal pathology despite a thorough post-mortem examination. It has long been discarded, but its memory is a monument to the fact that sudden deaths in young adults may be as obscure as are cot deaths in infants. Such a situation arises not infrequently in fit young men who have recently taken part in athletic pursuits. In my experience, the only common feature appears to be an enlargement of the spleen suggesting convalescence from a recent infection. Microbiological studies are, however, consistently negative, and the cases remain as a distressingly inexplicable group. Rather than certify death on extremely tenuous grounds in order to satisfy the Registrar, it would be better to classify such cases under, say, 'sudden unexplained death in young adults'; such a policy would at least serve to stimulate research into an unexplored field.

In later years

Sudden death in late middle age is dominated by degenerative changes in the vessels of the cardiovascular system.

The main degenerative change is atheroma, in which the wall of the vessel is replaced by fatty material which, breaking down, leaves a greatly weakened structure. In the absence of surrounding support, the tendency is for such a diseased vessel to dilate—an aneurysm is formed. The commonest site is in the abdominal aorta—rupture is progressive but death is eventually very rapid as the blood intended for the lower limbs is poured into the abdominal cavity. Almost instantaneous death may result from a rather similar process—known as 'dissecting aneurysm' because the blood passes within the wall of the vessel—which occurs predominantly at the origin of the aorta; the blood may sometimes be forced back into the pericardial sac and sudden death is due to cardiac tamponade. Deep vessels in the brain may be weakened by atheroma and, in the event of rupture, will cause intracerebral haemorrhage while massive haemorrhage into the intestine may follow erosion of a vessel at the base of an ulcer in the stomach or duodenum; such deaths are only occasionally entirely unheralded.

Rupture of vessels is more likely in the presence of a raised blood pressure—hypertensive heart disease is a potent cause of sudden death in this age group. Apart from the peripheral catastrophes that may occur, the heart itself—which enlarges in order to perform more work—may 'outgrow its strength' and suddenly fail, a mechanism that is discussed below. High blood pressure is not, however, the only cause of steady enlargement of the heart; disease of the heart valves—in particular narrowing (*stenosis*) or incompetence of the aortic valve—may provoke the same effects.

Coronary heart disease

The subject of coronary heart disease has been left till last because its ability to kill is almost all-embracing in its age span—deaths from this cause have been reported in men aged 19 and, indeed, the younger the subject, the more likely is the first 'coronary attack' to be fatal. Death from coronary heart disease is, however, most common in the period of life from age 45 onwards and, from that point, becomes the commonest single cause of death in most industrialized countries. It is by far the most important cause of sudden death and is almost the only cause of instantaneous death. Inevitably, a high proportion of such cases are reported to the Coroner or the Fiscal. Some understanding of the disease process is essential to the lawyer because of its frequent appearance in pathology reports; the disease also has important associations with accidents, particularly of industrial or vehicular type, and many insurance companies attach much significance to coronary artery disease in relation to life expectation and compensation.

The heart, like any other muscle, depends on an efficient blood supply to provide it with energy. But, whereas most muscles have a comparatively simple action, the heart must contract constantly and rhythmically. This sophisticated action is controlled by aggregations of nerve tissue known as 'nodes', from which extend 'bundles' of conducting tissue; if any of these specialized areas are deprived of oxygen, the muscle as a whole will beat in an arrhythmic fashion—ventricular fibrillation is established and efficient pumping action ceases. It follows that localized ischaemia of the heart muscle may cause instantaneous death. Deprivation of oxygen in other than an essential area will cause localized ischaemic death of muscle but, very often, this dead area can be repaired by the process of fibrosis or scar formation. A 'coronary attack' has been survived, but the heart wall may be thinned and dangerously short of blood—a pathological process that has struck once is likely to do so again; a person in this situation is therefore a bad risk in respect of certain occupations. Oxygen deprivation of a large area of muscle is likely to be fatal because insufficient useful tissue remains; death in such circumstances may be less instantaneous than it is when a vital area is involved.

The blood supply to the heart is carried by the left and right coronary arteries which normally are of adequate bore. But, for reasons that are not entirely understood, most persons' coronary arteries silt up as a natural process of ageing—the condition is that of progressive coronary atheroma. The process is something like the furring of hot-water pipes but, in the case of the arteries, the atheromatous material is laid down within the lining of the vessel. The body's main defence against the process lies in the establishment of a collateral circulation (see page 71) which is effective so long as the occlusive process is slow. But this may not always be so. The thick atheromatous plaques require a blood supply of their own and, not infrequently, the walls of the minute vessels will give way—the condition of *intramural haemorrhage* is established and the bore or lumen of the vessel is *suddenly* occluded. Very often, the plaques degenerate without haemorrhage and a necrotic 'abscess' forms which may itself rupture, leading to sudden *atheromatous restriction* of the lumen; in each case, bursting results in *disruption of the intima* which may form a valve-like obstruction to the flow of blood. Finally, the blood in contact with a diseased area tends to clot *in situ* and the process of *coronary thrombosis* is superimposed on coronary atheroma. The significance of thrombosis in sudden cardiac death is to some extent controversial. Although it is common lay practice to speak of coronary occlusion as thrombosis, the two conditions do not necessarily go hand in hand. It has been stated that thrombi are found less commonly in cases reported to the Coroner or Fiscal than in those dying in hospital, but the degree of disparity depends on such variables as preselection of cases for dissection. Thrombosis is, however, not *essential* to the post-mortem diagnosis of a coronary death—many of these are physiological in nature and may be due to localized spasm of the arteries. Similarly, the result of ischaemia of the muscle—infarction—is not always seen at autopsy; death due to ventricular fibrillation may have been too rapid for the formation of visible changes.

The above description refers to acute coronary insufficiency arising at a specific point in the arterial tree. An equally common situation is that in which a sudden increase in cardiac effort is demanded—due either to a physical or to an emotional stimulus—and in which the diseased circulation is unable to expand so as to satisfy the immediate need for increased oxygen. Inadequacy of this type is particularly prevalent in those in whom the atheromatous process has advanced to calcification, with consequent rigidity of the arterial walls, and in those whose arteries have been severely affected by heavy smoking. These cases pose a difficulty in pathological interpretation—death is due to a failure of response, and the circulation will have the same appearance after death as it would have done had it been possible to examine it in life; much of the diagnosis must rest, therefore, on the circumstantial evidence or, if none is available, on the absence of any other cause of death.

This physiological type of coronary death relates in the main to inadequate arteries supplying a heart of normal size. Much the same situation will obtain if normal-sized arteries are required to maintain a heart of abnormally increased bulk. Potential examples of this have already been noted—the heart in hypertension, suffering from the effects of valvular disease or enlarged due to cardiomyopathy. Persons so affected are living dangerously, because a sudden requirement for oxygen may be beyond the immediate capacity of the relatively small vessels. Sudden death can result but, again, the findings at autopsy will need careful interpretation. The processes are illustrated in *Figure 7.2*.

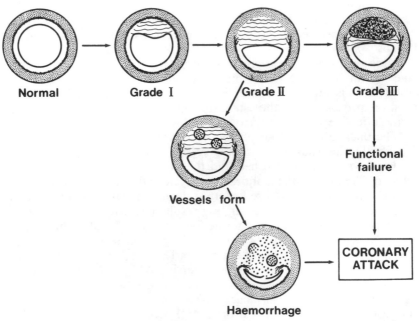

Figure 7.2 Development of a coronary attack. Atheroma forms, Grade II disease representing more than 50 per cent restriction of the lumen. The plaque becomes vascularized and haemorrhage results in sudden occlusion. Alternatively, calcified arteries may not be able to dilate to satisfy an urgent need for increased blood supply. It should be noted that simple Grade II disease may lead to insufficiency if the muscle mass of the heart increases without an increase in vessels.

Many of the natural sudden deaths described thus far are precipitated by the need for increased cardiac output. Major forensic significance therefore attaches to the conditions leading to that demand because these must be regarded as the basic cause of dying. Thus, the association of disease and death at work is of far-reaching importance in relation to benefits under the Social Security Act; this is discussed in Chapter 15. Disease may also cause vehicular accidents which are discussed in Chapter 10, but falls in the house, drowning and many other types of apparently violent death may be precipitated by natural disease. Natural disease is clearly of importance in the evaluation of homicide. Severe disease discovered in a man dying during a fracas may provide grounds for a plea to reduce a charge of murder to one of manslaughter or culpable homicide. It may, contrariwise, aggravate an offence. In a case seen by the author, a man seated in a locked parked car was threatened by a passer-by—he died suddenly and autopsy revealed extensive coronary disease with fibrosis of the heart muscle; although there had been no physical contact, the assailant was convicted of culpable homicide.

If the foregoing represents the normal sequence of events, it might be asked, 'Why do so many coronary deaths occur during sleep?' The answer is unclear. It has been suggested that lowering of the blood pressure, which occurs during the early stages of sleep, may predispose to the formation of thrombi (or clots) within diseased and narrowed vessels. But it has also been shown that the blood pressure rises erratically during sleep, possibly associated with dreams, and the effect is a subconscious demand for increased oxygen supply. Such cases do not invalidate the general hypothesis.

Causes of sudden death other than cardiovascular in adults

In practice, only two conditions merit space under this heading.

Asthma can undoubtedly cause sudden death. Severely affected persons may enter a condition of grave respiratory difficulty known as *status asthmaticus*. This may occur, but it is not essential to the valid attribution of death to asthma as sufferers seem to be unduly susceptible to sudden collapse. It has been suggested that these deaths may, in fact, be due to the general use of potent drug therapy, and certainly this is an aspect that should be investigated whenever such a case presents.

Epilepsy is in a rather similar category. *Status epilepticus*, a long-sustained epileptic attack, is a well-known cause of death but, again, epileptics are subject to sudden death in the absence of such obvious symptoms. This is additional to the extrinsic dangers of an epileptic attack, such as falling from a height or drowning.

8

Wounding

The law

From the purely medical aspect, anything that entails damage to the body tissues can be described as a wound, but it is more colloquial to speak of an accidental wound—or any wound caused other than by an instrument—as an injury. Medically speaking, wounds and injuries are a single pathological entity. A division of injuries on legal grounds is to some extent artificial and—since the basic problem in the pathology of violence is to distinguish between accident, suicide and homicide—it is almost impossible to discuss one category to the exclusion of the other two. For the purpose of this chapter, wounds are defined as injuries arising from an assault. So far as is possible, suicide and accidents will be discussed only in relation to differential diagnosis; some overlap is, however, inevitable.

The law on wounding in England is governed by the Offences Against the Person Act 1861 which itemizes various offences.

Wounding or causing grievous bodily harm and shooting with intent to maim or resist arrest are considered in s. 18, while s. 20 describes the offence of maliciously wounding or inflicting grievous bodily harm either with or without any weapon or instrument; assault occasioning actual bodily harm and common assault are the subject of ss. 42, 43 and 47. The nature of a wound is not defined, but there is case law[1] to indicate that a wound must involve a break in the whole skin, which would include a similar injury to a contiguous mucous membrane[2]. The point is relatively unimportant, as the alternative charges of causing actual or grievous bodily harm will cover bruising or more serious injuries such as may result in fracture without skin damage[3].

In Scotland, an attack on the person of another is an assault for which punishment is not specified in any rule. An assault is, however, aggravated, for example, by the use of firearms, stabbing or by throwing corrosive substances. An assault that causes injury is likely to be more severely punished than is one that does not. Assault 'to severe injury' may be libelled, i.e. specified in the indictment, and it is a very severe aggravation to assault 'to the danger of life'[4].

[1] R. v. M'Loughlin (1838) 8 C. & P. 635.
[2] Confirmed in JJC (a minor) v. Eisenhower [1983] 3 All E.R. 230.
[3] Polson, C. J., Gee, D. J. and Knight, B. (1985). *Essentials of Forensic Medicine*, 4th edn., p. 92. Oxford; Pergamon Press.
[4] Gordon, G. H. (1978). *The Criminal Law of Scotland*, 2nd edn., p. 817. Edinburgh; W. Green & Son.

Murder—the ultimate in wounding—is defined in England as the unlawful killing of a reasonable creature in being with malice aforethought, either express or implied, the death following within a year and a day. In Scotland, voluntary murder is not so confined and is simply murder committed intentionally. The English concept of 'constructive malice'—that is, unintentional killing while committing some other offence—has been abolished[5] and the offence is now that of manslaughter. In Scotland, the difference between involuntary murder—that is murder committed without the intention to kill—and culpable homicide is blurred; it would seem that the former must be accompanied by 'wicked recklessness'—unintentional killing short of this is culpable homicide. This chapter is concerned, however, not so much with the law on homicidal wounding as with the general, non-specific, body responses and pathological evidence that may follow wounding or injury; specialized injuries, such as those due to heat or gunshot, are discussed separately.

Bruises

Even though the skin is not broken, the subcutaneous tissues—those beneath the skin—may be damaged by blunt violence; the resulting extravasation of blood from broken vessels constitutes a bruise.

Bruising comprises bleeding into the tissues. A clean cut with a knife seldom causes a bruise as the blood escapes through vessels that are damaged only on the edges of the cut. Bruising can, however, surround a laceration of the skin if that breach has been caused by a blunt object; in that case, there may be damage to the vessels internal to the cut surface and blood will escape in both directions. The extent of bruising is, in general, inversely proportional to the sharpness of the object inflicting a wound.

The appearances of bruising without laceration of the skin are not uniform and depend on several factors. First, the part involved is important—the more lax the tissue, the easier it is for the blood to spread; the tissues around the eye will bruise far more readily than will the firm tissues of the back. Secondly, there is the age of the person—blow for blow, children and old people bruise more easily than do young adults or the middle aged; an assessment of the force involved must take these factors into consideration. Thirdly, extravasated blood will move along the tissue lines of least resistance under the influence of either pressure or gravity; the shape of a bruise may thus have, and probably will have, little relation to the agent causing it and its shape may change with time.

Not only the shape but the external evidence of bruising may alter; it is often most valuable to re-examine the victim of an alleged assault some 24 hours after an inspection made shortly after the event—bruises that were indistinct or even invisible may, by then, have become quite defined. Some bruises may not appear on the surface—this is particularly true over flat bones such as the skull when, should the head strike or be struck by a relatively soft structure, maximum damage to the vessels may be effected against the hard underlying bone and bleeding will be internal rather than visible; the extent of a head injury must not be assumed on the basis of an external examination alone.

The degree of bruising is further influenced by the physical state of the injured person irrespective of age. The physiological limit to a bruise is set by the body's

---

[5] Homicide Act 1957, s. 1.

capacity to plug the injured vessels and to clot the escaping blood. Persons with inborn coagulation factor deficiences, of which haemophilia, itself rare, is the best-known form, or with a diminished number of platelets, with abnormalities of the small blood vessels or with liver disease will bleed more readily than normal and may give a false impression of the severity of injury.

Capillary blood is dark red; recent bruises will be purple in colour. The tint darkens and browns as oxygen is removed and, soon, the enzymes of the body begin to change the haemoglobin into bile pigments; as a consequence the bruise of a few days' age takes on a greenish hue which, as it disperses, changes to yellow. It is often stated that the cycle takes about 1 week, but this is so dependent upon the size of the extravasation and upon the factors discussed above that accurate 'dating' of a single bruise is by no means a simple matter. The medical witness will be able to provide far more valuable evidence as to timing when this is of a comparative nature—it is often perfectly possible to state that a given bruise or set of bruises is older than another. This is of obvious importance in cases of alleged assault in which it is important to eliminate those injuries that are of no immediate concern: such comparative evidence reaches greatest importance in the analysis of injured children (see Chapter 20). A feature of the natural elimination of bruises is that some free iron is commonly left in the area, and this is readily demonstrable under the microscope. Thus, a more objective method of ageing bruising—and wounds of all types involving haemorrhage—is theoretically available after post-mortem dissection. Unfortunately, the appearances are again variable, and it is scarcely possible to do more than generalize—'it is probably safe to say that it is not usual to find iron-containing pigment in less than 12–24 hours'[6]. The method is of some value in distinguishing cerebral haemorrhage that is the result of an accident from natural haemorrhage—which could have been accruing for some time and which may have caused the accident.

Bruises occurring in the subcutaneous tissue seldom cause significant damage unless they become infected. Bruising may, however, affect the deeper tissue. Thus, a bruise within the eyeball may cause permanent blindness and the possible fibrous reactions to bruises of vital organs—say, for example, bruising involving the coronary circulation of the heart—may cause physical effects some time after the original injury; the significance of such lesions is discussed in Chapter 10. Deep bruises which, by virtue of the size of the vessels involved, amount to frank haemorrhage may have severe immediate and long-term effects which are also influenced by the function of the structure involved—bleeding into the brain, for example, may cause irrecoverable damage to the nerve cells.

All authorities are agreed that bruises can be produced after death. Such bruises will probably be of small size and, in the event of doubt, microscopic studies designed to demonstrate the persistence or absence of enzymatic processes may on occasion distinguish ante- from post-mortem lesions. It is often only possible to say that such bruising occurred 'at or about the time of death'.

Abrasions

An abrasion occurs when the outer skin is damaged but the deeper layers remain intact. Although little harm is caused to the body as a whole, rupture of vessels of

---

[6] In Simpson, K. (ed.) (1965), *Taylor's Principles and Practice of Medical Jurisprudence*, Vol. 1, 12th edn., p. 189. London; Churchill.

minute size may result in permanent and relatively faithful reproduction of the object causing the abrasion; it follows that such injuries are of major diagnostic importance[7].

Abrasions may be due to a frictional movement between the skin and an object or to simple pressure on the skin; in either case, the damage may be *ante mortem* or *post mortem*.

Moving abrasions will not replicate the pattern of the offending object but will give evidence, first, of the direction of the abrasive force. Thus, by visualizing the 'pile-up' of epidermis at the far end of an abrasion, the pathologist can give evidence as to the direction of a blow or of contact with the ground in, say, a pedestrian street accident. Parallel, linear abrasions are suggestive of having been caused by finger-nails; they may confirm the fact of an assault, they may give evidence as to the relative positions of attacker and attacked and they may serve to identify or exclude a suspect by demonstrating finger span or abnormalities of the fingers or finger-nails. These abrasions must be distinguished from 'knife-point' abrasions, which may also be made, for example, by gem stones. Such markings are thin, generally straight and often in criss-cross pattern. They may be self-inflicted, with a sexual motivation, in which case they are of remarkably uniform depth; it is, however, surprising how such injuries inflicted as part of an assault can simulate self-infliction.

Impact abrasions, without relative movement, often reproduce closely the object causing the injury. Examples include the imprints of weapons, boots or parts of an automobile; even if clothing intervenes and makes it own imprint, the shape of the abrasions may indicate its cause. An outline of a contact object will appear when skin having loose underlying connective tissue is struck; the abrasion is then caused, in effect, by the differential movement of the skin at the edges of the instrument.

Abrasions inflicted coincidentally with or after death merit special mention. They are devoid of vital reaction and take on the appearance and texture of parchment; wide areas of 'parchmenting' may result from contact with a flat object. Such post-mortem 'pressure' abrasions are very common in vehicular accidents, and are found in bodies recovered from the sea that have been pounded on the rocks. They must be distinguished from the rather similar appearance produced by the post-mortem application of heat or other forms of localized desiccation.

Lacerations

Strictly speaking, any breach in the whole skin thickness is a laceration. It is customary, however, to confine the term to a breach of the skin caused by direct blunt injury or by tearing or shearing forces; a laceration caused by a sharp object is an incised wound or a stab wound (*see* below).

Lacerations resulting from blunt force must involve crushing of the skin as a prelude to splitting. They generally occur over a bone that lies close to the skin with little intervening soft tissue, e.g in the scalp. A blow over the cheek bone may result in a laceration; an identical blow 2·5 cm (1 in) below on the cheek itself might well cause no more than a bruise. Perhaps the classic laceration due to blunt injury is the boxer's 'cut eye', which is found in the eyebrow area.

The essential features that define a laceration due to blunt injury are the presence

---

[7] Even in the absence of skin damage, ante-mortem 'blushing' of the vessels beneath a pressure point may leave a distinct pattern, e.g. following a slap.

of associated bruising, the irregularity of the split and the manifest crushing or tearing damage to structures *within* the split—an incised wound will merely divide them neatly. A laceration cannot, therefore, give as much evidence as to the shape of the causative instrument as can an abrasion; the two may, however, often coexist. The presence of multiple lacerations of generally similar type, particularly if they are closely grouped but not identical in direction, must raise the suspicion of foul play. Lacerations as here defined can seldom be suicidal unless they result from a fall; remarkable motivation would be needed to produce self-inflicted lacerations with blunt instruments—but this has been seen.

Lacerations due to kicking are generally multiple and are concentrated around the ear and side of the neck. Other selective sites for kicking, such as the abdomen, may well not show skin breaks. Whatever the site, the characteristic feature is the unusual extent of associated deep bruising.

Lacerations due to tearing or shearing are characteristic of vehicular accidents. They are often accompanied by severe damage to the underlying muscle or even bone. The extreme example is the very frequent spiral laceration of the leg involving all the tissues, which is caused by savage twisting of the limb held firm while the torso is free to move.

Incised wounds

Incised wounds result from the use of a knife-edge of any type including, for example, glass. The danger of such a wound depends upon the position and its depth; a deep incision of the buttock may cause little more than discomfort whereas a comparatively superficial cut in the wrist may prove fatal due to division of a major artery.

Incised wounds may be accidental but, as such, are seldom serious. A most common problem, however, is to distinguish cutting injuries that are self-inflicted with suicidal intent from similar dangerous injuries sustained as a result of an aggravated assault. The major points of distinction include:

1. The position of the incision. The neck is the most common site for both homicidal and suicidal incisions. Those in the wrist are, however, almost diagnostic of suicide.
2. Suicidal injuries to the neck are nearly always multiple and show evidence of altering determination, some incisions being superficial while one, or perhaps two, are deep and lethal. True, a suicide may be resolute at first attempt but the murderer is unlikely to be tentative; homicidal incised wounds are, therefore, commonly both severe and of similar depths.

Incised wounds are not infrequently inflicted for the purpose of maiming or disfiguring rather than killing. Intended as punishment, they are nearly always made on the face; deep self-inflicted wounds in this location are very rare save in the presence of severe mental derangement or as a form of ritual disfigurement. A specific incised wound of different type may be found on the fingers or palm of the hand; such injuries, often irregular in distribution and depth, commonly represent attempts at self-defence, and strongly indicate that other wounds on the body are homicidal in nature. Similar 'defence injuries' may be found on the forearm, although in this situation they are more likely to be in the form of lacerations or bruises.

Pathological findings designed to demonstrate the direction of the cut are often difficult to interpret. The 'exit' portion is almost bound to be shelving; the 'entry' wound may well be precipitously deep in homicide or shelving towards the centre when self-inflicted, but the appearances must be very variable and will also be modified by the shape of the part that is cut.

Penetrating wounds

A wound can be described as penetrating if its depth exceeds its width. When the superficial characteristics of such an injury are those of an incised wound, it is a stab wound; it is customary to restrict the term to injuries inflicted by pointed instruments, e.g. a needle, a knife or a bayonet.

Accidental stab wounds arc invariably single unless the offending instrument has multiple penetrating points; an accidental fall on to the points of a garden fork or a spiked railing could provide multiple stab wounds of symmetrical pattern, identical direction and equal depth. It may be difficult to distinguish accident from suicide or homicide when there is evidence of only a single thrust. Much will depend upon the findings at the locus of death and on the position and direction of the wound. The site of a suicidal stab wound must have been accessible to the dead person and, in practice, the great majority of single suicidal stab wounds are in an elective site, occasionally deep in the neck, but more commonly following the path of the classic Japanese method of self-immolation running upwards from below the ribs to penetrate the heart. Single homicidal stab wounds are comparatively rare, as most wounds leave the victim capable of resistance for a measurable time during which the blow is repeated; single homicidal wounds are, therefore, often associated with a drugged, drunk or sleeping victim and are almost always aimed at the heart. Occasionally, single homicidal wounds may cause difficulty by reason of their unusualness. In a case seen by the author, a man's body was picked up from his front garden and treated as a supposed sudden natural death; it was not until the body was being undressed in the mortuary that a single stab wound was noted in the right loin—very rapid death had resulted from transfixion of the aorta. It may be reasonable in such atypical cases to question the intention to kill and to accept them as instances of involuntary murder, manslaughter or culpable homicide.

Multiple stab wounds are very strongly suggestive of voluntary murder. When a suicide inflicts several wounds upon himself, the earlier wounds are likely to be shallow—a close grouping of the injuries is likely unless the suicide results from religious frenzy or other mental imbalance. Multiple murderous stab wounds show, by contrast, a more uniform degree of force, several being potentially lethal—they are often widely spaced and of different directions unless the repeated stab wounds have been inflicted on an unconscious body.

Evidence will be drawn from the pathologist as to the nature and shape of the weapon, either to assist in the search for, or for purposes of comparison with, a suspect article. As with all wounds, the sharper the instrument, the less tissue damage and bruising will be found. A stab by a knife will produce a clean incised wound which, by virtue of the elasticity of the skin, will stretch into an ellipse. A double-edged weapon will normally produce a symmetrical surface pattern, whereas one with a single edge may show relative blunting, or 'fish-tailing', of one end of the entry slit; all authorities are agreed, however, that differential contraction of the skin and subcutaneous tissue may, on occasion, give a misleading impression. The maximum diameter of the wounds must be measured with the edges opposed. In general, the weapon—and, in particular, a knife—cannot be wider than this so long as the natural taper of the point is taken into consideration and the width is related to the depth of the wound; rocking or twisting the knife obviously may produce a wound that is larger than its maximum width. Similarly, the depth of the wound is unlikely to be longer than the full length of the weapon; a false indication of length may be obtained if the body surface has been compressed by the hilt, as may particularly be the case in wounds of the abdomen. Despite the obvious need for caution, the accurate measurement of a number of stab wounds in a single body may enable the pathologist to give a reasonably accurate description of the likely size and shape of the blade of the weapon used, especially if it was a knife (*see Figure 8.1*); different measurements may indicate that there was more than one assailant.

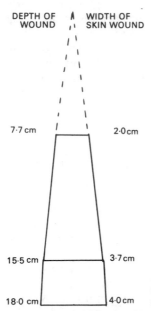

Figure 8.1 The shape of a knife assessed from the appearance of three stab wounds of different depth. The actual knife was of remarkably similar shape although the point was curved.

These measurements, together with an assessment of the direction of multiple stab wounds, may also enable the pathologist to establish how the knife was held, and to gauge the strength with which the blows were struck. The question of the 'force used' is often difficult to evaluate and an opinion must take into account the clothing of the victim. To find that the wounds penetrated 'up to the hilt'—often demonstrable by bruising at the edges of the wound—is to assess the results of force rather than its degree. Deep penetration of the tissue by a sharp, pointed instrument is surprisingly easy, and it would be within the power of practically any adult to inflict a lethal wound using the usual pattern of sheath knife which is freely saleable to persons of all ages[8].

    [8] 'Flick knives' may not be sold—nor, indeed, dealt in any way (Restriction of Offensive Weapons Acts 1959 and 1961).

The mode and cause of death after wounding

Rapid death resulting from incised or stab wounds is usually due either to haemorrhage or to damage to a structure that is vital to life; death may occasionally be caused by air entering a broken vein.

Haemorrhage is by far the most common of these and will be much more severe if an artery is penetrated than if only veins are affected; the speed of death will depend upon the size of the vessel involved and on the secondary effects of the accumulation of blood. It is difficult to inflict a stabbing injury of 15 cm (6 in) depth without lacerating an artery of at least moderate calibre, and the direction of most homicidal stab wounds results in their frequent termination in the heart, aorta or major pulmonary vessels. Death is often very rapid, but it pays to be cautious in interpretation as some remarkable periods of survival have been recorded. Haemorrhage from non-penetrating incised wounds need not be severe unless a major artery lies superficially at the site if injury—the most obvious example of such an area is on the flexor surface of the wrist which, accordingly, is a favourite site for suicidal incision.

Rapid death due to interference with the function of structures other than blood vessels is rare and is confined to special situations. Thus, stab wounds at the nape of the neck may result in near instantaneous death, with minimal haemorrhage, due to the destruction of the vital centres in the medulla of the brain stem. Incised wounds of the trachea or larynx may lead to collapse of the neck structures with valve-like obstruction of the main airway; more probably, the airway will be blocked by blood or impacted tisses. Incised wounds of the neck may, in fact, result in many modes of death—vagal inhibition of the heart, airway obstruction, air embolism, venous bleeding from the jugular veins or arterial bleeding from the carotid arteries; consequently, the length of the agonal period may be particularly difficult to assess.

Death attributable to wounds or injuries occurring some time after the event presents no special features. Among other complications, those of prolonged immobilization—pneumonia or pulmonary embolism—or of reduction in blood volume—in particular acute renal failure—may arise and must be regarded as logical sequences of the original assault in the absence of proof of intervening medical negligence, although even this may not affect the question of causation[9].

[9] R. v. Smith [1959] 2 Q.B. 35.

Injury and death due to firearms and explosives

The law

The law relating to firearms is statutory throughout Great Britain and is contained in the Firearms Act 1968[1]. A firearm is defined in s. 57(1) of the Act as any lethal barrelled weapon of any description from which any shot, bullet or other missile can be discharged. Excluding air weapons, personal firearms are of two categories—the smooth-bore weapon, or shotgun, and rifled weapons which include revolvers, 'automatic' pistols and rifles. The former were devised primarily for the sport of killing small animals; the latter, while being used in some forms of sport hunting, e.g. deer stalking, were mainly perfected for the killing of man. The regulations governing the possession and use of rifled weapons are, accordingly, far more strict than apply in the case of shotguns. Section 1 defines, by exclusion, those weapons that it is unlawful to possess without simultaneously holding a firearm certificate.

No one under the age of 14 may acquire or use any firearm or ammunition unless as a member of a recognized club, or when in a shooting gallery using miniature rifles or air weapons; but an airgun can be used under supervision by an adult over 21 in a private place. Persons over 14 may be given or lent an airgun, or a 'Section 1' firearm subject to the possession of a firearms certificate, but sale to a person below the age of 17 is prohibited; the possession of an assembled shotgun under the age of 15 is subject to supervision by an adult. The carriage of an airgun in a public place by a person under the age of 17 is prohibited unless the gun is securely covered.

Certificates to possess and use an airgun are not required; in addition to it being illegal to sell such a gun to anyone under the age of 17, it is also unlawful to present a young person under the age of 14 with an airgun for his possession. The relaxation of certification does not apply to 'specially dangerous air weapons'—defined as pump-action air rifles having a kinetic energy greater than 16 J (12 ft lb), or 8 J (6 ft lb) in the case of pistols—which are classified as 'Section 1' firearms. Smooth-bore guns having a barrel not less than 60 cm (24 in) long are not Section 1

---

[1] The use of other offensive weapons of discharge type, e.g. ammonia guns, is dealt with, under the Prevention of Crime Act 1953.

firearms, and their possession is regulated by the issue of shotgun certificates which are obtained from the local police; there are no further restrictions on the acquisition of shotguns by persons over the age of 17 and, in certain circumstances, shotguns can be used without a certificate being held—the most important of these being when the gun is borrowed from a person with a certificate and is used on his private property. It is an offence to shorten the barrel of a shotgun to less than 60 cm (24 in); the resultant 'sawn-off shotgun' would be a Section 1 weapon and its possession restricted to the granting of a firearm certificate.

Whereas it is generally only necessary to be 'of good character' to qualify for the issue of a shotgun licence, a person seeking a firearm certificate must not be of intemperate habits, of unsound mind or for any reason unfitted to be entrusted with firearms. The Chief Constable must be satisfied that the applicant has a good reason for acquiring a firearm and that its acquisition would not be prejudicial to public safety or to peace. Very few categories of person are exempt from firearm certificate requirements—the commonest are members of approved rifle clubs and cadet corps and race starters at athletic meetings: persons in the service of the Crown or in the Police are exempt although subject to rigid regulation by their parent authorities. The possession of certain weapons—e.g. automatic repeating rifles or weapons discharging a harmful liquid or gas—is prohibited without the specific authority of the Home Office or Scottish Home and Health Department in addition to the possession of a firearm certificate.

Shotguns are, therefore, widely distributed and despite the regulations, legally held firearms are responsible for a substantial number of deaths; the illegal possession of firearms, including the retention of 'war souvenirs', is fairly widespread. A number of specific offences relating to the use of firearms are created by the Firearms Act. These include:

1. The possession of a firearm or ammunition with intent to injure a person or to damage property.
2. Using a real or imitation firearm to resist arrest or possessing a firearm or imitation firearm at the time of committing (or being arrested for) a 'specified offence'.
3. Trespassing with a firearm.
4. Carrying in a public place without lawful authority or reasonable excuse a loaded shotgun or any other firearm whether loaded or not together with appropriate ammunition.

To wound or cause grevious bodily harm with intent to do so by any means—which includes shooting—is a statutory offence in England and Wales[2]. In Scotland, wounding by shooting is a serious aggravation of an assault.

Gunshot injuries are of major pathological interest in that they can be interpreted with considerable objectivity; the pathologist can often give opinions that are very well based and that are particularly valuable both to the police and to the lawyer.

Airgun injuries

Unless the pellet penetrates some vital spot, such as the eye or the brain, severe injuries from the normal airgun or air pistol are unlikely. The same is not true of the

---

[2] Offences Against the Person Act 1861, s. 18 as amended by the Criminal Law Act 1967, Schedule 3, Part III.

powerful air weapons described as especially dangerous, the effect of which may be comparable with a small bullet from a rifled firearm. Injuries due to air weapons do not merit a separate description.

Shotgun injuries

Shotguns may be single or double barrelled. The barrel of the former or one barrel of the latter may be tapered towards the muzzle—a manufacturing process known as *choking* which serves to lengthen the period during which the shot is restrained in a compact mass. The calibre of shotguns is expressed in unusual terms. When the diameter of the barrel is less than ½ in (1.25 cm), the calibre is given by that diameter—e.g. 'four-ten' means a barrel diameter of 0.410 in; guns larger than this are measured by 'bore'—or the number of spherical lead balls exactly fitting the barrel that go to make 1 lb. An 8-bore is therefore a larger and more powerful gun than is the common 12-bore[3].

The shotgun cartridge consists of a cardboard or plastic cylinder attached to a brass plate which contains the primer. The main powder charge is separated from the shot by a wad or washer. The shot is maintained in the cartridge by a distal wad. When fired, the shot—which consists of a large number of pellets of a size chosen for the particular sporting purpose intended—is propelled in a solid mass which begins to fan out as the compression by the wads is released. The propellant continues burning as the shot passes down the barrel and some powder always remains unburnt. The effective range of a sporting shotgun is approximately 50 yards (or metres), and the shot is rapidly halted within the tissues of the target.

The pathological evidence as to the distance from which the shot has been fired can be deduced from these principles, although it cannot be overstated that some variations occur in practice. A contact injury will show bruising due to the recoil of the gun and a perfect representation of the single or twin barrels may be formed on the skin; the shot will enter the body as a solid mass so that the entry wound will approximate to the bore of the barrel; however, explosive gases will also enter the wound so that the external wound may be ragged—the skull, for example, may be literally blown apart; an exit wound may be seen, except in the very thick torso, because the shot in a contact wound is in a solid mass. Shot in its diffuse form, as fired from a distance, has little penetrating power; exit wounds are, therefore, not a feature of shotgun injuries other than in the contact situation. At very short range, the appearances described above will be modified by the differing effects of the gases of combustion—these will not be forced into the wound but may still cause some irregularity of the entry hole. Unburnt powder will be discharged into the surrounding skin, leading to what is known as 'tattooing'; soot is likely to be deposited. The hot gases will burn the skin or clothing, either of which may be charred; in both contact and close-range wounds, any carbon monoxide contained in the gases of combustion may form local carboxyhaemoglobin which can be recognized by its pink colour.

These effects diminish as the distance from muzzle to wound increases. The critical distance is at about 2 yards (or metres) as, at this distance, tattooing is scarcely visible and the wads fail to penetrate the wound. The shot now begins to fan out and creates a pattern of entry in the clothing and on the skin. Although the

[3] These measurements can now be metricated (Gun Barrel Proof Act 1978, s.5).

inclination of the body to the line of flight of the shot will alter the appearances, ideally the pattern will be circular. The size of this circle depends to some extent on the degree of 'choking' of the gun, but the appearances are sufficiently standard to permit the use of a simple rule— the diameter of the shot pattern in centimetres is some 2.5–3.0 times the muzzle distance from the wound in metres (or the spread in inches is equivalent to the distance in yards)[4]; estimates derived in this way must be checked by test firing whenever possible. Fatal 12-bore shotgun injuries are unlikely at a range of over 20 yards (*see Figure 9.1*).

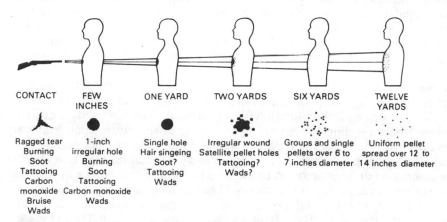

Figure 9.1 Effects of a shotgun injury related to distance. (Reproduced from Knight, B. (1982). *Legal Aspects of Medical Practice*, 3rd edn., p. 16. Edinburgh; Churchill Livingstone; reproduced by permission of the author.)

The majority of shotgun injuries are sustained at close range. The internal injuries are therefore due either to the violent expansion of gas within the body or to the penetrating effect of what is, essentially, a solid mass of lead more than ½ in (1.25 cm) in diameter; the former effect is well seen in the head and the latter in the heart which can be torn apart by a shot fired from within a range of 2 yards (metres). Otherwise, the effects of a shotgun injury are variable and depend upon the ability of individual pellets to penetrate either the heart or individual blood vessels or other organs liable to severe bleeding; the surgery of such an injury may present a formidable problem.

Rifled weapons

The main diagnostic difference between wounds due to shotguns and those due to rifled weapons rests on the fact that, whereas shot will certainly be found in the body, a bullet is likely to have exited; entry and exit wounds are, therefore, a feature of the latter.

Contact and close-range entry wounds due to rifle bullets will have much the same characteristics as those of a shotgun injury—bruising, blast effects, soot

[4] Attempts to improve the accuracy of this estimation by complicating the formula probably fail in their purpose and merely make the matter harder for juries to understand.

deposition and tattooing will be present, the last being found up to a range of some 1.0–1.3 m (3–4 ft).

If the range has not been so short as to cause explosive damage to the tissues, the characteristics of the entry wound will be governed by the gyroscopic stability of the bullet. In the early phase of its flight—up to some 50 m (yards) for a pistol or 150 m (yards) for a rifle—and towards the end of its effective range—of the order of 460 m (500 yards) for pistol and 2.4 km (1½ miles) for a rifle—there is considerable 'tail wag' which results in a relatively large and ragged entry wound. In the most efficient phase of flight, the bullet will enter the body neatly nose on and leave a regular, small hole which, because of the elasticity of the skin, may well not correspond exactly to the diameter of the missile. The entry wound will always show inverted edges and is likely to demonstrate 'soiling'—that is, contamination of its edge by the grease covering the bullet which is wiped off either by the clothing or by the skin.

As the bullet traverses the body, it may become deflected, it may be deformed and it may take with it fragments of tissue—particularly bone—to act as secondary missiles. The exit wound is therefore likely to be irregular, its edge will be everted and there will be no soiling—it cannot be smaller than the entry wound save at extremes of range. The modern, very high velocity rifle presents something of an exception. This weapon kills by virtue of the massive internal damage that results from the dissipation of large amounts of kinetic energy; the entry and exit wounds are, however, small and of closely similar size. The common tendency for the wound to enlarge from entry to exit is well shown in bone, particularly the bones of the skull, in which the penetrating wound bevels outwards to be of larger diameter on the exit side; this difference in size is useful in distinguishing a bullet wound from a surgical burr-hole in a skeletonized skull or fragment of skull bone presented for examination.

The pathologist is likely to be able to give a very good opinion as to the direction of an injury from a rifled weapon as compared with shotgun injuries but has less evidence on which to base an estimate of range. The recovery of a bullet from the body is, of course, of great importance to the investigation, as every weapon leaves a characteristic pattern of scorings on the surface of the bullet; test firing of suspected weapons may then result in a convincing identification by comparison. Equally good—if not better—comparative evidence can be derived from spent cartridges recovered at the scene of a shooting—marks of an individual nature are made by the firing pin and hammer, the ejection mechanism and during extraction; such methods of weapon identification are also open in the case of shotguns but lie in the province of the ballistics expert.

Bullets may kill by virtue of penetrating the heart, a major vessel or a vital centre of the brain. By far the greatest damage is, however, caused by 'cavitation' in the track of the missile, and by the discharge of energy which can tear vital tissues associated with, but removed from, the actual path of the bullet; widespread destruction may result from fragments of tissue which form 'secondary missiles'. Delayed death is likely if a solid organ with a large blood supply, such as the liver, is damaged; death from septic shock or simple sepsis may follow penetrating injuries of the bowel.

The nature of the wounding

The immediate need in any case of fatal firearm wounding is to distinguish between accident, suicide and homicide. The forensic doctor will often be able to give sound evidence as to the probability of suicide; the distinction between accident and homicide, is, however, a far more difficult problem. The medical evidence will rest, first, upon an examination of the locus and, second, on the post-mortem findings.

The scene of death will provide much evidence in relation to suicide. First, the weapon must be within reach and almost always will either be retained in the grasp or lie close to the hand of the dead person. A murderer may attempt to simulate suicide and it is most important that the doctor, called in to pronounce life extinct, takes full notes of the precise conditions. The presence of the rare cadaveric spasm is of importance; this is one post-mortem condition that cannot be artificially produced (*see* Chapter 4). Homicide is clearly indicated if the gun is found at the scene and is beyond reach of the deceased; the main exception rests in the possibility of a suicidal or accidental shot that is not immediately fatal—in which case, there may well be evidence of movement in the form of blood splashing and the like. Mention is generally made of suicide accomplished by means of a remote firing mechanism such as a pulley attached to the trigger; such contraptions are set for deep-seated psychological reasons, and not for the purpose of confusing the investigating officers—they rarely cause difficulty although, again, the possibility of an artefact rigged by an assailant has to be eliminated. The examining doctor should always confer with the police officer in charge as to the presence of spent cartridges; the firing of more than one shot is uncommon in suicide.

The post-mortem findings indicating suicide can be deduced from the previous pages. Findings indicative of a range within 1 m (yard)—in particular, the appearance of tattooing—are clearly consistent with suicide as this is the maximum distance it is possible to hold a pistol from the body; similarly, the absence of close-range characteristics in a shotgun or rifle wound will strongly militate against suicide as the barrel length of the gun approximates to that of the arm. In practice, it is extremely uncommon for suicidal wounds to be other than of a contact nature. They will also almost always be in a 'site of election'; these vary according to the weapon. A suicidal pistol wound is generally inflicted in the right temple (whether the person is right-handed or not)[5], and an exit wound is usual close to the opposite temple; an alternative is the centre of the forehead—the precise symmetry is classic and of diagnostic importance—while the roof of the mouth may be chosen. Rifle wounds are, again, common in the centre of the forehead and in the mouth; in either case, massive tissue damage may result. The rifle suicide may lean on the gun with the muzzle on the brow or over the heart, a situation that is not unusual with shotguns. The commonest suicidal shotgun wounds are, however, those in the roof of the mouth or in the centre of the forehead, just above the bridge of the nose; in either case, the head is torn asunder, often, again, in a characteristic, symmetrical fashion. The important general features of successful suicidal firearm wounds are that they are always so placed as to eliminate the possibility of failure, and that the entry point must be accessible. Other evidence of close contact with the gun, such as heat discolouration of the thighs where the barrel has been steadied, may also be present.

Accidental gunshot injuries may be 'self-inflicted', as in the classic 'cleaning the gun' situation, or involve a second party, as when a moving fellow hunter is mistaken for game. The former situation may closely simulate suicide, the essential differentiation being the asymmetry inherent in a random occurrence. The latter type of accidental injury, showing no more than the effect of a relatively long-range discharge, is indistinguishable from homicide on purely pathological grounds.

[5] I am indebted to the late Professor C. K. Simpson for this expression of his wide experience.

Certain features are strongly indicative of homicide—a single wound of contact or very close range type in an inaccessible position is an obvious example, the back, the nape of the neck or behind the ear being the commonest sites; similarly, the existence of more than one fatal injury will be very strong evidence against both suicide and accident—in circumstances of high emotional tension, such as marital brawls, a mixture of both non-fatal and fatal wounds may be found. The suspicion of homicide may, however, rest on the exclusion of suicide by the pathologist, coupled with the circumstantial evidence obtained by the police officers.

Examination of suspects

There is little or no valuable evidence that the forensic doctor can derive from the general medical examination of a suspected firearm assailant. The doctor may, however, provide specimens for analysis in the forensic science laboratory.

The older relevant tests are based on the assumption that residues of propellant will settle on the firing hand. Both gunpowder and modern smokeless powders contain nitrates which are readily detectable when present. It was the habit to remove skin-surface contaminants with paraffin and the test thus became incorrectly known as 'the paraffin test'. The identification of nitrates has since been regarded as non-specific and, in 1964, Interpol 'did not consider the traditional paraffin test to be of any value'[6].

Later work has concentrated on the identification on the hands of metallic residues derived from the primer contained in the percussion cap of the cartridge; mercury, antimony, barium and lead can be quantified in this 'dermal residue' test. The residues are removed by swabbing with moistened filter paper. Current work in Belgium has indicated certain drawbacks to a promising approach—for example, the 'natural' residue is strongly dependent on occupation and a negative result, even under experimental conditions, does not necessarily exclude the possibility of a firearm having been used; moreover, the residues are easily removed by washing. Tests of this type must be regarded as still subject to critical appraisal; hopefully, what may be a useful indicative test will not become discredited due to the exaggeration of improbable alternative interpretations.

Injuries and death due to explosion

Injury and death due to explosion may occur industrially or in the home—as, for example, when gas filling a room is ignited. The resulting injuries will be due, first, to the air blast itself and, secondly, to random impacts as the body is hurled against other solid objects. If the blast is due to a bomb, there will be added damage from the splintered casing.

The effects of blast are due to a combination of positive pressure, the blast wave itself and the subsequent negative pressure. The effects, which are exaggerated in an enclosed space, are seen particularly in those organs capable of elastic recoil and containing multiple gas/fluid or fluid/solid interfaces. Thus, the lungs in particular

---

[6] First International Criminal Police Organization Seminar (1964). *International Criminal and Police Review*, **174**, 28. Quoted by Cornelis, R. and Timperman, J. (1974); *Medicine, Science and the Law*, **14**, 98, where an interesting review is given.

are the subject of much disruption and haemorrhage; the ear-drums are also most sensitive to pressure changes. Blast effects are well transmitted in water; the hollow viscera are particularly vulnerable to underwater explosions and, since there are no injuries due to secondary impacts, those killed in these circumstances often present with little external but massive internal damage.

Bomb injuries[7] may approximate to disintegration of the body; short of this, the wounds are characterized by their multiplicity and by their association with foreign particles not all of which necessarily derive from the bomb itself—many fragments of glass, brick dust or even pieces of furniture will contaminate the wounds and will give a distinctive pattern of 'peppering' of the body.

As in all types of wounding, death due to bomb blast may be accidental, suicidal or homicidal. Accidental cases are of legitimate and illegitimate type. The former are confined to members of bomb disposal squads and to workers in authorized armouries—for example, in the armed forces. When the device involved is a small one, the track of metallic fragments can often be traced in the body so as to define the reconstruction of events with considerable accuracy. Accidental bomb injuries of an illegal character—e.g. occurring in those manufacturing bombs—are likely to be far more severe. Suicidal bomb injuries might occasionally be used as a form of political exhibitionism but are probably now relegated in history to the more bizarre aspects of the Second World War. Suicidal actions may be differentiated pathologically by the concentration of massive injuries in the abdominal region; the victims of random bomb attacks commonly show maximal injury in the legs. Homicidal bombing in a civilian context is a comparatively recent form of outrage; despite the fact that the conditions in which it occurs are so diverse, the pattern of injuries is surprisingly reproducible[8]. Burns associated with bombs are of two types—the 'flash burn' affecting persons close to the explosion from which clothing provides good protection, and ordinary thermal burns resulting either from the clothes or from the building catching fire.

The pathological diagnosis of bomb explosion is never in doubt unless associated with, say, an aircraft (see below). The important evidence to be obtained from post-mortem dissection lies in the recovered fragments of bomb casing, from which information of value to law enforcement can be derived, much as in the case of firearm wounds; the importance of X-ray study as a means of localizing such fragments cannot be overemphasized.

The deliberate destruction of commercial aircraft in flight introduces a currently interesting variation on the theme of homicidal bombing; the diagnosis of this crime—which world-wide occurs between once and twice a year on average—has civil medico-legal as well as criminal implications[9]. The nature of the event often results in extensive destruction of the aircraft due to the high forces sustained in the resultant crash, while the whole wreckage may be lost should the catastrophe occur over the sea; much may, therefore, depend upon the pathological evidence[10]. This

---

[7] The offence of causing an explosion likely to endanger life or cause serious injury to property is defined in the Explosive Substances Act 1883, s. 2, as amended by the Criminal Jurisdiction Act 1975, s. 7.

[8] *See* Marshall, T. K. (1978). Major Civil Disturbance. In *The Pathology of Violent Injury*. Ed. by J. K. Mason, ch. 5. London; Edward Arnold.

[9] In the event of sabotage being shown as the cause of an aircraft accident, responsibility for insurance passes from the 'All Risks' insurers to those underwriting 'War Risks'.

[10] In fact, there is a trend towards an increase in the number of cases of attempted sabotage with a decrease in the proportion of aircraft completely destroyed thereby. The saboteurs appear to be less professional than was once the case.

rests upon observations that derive from a full examination of all the human wreckage recovered. The pattern of injuries throughout the dead may indicate an abnormal accident situation; search must be made for the 'target' who may present as an 'odd man out', by reason either of his position relative to the other passengers or of his injuries. Radiological examination of all human tissue is essential—and must nowadays be undertaken in all unexplained catastrophes occurring at altitude until a credible alternative to sabotage is agreed; finally, any metallic fragments other than those that are clearly part of the aircraft structure must be subjected to expert examination. The investigation of such a case is, inevitably, time consuming and extremely costly[11]. The perpetrators of this form of mass murder have been found to be of various types—political motivation may be present, but possibly the commonest reason in the past has been pecuniary and related to life insurance policies; suicides have been suspected and instances have been traced to motives of almost incredible frivolity, such as the removal of an unwanted girlfriend. A main difficulty facing the investigators is to distinguish sabotage from explosive decompression due to structural failure of the airframe in flight[12].

[11] Two examples of the medical investigation of such cases are: (a) Dille, J. R. and Hasbrook, A. H. (1966), Injuries due to explosion, decompression and impact of a jet transport, *Aerospace Medicine*, **37**, 5; and (b) Mason, J. K. and Tarlton, S. W. (1969), Medical investigation of the loss of the Comet 4B aircraft, 1967, *Lancet* **i**, 431.

[12] Compare, for example, the case described in footnote[11] (b) with the loss of the Comet aircraft in 1954 (Armstrong, J. A. *et al*. (1955)). Interpretation of injuries in the Comet aircraft diasters. *Lancet* **i**, 1135.

10

Accidental injury and death due to deceleration and acceleration[1]

The nature of the injuries

Accidents may occur in the home, at work or at play, and some of these situations are covered elsewhere in this book. Transportation accidents are, however, not only the commonest single source of severe traumatic injury and death in the United Kingdom, but they are also likely to lead to litigation. The majority of significant injuries sustained in road-traffic accidents are of a decelerative or accelerative nature and the forces involved are applied in the horizontal plane. Injuries sustained in accidental falls essentially result from vertical deceleration. Aircraft accidents link these two conditions in that the injurious forces are a varying combination of the horizontal and the vertical. It is with these three categories of accident that this chapter is concerned.

As discussed in Chapter 8, accidental injuries are similar in character to wounds. Although a large proportion of injuries may appear non-specific, many abrasions and some bruises may be remarkably distinctive in both appearance and distribution, and may provide important evidence in accident reconstruction—this is particularly well shown in the pedestrian road-traffic death.

The source of abrasions discovered on killed pedestrians may be obvious. Examples include the pattern imprinted by radiator grilles or by tyres; on occasion, this may be so individual as to provide corroboration of a cause-and-effect relationship with a particular vehicle. The importance of scaled photography of such abrasions, particularly in the hit-and-run type of accident, cannot be overemphasized as a means of preserving valuable evidence.

Useful pathological information can often be derived from an assessment of the sequence in which the injuries were sustained. The time intervals are usually extremely short and an evaluation through appraisal of the degree of bruising or of vital reaction is often impossible. Nevertheless, an attempt to distinguish direct contact wounds from those due to abrading, and a division of the latter into those caused by sliding over the vehicle or along the ground—as shown by contained glass, paint or earth—may be of value both to the police and to other interested investigators; whenever possible, the autopsy should include an examination of the

[1] 'Deceleration' to the physiologists is a substitute term for 'negative acceleration'. But the word is used colloquially and it is in this sense that it is introduced here.

clothing *in situ*—the correlation of clothing damage and bodily injury is one of the most useful examinations in the vehicular accident.

Abrasions in the occupants of cars who are killed in an accident are of particular importance, not only in indicating the identity of the driver—through the characteristic 'steering wheel' abrasions so often imprinted on the chest with underlying fracture of the sternum—but also in relation to the use of seat-belt restraint. This has important practical applications; an increasing number of insurance companies are tying the amount of indemnity to the use of or failure to use restraining harnesses, while judgements for damages for injuries sustained now take this factor into account[2]. It is clear that, in future, a plaintiff's (or pursuer's) damages will be reduced in part-proportion to the extent that his injuries were caused or aggravated by failure to use a seat belt—generally assessed as 20–25 per cent—and that this will apply even when the plaintiff is entirely blameless[3]. The pathologist may therefore properly be asked for evidence on this point which may be of even greater significance when the regulations resulting from the Transport Act 1981, s. 27 are promulgated. Although there will often be no residual evidence even though the equipment was used, bruising may be found in accidents involving relatively low force; the shape may be specific to the belt but any fine pattern will be that of the clothing closest to the skin. In accidents of severer type, the abrasion is more likely to be of the parchmented pressure type without pattern or vital reaction. The reflection of belt restraint in more serious injuries of internal type is discussed on page 99.

Lacerations may have a 'general' specificity. Thus, notes should be available of damage to the legs of pedestrians that is characteristically caused by car bumpers and which may provide excellent evidence as to the positional relationship at the time of impact; very similar injuries are common in pedal cyclists knocked down by motor cars. Multiple lacerations due to fragmented glass are common in killed car occupants, particularly those in the front passenger seat; the distinction between those who have been so injured because they were not restrained by a seat belt and those who suffered injury when their belts failed can often by made by a simultaneous appraisal of abrasions in the harness area. On the other hand, lacerations may be very specific and diagnostic as to causation—this applies both in automobiles and in light aircraft. The importance of photography in the accident autopsy cannot be overemphasized; photographs serve not only as *aides-mémoire* but may also draw attention to a previously unnoted correlation between an injury and its cause.

Internal injury without external evidence

Severe or fatal deceleration injury may be transmitted to the internal organs without corresponding visible external damage. The two common circumstances are compression of the chest or abdomen and accelerative displacement of the viscera.

Compression of the chest may result from impaction against some object, such as the steering wheel of a car; superficial abrasive evidence may then be found and the

[2] For an interesting review of the early cases *see British Medical Journal* (1974), Seat belts and damages; **ii**, 454.

[3] Froom and others v. Butcher [1975] 3 All E.R.520. The case and its interpretation are discussed in *British Medical Journal* (1975). Seat belts and negligence, **iii**, 315. The importance of the merits of the individual case are emphasized in Owens v. Brimell [1976] 3 All E.R.765.

breastbone (sternum) and ribs can be bruised or fractured. Alternatively, compression may be due simply to forceful flexion of the upper torso—the head and knees being thrown towards each other. This often occurs in motor cars when the abdomen is restrained by a belt; the legs and arms are flung forward with the body compressed into a shallow C-shape. The condition is even more apparent in aircraft accidents when the severe vertical component of force exaggerates the deformity. The heart may burst like a blown-up paper bag if it is crushed between the breastbone and the spine. The weakest areas lie in the atria, especially at the entry points of the great veins[4], but, often, the compression is such as to lacerate the muscular walls of the ventricles. There may be important residua if the forces have been severe yet insufficient to rupture the heart on impact. A lowering of the arterial blood pressure is an almost inevitable immediate physiological reaction to severe injury; areas of the heart that have been damaged in the accident may be unable to withstand the increase in pressure that accompanies the phase of recovery, and delayed rupture of the heart may occur within minutes or hours. Additionally, the process of rupture, which often runs from within the heart to the outside, may cause laceration of only a partial thickness of the muscle; the wall in the area where the inner lining is thus damaged is weakened and may rupture some considerable time after the event; a cause-and-effect relationship may then be difficult to establish.

The heart will be displaced downwards if the major compression between the sternum and spine occurs just above its base (or upper border); the aorta is, however, tethered to the tissues surrounding the spine and is unable to move. As a result, the heart is torn from its major blood vessel much as one squeezes a cherry from its stalk; the effect is similar to rupture of the heart itself. This sequence is even more probable if the heart is, itself, displaced downwards under the influence of a vertical force as occurs in falls or in aircraft accidents. The injury is common in both situations and, again, an incomplete laceration may result in delayed full-thickness rupture (*see Figure 10.1*).

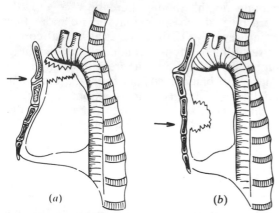

(*a*)   (*b*)

Figure 10.1 Major rupture of the cardiovascular system. (*a*) The heart will be torn from the aorta if the pressure on the breastbone is high. (*b*) If the point of pressure is lower, the heart will burst like a paper bag.

[4] Damage at these points may also be due to sudden increase in pressure in the venous system due to compression of the legs or abdomen.

Injuries of broadly similar type may be inflicted on the organs in the abdomen. These, by virtue of the organs' functions, may be of less catastrophic nature and prompt surgical intervention may be life saving.

The great bulk of the liver renders it particularly susceptible to blunt injury. It is easily ruptured by bending and stretching of the upper surface during severe body flexion, while its solid structure is particularly vulnerable to the high-frequency oscillations that are set up in a severe accident. Hepatic damage may well be fatal because bleeding from the organ is hard to stop and the liver, being essential to life, cannot be removed *in toto*. The almost equally common rupture of the spleen—which is a disposable organ as far as the body is concerned—or of one of the kidneys can be treated by removal of the damaged part; the important feature is awareness of the possibility that such injuries can be present despite the absence of external damage. Although rupture of the bowel itself is comparatively rare, compressive damage to its nutrient blood vessels as they traverse the mesentery is not uncommon in car accidents and occurs frequently in aircraft accidents; it may result from violent flexion alone but is more likely when this is combined with sudden and severe pressure on a simple lap belt.

The spine is under considerable strain in those conditions that produce sudden body flexion and, in practice, fracture of the thoracic spine is very common both in car and in aircraft accidents. There are two primarily vulnerable points; first in the upper spine if the torso is restrained by a full harness—in which case the forces are likely to be beyond the tolerance of the body as a whole—and, secondly, at the midpoint due to flexion over a lap belt. If severe vertical force is applied to the buttocks, as in a fall, an aircraft accident or, occasionally, in the unusual situation of ejection from a military aircraft, the spine is weakest at the junction of the thoracic and lumbar portions. Very severe vertical force will cause fracture of the pelvis. The pelvis is also especially liable to damage from a direct lateral blow and fracture is common in pedestrian or cycling victims of road-traffic accidents.

If the spine or pelvis are severely damaged, the sum of bodily injury may well have been sufficient to cause immediate death. Should there be recovery, the long-term disability resulting from fracture of the spine may be no more than stiffness and spasmodic pain of varying severity. If, however, the spinal cord is irrevocably injured, the extent of the resulting paralysis is related to the 'height' of the injury site in the spine; the common lower thoracic fracture is associated with paraplegia, that is paralysis of the legs and bladder. Apart from the extremely severe disability, there is an increased danger of death due to infection, particularly infection of the urinary tract. The additional disability related to childbirth that may result from fracture of the pelvis in women also requires special consideration as to compensation accruing from an accident.

The condition of fat embolism

Fat embolism is a form of death, nearly always associated with accidents, which is of sufficient medico-legal interest to deserve individual consideration. It is closely correlated with fractures of the long bones, spine or chest cage though, theoretically at least, it may result from severe injury to fatty tissue of any sort. Following fracture, there is a release of fat from the marrow cavity; this fat is passed into the venous system where, being particulate, it is caught up in the sieve of the pulmonary capillaries—the condition of pulmonary fat embolism is established.

Pulmonary fat embolism is of no clinical significance except in the aged with incipient heart failure; its main importance as a post-mortem finding is that it may be indicative of the time of survival between fracture and death (*see* page 106). But in a proportion of fracture cases, the fat appears to pass through the lungs and lodges in the capillaries of the brain and kidneys; the potentially fatal condition of systemic fat embolism is established[5]. Some 24 hours after injury the patient's temperature rises and, in severe cases, fatal coma supervenes; treatment of the established condition is unsatisfactory. It is only fair to say that this précis is a gross oversimplification, and the development of the clinical syndrome of systematic fat embolism probably depends on many interrelated factors including, particularly, the presence of surgical shock. Whatever the precise mechanism may be, two considerations are unaffected. First, the condition is associated with injury in all but a handful of very unusual conditions; consequently, it always has medico-legal connotations. Secondly, despite a tendency to an association with manipulation of fractures under anaesthesia, fat embolism is an unfortunate but natural complication of injury. These deaths are in no way associated with medical negligence.

Pathological appraisal of safety equipment

A correlation between the pathological findings and the safety equipment provided—whether the fatal accident results from the use of a vehicle or is of industrial type—is important for several reasons. First, there is the problem of the assessment of damages in car accidents which has been discussed above. Secondly, dependants of an employee killed at work are entitled to any evidence that indicates failure on the part of the management to provide an adequate safety environment; the employer must also be provided with any evidence that might limit his liability as to civil damages. Thirdly, this aspect of his work must be of major professional interest to the pathologist in that the function of any doctor is to save lives; the autopsy following an accidental death provides an almost unique opportunity for the forensic pathologist in this respect—by applying his findings so as to convert fatal accidents to those of non-fatal type, he is practising good preventive medicine. This was, and still is, a main function of a Coroner's Inquest or an inquiry under the Fatal Accidents and Sudden Deaths Inquiry (Scotland) Act 1976.

Pathological evidence on this score should be available both when safety equipment was provided and when it was not.

In the former case, the pathologist is certainly not the best person to evaluate the equipment as, by definition, he is dealing with a case in which it has failed to preserve life. The question often arises, however, as to whether the equipment actually contributed to death; an objective assessment, taking all the circumstances into account, is then essential. A number of road-traffic accident investigations describe 'seat belt syndromes' and there is no doubt that the seat belt, especially of the lap-strap-only type, can cause rupture of the mesentery, bowel or even major solid viscera. But the alternative to such a syndrome is likely to be death, and an operable rupture of the bowel is a small price to pay for a life saved. If the accident

---

[5] Precisely how often this occurs is difficult to assess. *Significant* systemic embolism occurs in perhaps as many as 1 per cent of fracture cases.

results in death from multiple injuries, the presence of lesions attributable to seat belts is no more than a part of the pattern of non-survivable loads on the body; but an isolated fatal injury positively associated with an intended safety device is of major concern. Thus, a number of fatalities have occured in light aircraft due to the subject 'submarining' through the harness and sustaining injuries similar to those of the old judicial hanging—such accidents clearly indicate the need for incorporation of a crutch strap; it seems at least possible that the *combination* in a car of a diagonal torso harness *and* a markedly reclined driving seat might produce the same effect.

The pathologist should be able to answer the closely related problem of whether safety equipment that failed to save life could be so modified as to be of greater value in similar circumstances in the future. One example of such research, again stemming from light-aircraft accidents, showed that approximately one-third of fatal head injuries discovered at post-mortem were in such a position as not to be preventable by the standard form of 'crash helmet', but the incorporation of an efficient visor skeleton would probably improve the survival rate appreciably[6].

It should be emphasized that no item of personal safety equipment can be expected to be effective in all possible circumstances. Its design is a matter of compromise—'child-proof' door locks on cars are, for example, potentially life saving in ordinary travel but may be positively detrimental to survival in the event of fire after a crash; it is a matter of calculating the risks involved and providing accordingly, the important feature being that a positive assessment has been made and a reasonable decision taken. Escape by traditional means from an aircraft in flight provides another good example of the dilemma—the provision of a bulky dinghy pack must complicate easy egress but, without a dinghy, survival after a descent into water is compromised; the decision to provide a dinghy would, therefore, depend upon whether the aircraft was operating predominantly over land or over water.

If death occurred when no equipment was provided the pathologist can only surmise as to the likely effect of the omission; an attempt must be made because important questions relating to liability may be raised. In cases in which the material was lost or damaged, it would also be proper to seek pathological evidence as to whether equipment that had been provided was, in fact, used.

It is not out of place to conclude this section with a brief review of the significance of the long-awaited introduction of compulsory seat harnessing under the Transport Act 1981. The medical and pathological evidence for the efficacy of a well-adjusted and well-designed harness, which excludes a simple lap-belt, is convincing[7]; a 25 per cent reduction in mortality can be anticipated if the law is properly enforced. Fire after motor-car accidents is in itself rare, and the chances of dying from such incineration are in the region of 1 in 500 fatal accidents; to this should be added the reduction in concussion, and consequent failure to escape the fire environment, offered by restraining harnesses. Moreover, the consequences of being thrown clear from a car involved in an accident are capricious and certainly not generally advantageous. Regulations governing exemption on medical grounds have been laid[7a]. The need for such exceptions is probably small, particularly when assessed in relation to fitness to drive, and, perhaps of greatest importance, there is no

[6] See Cullen, S.A. (1973), in *Aerospace Pathology*. Ed. by J. K. Mason and W. J. Reals, ch. 12. Chicago; College of American Pathologists Foundation.
[7] Seat belts: The overwhelming evidence. *British Medical Journal* (1977), i 593.
[7a] Motor Vehicles (Wearing of Seat Belts) Regulations 1982 (S.I. 1982/1203).

country in which pregnancy is an automatic ground for exemption from seat-harness law; the chances of a fetus being injured in a car accident are very much greater when the mother is unrestrained than when she is wearing a well-fitting harness[8]. The point is of considerable importance in the context of the Congenital Disabilities (Civil Liability) Act 1976, s. 2, which refers to the responsibilities of a pregnant woman driver to her unborn child.

The interrelationship of disease and accidents

Natural disease may cause varying degrees of incapacitation in the operator of a vehicle and may thus precipitate an accident; such disability is likely to be of more serious consequence in pilots than it is in drivers[9]. Further, the driver or pilot may die from sudden natural causes while at the controls, and it is at least theoretically possible that a passenger might die in the same way while under the stress of an impending catastrophe. The precise relationship between discovered disease and a fatal accident is of medico-legal importance on two main counts—first, a suspicion of negligence may be raised either on the part of the operator, in that he was driving or piloting while he knew himself to be unfit, or on the part of those scheduling the task without apparently ensuring adequate medical supervision; secondly, questions may be raised as to the entitlement of indemnity under an insurance policy against accidental death in the event of a natural death being followed by multiple injuries.

Disease of any sort discovered after an accident may be causative of, contributory to, or merely incidental to that accident. The distinction is often difficult to make; this is for two main reasons which are particularly well illustrated by coronary disease (see page 74). First, there is the simple 'population' problem illustrated in Table 10.1; a random search of persons killed accidentally will demonstrate a high proportion with potentially lethal disease of the coronary arteries yet in few, if any, of the cases could there have been more than an incidental association. Secondly, there is the technical problem arising from the fact that the disease process may need to do no more than cause symptoms for it to precipitate a crash; death is them due to injuries and the pathologist is confronted with appearances in the heart that stop short of those that are seen in natural death—the interpretation of events then rests on an opinion as to cause and effect which has to be given with what must sometimes seem to be undue reservation. There is often less difficulty in automobile cases in which the findings may be those that are normally accepted as good evidence of a coronary 'heart attack', but these may then have to be distinguished from appearances resulting from injury to the heart—a problem that is also relevant to aircraft accidents.

In making his assessment, the pathologist must consider, on the one hand, the special quality of his autopsy findings that might distinguish significant from asymptomatic disease[10] and, on the other, the circumstantial details of the accident.

[8] The whole subject is well reviewed by Cullen, S.A. (1978), The prevention of injury in vehicular accidents in *The Pathology of Violent Injury*, Ed. by J. K. Mason, ch. 2. London; Edward Arnold.

[9] Mason, J. K. (1974). Comparative medical requirements for drivers and pilots. *Journal of Traffic Medicine*, **2**, 58.

[10] These include evidence of previous damage to the heart muscle (fibrosis), calcification of the coronary vessels and evidence of activity of the disease in the form of infiltration of the vessel's coat by white blood cells (adventitial lymphocytosis).

He must also know the extent of the disease in the particular group of persons, e.g. drivers or pilots, concerned. Having all this information, he can ascribe the accident to disease in the operator on the basis of probability ranging from say, a significant association that is just possible (+) to a very probable association (+ + + +). It is doubtful, however, if he should often be more definite. An account of how these problems of interpretation can be argued was given at the Inquiry into the accident at Staines involving a Trident aircraft in 1972[11]. A further interesting fatal aircraft accident was reported in which a faulty instrument was discovered coincidentally with inflammation of the pilot's heart. The division of responsibility between the airline and the instrument manufacturers was of obvious significance; in the event, the case was decided out of court[12].

The extent of the problem of disease as a cause of accidents deserves careful evaluation. The threat is clearly very real in the case of aircraft pilots who, accordingly, are stringently screened for fitness—screening includes, in particular, periodic electrocardiography (ECG). But, by and large, disease of the coronary arteries and experience go in hand. In the long run, therefore, greater safety may be achieved by 'double crewing' than by intensive medical selection. Similarly, the potential danger to the public dictates that drivers of public services vehicles should be subject to medical examination but, in practice, serious motor-vehicle accidents of any sort due to disease in the driver are rare—there is a 'fail-safe' mechanism as the foot comes off the accelerator and, before this, most drivers will be able to pull into the side on feeling the premonitory symptoms of a heart attack. Epilepsy is, therefore, a more significant disease in relation to road-traffic accidents and is further discussed in Chapter 30. Diseases likely to lead to accidental death in pedestrians are of a different type and are scarcely amenable to detection at autopsy—in particular, disease of the locomotor system or of the special senses. Fatal accidents in the home are especially common in the elderly and, as a logical corollary, are very largely associated with disease, much of it having a causative or contributory role.

TABLE 10.1 Prevalence of coronary artery disease in UK aviators. Results are given as numbers of cases, with percentage of group in parenthesis*

Grade of disease	Military	Civilian	Total
0	114 (40)	38 (34)	152 (38)
I	103 (36)	48 (43)	151 (38)
II	46 (16)	16 (14)	62 (15·5)
III	23 (8)	10 (9)	33 (8.5)
Mean age (years)	27.6	34.9	29.7

* In the UK, almost a quarter of persons subject to relatively strict medical surveillance show restriction of 50 per cent or more of the lumen of a main coronary vessel without accompanying symptoms (Grades II and III).

Toxicological factors in vehicular accidents

Toxic substances contributing to vehicular accidents may be deliberately ingested or accidentally inhaled. Alcohol is the outstanding example of the first category

[11] *Report of the Public Inquiry into the Causes and Circumstances of the Accident near Staines on 18 June 1972.* Civil Aircraft Accident Report 4/73. London; HMSO.
[12] For details, *see* Stevens, P.J. (1970), *Fatal Civil Aircraft Accidents,* p. 19. Bristol; Wright.

and is discussed in detail in Chapter 25. Other drugs do play a part, their extent at present undetermined. To be significant in accident causation, a drug must be readily available, it must be used generally for the treatment of common ailments, and it must have a deleterious effect on concentration and performance; the antihistamines—widely used as cold cures—fulfil this specification outstandingly. Most of these drugs are available as pharmacy-sale drugs (*see* Chapter 23), but when they are sold their labels must indicate not only that they may cause drowsiness but must also include warnings not to drive, operate machinery or consume alcohol. Amphetamines used to be a potential cause of accidents, particularly when used to excess in night driving or as weight controllers without appreciation of their effect on function; this group is now controlled under the Misuse of Drugs Act 1971. Other commonly prescribed drugs, e.g. of the tranquillizer groups, may cause accidents by virtue of the taker being unaware of their intrinsic effect on driving or, more commonly, of the potentiating effect of combinations of drugs, particularly those that include alcohol. There are two major difficulties in assessing the role of such drugs in accident causation. First, there is the technological problem of searching *post mortem* for the presence of virtually unknown substances in near therapeutic concentrations; to do so is generally beyond the laboratory's resources in manpower and finance. Secondly, there is again the problem of interpretation. Who, for example, is to say that a light-aircraft pilot is any less safe when on a recognized dose of antinauseants than is the same pilot suffering from air sickness? And if traces of the drug are found at post-mortem, how is one to distinguish with certainty between a causal and an incidental association with the accident?

Barbiturates, which are so commonly the cause of accidental poisoning in the home, are not thought to be a potent cause of vehicular accidents. Together with other drugs they may, however, be a significant indicator of psychiatric or other nervous disease that is not demonstrable by standard post-mortem techniques—the prime example being epilepsy. Regulations are in force to prevent epileptics from obtaining either an unrestricted driving licence or a pilot's licence, but it is not difficult in present conditions for these to be bypassed. A search for barbiturates or anticonvulsants may, therefore, yield useful clues in indicating the basic cause of an apparently inexplicable accident.

Of the gaseous toxic factors in vehicular accident causation, only carbon monoxide deserves emphasis. A natural product of the internal combustion engine, it may leak into the cabin of the car through a faulty exhaust system or into an aircraft cockpit via a defective cockpit heater; carbon monoxide may also be drawn in from the exhausts of other cars if a car heater fan is connected in heavy traffic conditions.

Fatal levels of carbon monoxide in the blood are unlikely to be discovered in accidental deaths involving cars or aeroplanes; only a level sufficient to cause lack of concentration is required to cause an accident. Levels of 20–30 per cent carboxyhaemoglobin[13] are commonly associated with symptoms of dizziness and headache, but there are two reasons why even lower levels may be of significance in drivers and pilots. First, fine judgement is certainly affected at much lower levels. Secondly, a synergistic effect may result from the interaction of carbon monoxide, alcohol, fatigue or hunger while, in aviation, the effect of even slight oxygen lack due to altitude may be compounded to produce a most dangerous situation.

True intoxication of the operator is not the only possible cause of a raised carboxy-

[13] That is, 20–30 per cent of the normal respiratory haemoglobin of the blood is combined with carbon monoxide and is not available for the transport of oxygen.

haemoglobin level discovered in the blood after a fatal vehicular accident. Survival in a fire after the crash is by far the commonest cause (*see* page 141). Low levels, particularly in aircraft, may indicate an engine defect rather than an effect on the pilot, while the 'natural background' of carboxyhaemoglobin—which may reach 8 per cent in heavy smokers—must be considered in the interpretation of resuls.

Ideally, an analysis for carboxyhaemoglobin should be an integral part of the investigation of any vehicular death but, since levels of less than 20 per cent saturation may be of significance in an accident, the methodology must be adequate for the purpose. The methodology should, indeed, be considered whenever a scientific result is obtained for medico-legal purposes. The technical method used must be shown to have adequate sensitivity and specificity at the range of the levels required, and it must also be related both to the quantity of the specimen and to its quality—a method useful for examining good samples of blood taken from a living person may be quite inadequate when applied to a partially decomposed post-mortem specimen. The laboratory must be able to state its range of normal values when these factors are taken into consideration.

Accidents as a cause of disease

Although discussion has thus far centred on disease as a cause of accidents, the converse proposition is also of medico-legal importance.

Much of the debate on this subject has centred on the induction of cancer by injury; there is no doubt that this can occur, the most obvious examples being the growth of a tumour in scar tissue—especially in scars resulting from burning. Skin cancer is relatively obvious and its topographical associations are clear. The attribution of cancer of the deep tissues to previous trauma is a far less certain matter due, in the main, to the time lapse between any precipitating injury and the clinical recognition of the tumour. Most interest has lain in the possible association of tumours of the brain with head injury, although cancer of other tissues—for example, the breast—might well be related to injury. But accidental injury, albeit slight, to the head is commonplace while brain tumours are rare; moreover, even were it suggested that *all* such tumours were precipitated by injury—and it most certainly is not—the time interval would be such as to make it very difficult to decide which particular traumatic incident during that time represented the trigger mechanism. In an attempt to reconcile these difficulties, a set of rules, commonly known as 'Ewing's postulates', has been developed. These lay down that, before a tumour can be reasonably attributed to injury:

1. There must be evidence of previous normality of the part.
2. The injury must have been substantial.
3. The interval during which the tumour matured must have been of reasonable length.
4. The tumour must have developed at the site of injury.
5. The nature of the tumour must be scientifically proved.

Even accepting these premises, the attribution of a tumour to a previous traumatic incident is a matter of probability and there may be room for appreciable divergence of expert opinion[14].

[14] As an example, see Barty-King and another v. Ministry of Defence [1979] 2 All E.R. 80, where death in 1967 from cancer developing in a wound sustained in 1944 was held to be attributable to war service—a matter of great importance in relation to estate duty.

Similar reasoning can be applied to other types of disease that may be associated with trauma. Very often, there is little ground for disagreement. Thus, it would not be disputed that acute inflammation can be set up in a broken bone if virulent bacteria are present in the bloodstream at the time of injury. Or, if a man's pelvis were fractured in a car accident and his bladder was repeatedly catheterized, subsequent damage to the kidneys due to ascending infection would clearly bear a cause-and-effect relationship with the accident.

More difficulty arises in relation to the repair of injury—scar tissue is inherently weak and the effect of its substitution for normal connective or muscle tissue in an organ may appear only some considerable time after the original incident. It has been noted above that the inner lining and associated muscle of the heart may be lacerated during a severe fall or vehicular accident; in the event of survival, such areas must be permanently weakened and liable to rupture. Similarly, bruising and local damage to the muscle fibres of the heart may be caused by direct injury to the chest wall—the area when repaired is likely to be of less than normal strength. The same type of blunt injury causes haemorrhage into the wall of, or into the tissues surrounding, the coronary arteries. In either case, the reparative fibrosis may cause restriction of the blood flow and a coronary 'heart attack' at an unpredictable point in the future. Relationships of this type are very much open to argument, though few would deny the possibility of such a sequence of events occurring; as a consequence, expert opinions are likely to be very guarded.

Simultaneous death

Prior to the late nineteenth century, the establishment of the precise order of death in relation to the disposal of estates seldom gave rise to difficulty. The advent of the steamship, the train and the increasing risk of major conflagrations then exaggerated the problem. By now, however, the increasing safety measures taken have greatly reduced the incidence of simultanous death in close relatives; the solution of *commorientes* is virtually a problem of fatal motor car and aircraft accidents with occasional cases arising from hotel fires.

The legal solutions to simultaneous death are, basically, of two types. That operating in England and Wales states in general that, in the event of two (or more) persons dying in circumstances that make the order of death uncertain, the younger will be presumed to have survived the older[15]. In America, it is presumed that neither survived the other[16], and this rule is adopted by most central European and Scandinavian countries. France and Belgium include clauses in their codes to allow for extremes of age and for the legalistic nicety that, in similar adversity, the female is weaker than the male[17]. Since most wives are not only younger but are also less wealthy than their husbands, the clear defect of the English system is that it introduces a strong possibility that a finding of uncertainty as to which of the husband and wife survived the other may result in the male estate being diverted in ways that neither husband nor wife anticipated. This is because the test in deciding if s. 184 of the 1925 Act applies is not whether there *was* a simultaneous death, but whether there was uncertainty as to which of two or more persons survived the

---

[15] Law of Property Act 1925, s. 184.
[16] Uniform Simultaneous Death Act, 8 Uniform Laws Annotated 608.
[17] *Code Civil*, Art. 720–722.

others and the Courts appear to take the view that simultaneous death cannot be proved pathologically[18]. However, if the words 'simultaneous death' are used in a will, it is unlikely that the Courts will engage in metaphysical argument, but will decide on common-sense principles and on the medical evidence[19]. Scots law has recognized this imperfection and, while generally following that of England, has excluded 'spouse commorientes' from the general rule[20]. In fact, it would seem that, whenever possible, opportunity has been taken to adopt the American system—if, in England, one of the commorientes is intestate, then the estates devolve as if neither had survived the other[21]. Australia and New Zealand both followed the basic English system, but New Zealand effectively reverted to the American code in 1958[22]; it is possible that legislation was precipitated when the law's manifest unfairness was demonstrated after the disastrous eruption of Mount Ruapehu the year before.

From the aspect of forensic medicine, however, it is not the differences in the systems that matter so much as that all have it in common that the presumption of simultaneous death is rebuttable by the evidence and that evidence of survival will be taken into consideration by the Courts; such evidence must be provided mainly by the forensic pathologist whose difficulties are compounded by the fact that no limit of time is set—survival for seconds is as significant in law as is survival for days.

Taking the commercial-aircraft accident as a typical example, the useful pathological evidence may be of several types and of varying sophistication. First, there is the precise cause of death. Thus it could well be assumed that a person who had survived the crash only to die from burning would have survived longer than another who had sustained a rupture of the cardiovascular system. Such evidence should not, however, be accepted uncritically. Delayed rupture of the cardiovascular system—particularly of the atria or of the aorta—is a well-documented phenomenon (*see* page 97). Moreover, the modes of death must be markedly dissimilar to be of good evidential value; thus, while the example above might well be valid, it would not be reasonable to suppose that a person with severe head injury had survived for a longer or shorter period than one with severe heart damage in the absence of other corroboration. Nor would it be right to assume that a person who had a greater overall degree of injury had necessarily predeceased someone with a single fatal injury.

The finding of carbon monoxide in the blood is objective evidence of an asphyxial death due to burning (*see* page 141). A raised carboxyhaemoglobin in X compared with a negative result in Y could be taken to imply that X sustained a longer agonal period than did Y; but it would be wrong to reach the same conclusion if both showed raised values, but X's level of carboxyhaemoglobin was higher than that of Y—such a difference could be related to the precise environment in which each died and to the air intake of each, which could be affected by disease, by activity and by other factors.

Further evidence of survival for a limited time may be provided in persons with fractured bones by the microscopical finding of particles of fat or of bone marrow in

[18] Hickman v. Peacey [1945] A.C. 304 H.L.
[19] Pringle, In *re* Baker v. Matheson [1946] Ch. 124, per Cohen J., at pp. 126, 129–131.
[20] Succession (Scotland) Act 1964, s. 31.
[21] Intestates' Estates Act 1952, s. 1(4).
[22] Simultaneous Deaths Act 1958.

the lungs. Both these types of particle reach the lungs, as described on page 98; bone marrow particles provide the more unequivocal evidence because their structure indicates their origin beyond dispute. None the less, bone marrow emboli are often difficult to find, and a negative result might mean no more than that fragments that were present were not detected by the pathologist. Only a positive finding in indicating a definite time interval between injury and death is of true evidential value. Moreover, the *degree* of involvement of the lung in two persons cannot be used comparatively to assess the length of the survival period and anomalous cases, of both positive and negative type, occur[23].

The pathological observations designed to distinguish in time between apparent simultaneous accidental deaths thus require very careful analysis. But they cannot be interpreted unless they are sought; this implies the need for post-mortem dissection and for time-consuming and technically difficult follow-up investigations in the toxicological and microscopic fields—a daunting prospect with up to 150 families possibly involved in a single incident. Quite opposing results as to the likelihood of relative survival may be obtained depending on the diligence and motivation of individual medical examiners. If justice is to be even in this sphere, the standards of autopsy must also be even—and this is unlikely to be so, particularly on an international scale. The disposal of a family estate may depend to a large extent on the precise geographical location of an aircraft crash, and the routine use of 'survival' clauses in wills is therefore particularly important.

Novus actus interveniens

It is a clear principle that a person is responsible not only for his actions but also for the logical consequences of those actions. This applies both in aggravated assault and in accidental injury. It is logical to assume that competent medical treatment will be available, if sought, for any injuries sustained. Should such treatment—or lack of it—be negligent and should that negligence result in a deviation from the logical sequence of events, then the responsibility for the subsequent disability or death may pass from the original incident to the later negligent action—this by virtue of *novus actus interveniens* (an unrelated action intervening). The majority of such interventions will be of a medical nature and the pathologist must provide evidence on this point in relevant cases.

The possible variations of *novus actus interveniens* are legion and no purpose would be served in listing potential causes—some may be obvious as, for example, the leaving of a surgical instrument in the abdomen after the repair of a treatable internal injury, while some may be more subtle. The most vivid example in the author's experience was the accidental substitution of poisonous potassium chloride for the innocuous sodium chloride during treatment by the artificial kidney of a man injured in a road-traffic accident.

Special problems associated with organ transplantation are referred to in Chapter 12. An element of negligence is essential to a plea of *novus actus;* an unforeseeable complication or a failure of a recognized form of treatment could not

---

[23] Recent work has, in fact, emphasized the difficulties of interpretation. *See* Buchanan, D. and Mason, J. K. (1982) Occurrence of pulmonary fat and bone marrow embolism; *American Journal of Forensic Medicine and Pathology*, **3**, 73.

be so categorized. *Novus actus* often presents a difficult pathological problem and differences in expert opinion may be well held on such questions as the proportionate contribution to death of the original and the new events, or as to whether an admitted error in treatment did, in fact, affect an inevitable outcome. It would appear that, in practice, the plea of *novus actus* is rarely accepted by the Courts[24].

[24] Certainly this is so in the Criminal Courts. In R. v. Smith [1959] 2 QB 35, a stabbed man was dropped twice by the attendants and not given a life-saving blood transfusion; in R. v. Blaue [1975] 1 W.L.R. 1411, a stabbed woman refused a blood transfusion on religious grounds and died 5 hours later. It was concluded in both cases that death was caused by the original wound. The contrary case of R. v. Jordan is noted in Chapter 31. *See* also R. v. Vickers (*Daily Telegraph* (1981), 9th Oct., p. 3), where a man was acquitted of manslaughter on the basis of a faulty anaesthetic having been given to the victim. The paucity of material in the civil field may well result from the most blatant cases being settled out of court.

11

Head injury

The mechanics of head injury

The common head injuries which may occur either singly or in combination are
bruising or laceration of the scalp; fractures of the skull—which must be divided
into those involving the vault, which covers the upper and outer surfaces of the
brain, or the base, on which the brain rests and through which the cranial nerves
and the spinal cord pass; intracranial haemorrhage—which may be extradural,
subdural or subarachnoid (see page 13); laceration of the brain; and intracerebral
haemorrhage. These injuries may be produced by sharp weapons or by blunt force;
they may be homicidal, suicidal or accidental in origin. For practical purposes,
suicidal head injuries, which will generally result from falls from a height, will be
similar in nature to those of accidental origin; homicidal head injuries have only a
few characteristics that distinguish them from such wounds elsewhere and will be
discussed first; the bulk of this section will be concerned with accidental injuries.

The tissues of the scalp are comparatively dense and are lined internally by firm
but very vascular fibrous tissue. Direct violence to the scalp which lies on the rigid
vault of the skull results in a unique form of crushing between two hard objects. If
the crush is of minor nature, a contusion or bruise will be produced; tracking of
blood is likely to be slight in the dense connective tissue and, although bruising will
usually be evident on both the outer and inner surfaces, it will commonly be more
apparent on the deep aspect of the scalp. At the same time, since the scalp is held
firmly over the skull, it is not unusual for the outer surface to reproduce the pattern
of the weapon or object responsible for the violence. The skin will split when the
compressive force is greater—the scalp is the classic place for lacerated wounds to
be produced by blunt force; because the skull is convex, such lacerations may well
be of linear type even when the object with which contact was made—for example,
the roadway—was flat.

With the application of greater force, the underlying skull will fracture. The skull
is not uniformly solid but is composed of two layers or tables of bone separated by
spongy tissue. When struck, the skull will deform to some extent depending largely
upon its age. A child's skull will bend before breaking; but since blood vessels will
be torn in the process, head injury in children often shows a surprising degree of
haemorrhage when compared with the relative lack of damage to the skull. Once
the bounds of moulding are passed, the bone will break. In the adult direct trauma
could theoretically break only the outer table, and in these circumstances a

relatively perfect impression of the striking object would be reproduced; such a condition is very rare in practice, More usually, lines of stress fracture radiate from the point of contact while that part of the skull struck is depressed—a situation almost exactly comparable with striking the shell of a hard-boiled egg. These radiating fractures may damage blood vessels over a wide area, thus explaining why death results from what seemed to be a relatively mild impact injury.

The membranes of the brain, with their accompanying blood vessels, may be crushed or torn beneath a depressed fracture; more seriously, the brain itself may be lacerated either by the instrument causing the external injury, or by the fragments of bone that are forced inwards.

The above description illustrates the characteristics of homicidal head injuries. These may be modified by the precise type of weapon used—for instance, as between a cleaver and a baseball bat—and they may well be multiple, a factor that clearly provides evidence as to intent. Essentially, the injuries are local, are strongly related to the shape and size of the weapon and are not difficult to understand.

Head injury predominantly related to accident

Fracture of the base of the skull is particularly dangerous not only because dissipation of the force needed to cause such an injury produces general effects on the brain, but also because of local and indirect damage done to the blood vessels as they pass through the bone on their way to the vital centres controlling the life processes; these vessels are concentrated close to the tentorium and to the foramen magnum—the apertures through which the hindbrain and the spinal cord pass.

Fractures of the base may be continuous with those originating in and radiating from the vault of the skull. Thus, a blow to the front of the head, such as that sustained by an unrestrained front-seat passenger in a car crash, may fracture the frontal bones and radiate into the anterior fossae—this is a specially dangerous injury because, in breaking into the frontal air sinuses, direct communication is established between the brain coverings and the outside air (see below); a blow to the side of the head, fracturing the temporal bone, is likely to radiate into the middle fossa of the base; a blow to the back of the head, as sustained in falling or being pushed over backwards, may produce a fracture that radiates into the posterior fossa and involves the foramen magnum. These fractures may be multiple and cause extensive 'comminution' or fragmentation of the bone.

Accidental force transmitted to the base of the skull is generally of two types. The commonest is that transmitted through the spine when the body falls heavily on the feet or buttocks; a fracture may be formed that surrounds the foramen magnum in a 'ring' and, in very severe cases, the spine may be driven into the skull cavity. The vault of the skull may then be burst open, giving the impression of an original massive fracture in that area. The distinction of this type of injury is of importance in forensic medicine as a similar ring fracture of the base can be caused by a severe blow to the vertex—in this case, however, the accompanying fracture of the vault will be depressed rather than of 'explosive' type. The second important transmitted fracture stems from the point of the chin—force is applied through the lower jaw to the base of the skull in the region of each ear and the middle fossae of the base shatter. Such an injury rarely results from a fist blow but is common when, say, a person falls on the chin in the roadway or when the chin is impacted on the instrument fascia of a car or light aircraft. The essential feature is the hardness of the object struck, which influences the 'jolt' or rate of application of force.

Cerebral concussion

Head injury of more than minor severity will commonly be associated with loss of consciousness—in its simplest, short-lived, recoverable form this is known as concussion, a condition that is generally more severe when damage is caused to the moving head (i.e. decelerative injury) rather than when it results from blows to the skull. In addition to losing consciousness, the patient enters a state of surgical shock (see page 353), the severity of which greatly influences the rate of, or failure of, recovery. The precise cause of concussion is still disputed but is generally attributed to 'diffuse neuronal injury', which represents a functional abnormality of the nerve cells and of their connections rather than one with demonstrable pathological alterations in structure. The fact that no lesion can be shown is not, in itself, proof that none has been sustained; most would agree that some damage, in real terms, has been done and that this accounts for the late ill effects of concussion from which an apparently good recovery has been made.

Concussion has several important medico-legal connotations. In the first place, it commonly produces a genuine state of retrograde amnesia for events immediately before injury—a concussed person is likely to be an unsatisfactory witness; secondly, the sufferer may be left with sequelae of varying severity which will be mentioned later; perhaps of greatest immediate importance, concussion is a signal of potentially severe intracranial injury—it is an indication for examining the skull by X-ray and for retaining the patient under observation lest he develop an intracranial haemorrhage. Failure in these respects constitutes one of the more common bases of actions for negligence[1].

Intracranial haemorrhage (see Figure 11.1)

Intracranial haemorrhage can be divided into extradural, subdural, subarachnoid and intracerebral types. The loss of blood is insignificant in comparison with the effects of the resultant raised pressure on the brain itself; this can act directly or indirectly and may result in extensive destruction of tissue. It is for this reason that the quantity and the type of bleeding—arterial or venous—are of major importance to the outcome.

Extradural haemorrhage refers to bleeding between the skull itself and the outer covering of the brain. It is very commonly, but not always, associated with fracture of the skull. Venous extradural haemorrhage may be due to disruption of small veins and, occasionally, one of the large sinuses may give way. Tearing of a meningeal artery is, however, by far the commonest cause of this type of bleeding. About half the cases are complicated by intracerebral bleeding which often affects the opposite side of the brain (see below). Extradural haemorrhage is of particular

[1] But, overall, a fracture is present in only some 30 per cent of cases of concussion. X-ray examination, particularly in mild cases, might well be regarded as a form of insurance rather than as good medical economics. See Jennett, B. (1976), Some medicolegal aspects of the management of acute head injury, British Medical Journal, i, 1383, for a discussion of the dilemma and the importance of a genuine medical need to justify X-ray examination.

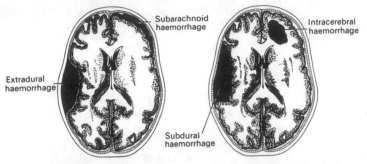

Figure 11.1 Four forms of intracranial haemorrhage. The dura is hatched; the arachnoid is shown as a solid black line. (The central structure is the normal ventricle of the brain.)

medico-legal importance in two respects. First, it is reasonably easy to treat and deaths from this cause should be rare. Secondly, there is typically an interval between injury and the onset of symptoms during which the patient, after an initial period of concussion, is perfectly normal; there is, therefore, a tendency for patients to be discharged to home and for the onset of symptoms there to be unappreciated—it may be 12 hours before the injured person is returned to hospital, by which time severe cerebral compression and brain damage may have occurred. The importance of observing a patient who has been concussed is again stressed, as is the frequent concurrence of this type of head injury with alcoholic intoxication—or the mimicry of the latter by the former; the death of such a case in a police cell is a tragedy that occurs not infrequently. If operative treatment of extradural haemorrhage is delayed, recovery may be complicated by emotional and intellectual disability.

Subdural haemorrhage occurs in the space between the dura and the arachnoid membrane. A large venous sinus may occasionally be lacerated but, commonly, the vessels torn are veins that are so small that no main bleeding point can be discovered either at operation or at post-mortem. This type of bleeding is not necessarily associated with fracture and results particularly from movement of the brain in relation to bone and to the relatively fixed dura matter. By its nature, subdural bleeding will take some time to produce symptoms; generally this is a matter of hours, but the effect of bleeding is aggravated by concurrent respiratory embarrassment and the consequent hypoxia. This 'latent interval' may be of very great importance in the assessment of non-accidental head injury in children; at post-mortem in such cases, it is often clear that blood has been collecting over a long period. Subdural bleeding is a common accompaniment of birth injury (*see* Chapter 20).

A chronic form of subdural haemorrhage may occur, particularly in children and the aged. Although these cases may represent the long-term effects of trauma, evidence of previous injury is lacking in the majority. Bleeding from small veins is slow; the body manages to contain the extravasations, which then become fixed to the underside of the dura by granulation and fibrous tissue. The lesions are very often symptomless or do no more than cause a general confusion of the intellect which is attributable to 'being a bit slow' or 'getting on in years'. Haemorrhage may, however, continue intermittently and severe symptoms may result from compression of the brain. It may then be difficult to decide whether there is a cause-and-effect relationship with injury that may have been sustained a long time past.

Subarachnoid haemorrhage has been noted in Chapter 7 as a fairly common form of sudden natural death; it is also a frequent sequel to injury. Subarachnoid haemorrhage occurring alone must be suspected of being due to spontaneous rupture of a congenital aneurysm, or of having been caused by injury to a vessel that was already weakened by aneurysmal changes. Another explanation, which has been recognized only relatively recently, is that the haemorrhage may result from damage to the vertebral artery arising as part of injury to the neck rather than to the head—the importance of this both in relation to the history of the case and to the post-mortem examination is obvious. The common indicative finding is bruising in the muscles close to the base of the skull and the mastoid process which lies behind the ear. A fracture of the first cervical (*atlas*) bone is found in about half the cases but is no more than confirmatory of trauma in the area; the fractures are demonstrable only by X-ray, and then often only after cleaning of the bone. Haemorrhage is attributed to tearing of the vertebral artery as it passes from the spinal column to the base of the brain, but it is technically difficult to demonstrate a bleeding point. Ideally, this should be done using radio-opaque injections which implies the availability of a radiologist with equipment and, also, some foresight on the part of the pathologist. An association with drunkenness has been noted in these cases but this may be no more than a reflection of the environment in which such injuries are sustained. Death may be very rapid and may be complicated by inhalation of vomit[2]. Otherwise, subarachnoid haemorrhage after injury is usually seen in combination with bleeding in other sites. In particular, there is usually some contusion of the brain, the generalized haemorrhage being due to local rupture of small vessels. Alternatively, massive subarachnoid haemorrhage may be no more than an extension of a severe intracerebral haemorrhage.

Intracerebral haemorrhage may be of two types. The first represents only contusion of the superficial areas of the brain. The distribution of such contusions as related either to bruising of the scalp or to fracture of the skull is of major importance. Injury to the brain may be local and direct—thus, if the skull is struck with a weapon and a depressed fracture is caused, the brain will be contused or lacerated at the point of impact. But brain damage as a whole—and particularly that resulting from accidents—requires a more subtle explanation which is based on the fact that, when the skull is accelerated or decelerated, the contained brain tends to continue moving; since it is attached more securely at some points than at others, it will be damaged elsewhere than at the point of application of external force. If the acceleration is rotational, sheer forces will be set up; if deceleration is linear, 'cavitation' will occur between the brain and skull as the brain tends to 'pile up' in its rigid covering. The results will be tissue damage and extravasation of blood at a distance from the point of impact and skull fracture. The cerebral contusion associated with a moving head—as, for example, one that strikes the roadway after a fall or one that impacts the windscreen in a car crash—will appear characteristically at the site precisely opposite to that of primary impact; this is known as 'contrecoup' haemorrhage. The important diagnostic feature is that the finding of internal bruising remote from the primary external injury clearly indicates *motion* of the head at the time it was sustained.

[2] An excellent review of this interesting condition is to be found in Harland, W. A. *et al.* (1983) Subarachnoid haemorrhage due to upper cervical trauma. *Journal of Clinical Pathology*, **36**, 1335.

Deep intracranial haemorrhages are also caused by indirect injury; they are also particularly associated with movement of the head and, therefore, with road-traffic accidents. The lesions result from tearing of the deep arterioles—again, usually those that are the most common sites of natural haemorrhage due to disease; the distinction between haemorrhage that results from an accident and that which causes an accident may be difficult to make (*see* Chapter 10). The incompressible brain resists the extension of such haemorrhages, and death may be delayed—but consciousness is not regained as so often occurs when extradural haemorrhage follows head injury. Deep haemorrhage in the absence of severe external damage is particularly common in young persons. Intracerebral haemorrhage is always serious but is almost inevitably fatal when it occurs in the brain stem, the site of the centres vital to life. Brain-stem haemorrhage may be primary—that is, caused during the traumatic event; it may also be secondary to raised intracranial pressure from other causes and often underlies delayed death after head injury.

Cerebral laceration

Cerebral laceration may be caused directly, either by an object that penetrates the skull or by fragments of bone that are driven inwards. In the event of widely radiating fractures with extensive isolation of skull fragments, there may be equivalent tears in the superficial substance of the brain.

Alternatively, severe *'contrecoup'* forces may cause laceration opposite the point of impact while rotational forces may drive the brain substance into the natural ridges that are found in the base of the skull. There is less restraint on the movement of the brain if the skull is fractured and, in these circumstances, the cerebrum or cerebellum may be torn from the brain stem.

The effect of cerebral laceration must vary with its location. Thus, a small laceration in the brain stem may well be fatal, while comparatively major damage in the frontal area may provoke no serious sequelae in the absence of haemorrhage. In practice, laceration of the brain is commonest in the frontal and temporal lobes.

Cerebral oedema

After trauma to the head, the patient very often falls into progressively deeper coma despite the fact that no localized haemorrhage is present; the condition of cerebral oedema, or swelling of the brain, is established.

The precise cause of this condition is uncertain. The effect is that the veins, rather than the arteries, are first compressed as the size of the brain increases while the circulation of cerebrospinal fluid is also compromised—the condition is therefore self-perpetuating and can cause death in its own right.

The pathological evidence of such swelling will often be referred to in the post-mortem report as 'herniation of brain substance'. The increase in pressure may force the undersurface of the temporal lobe through the tentorial opening at each side of the midbrain ('tentorial' or 'uncal' herniation), or the cerebellum may be pushed through the foramen magnum ('tonsillar' herniation). A further form of herniation that may be described in the pathologist's report results from escape of brain tissue through burr holes made in the skull in an attempt to relieve the condition.

The main significance of cerebral oedema, other than as a direct cause of death, lies in the secondary effects of brain-stem compression associated with 'tentorial herniation'. The interference with the cerebral blood flow that results may destroy the higher cortical centres while leaving those responsible for vital functions intact—the result can be a decerebrate person existing reflexly and without apparent awareness or volition.

Although oedema is a common cause of the compression syndrome, similar effects can be produced by a large haemorrhage or other lesion that occupies space in the cranial cavity.

Long-term effects of head injury

If a portion of brain is damaged by injury there will be localized effects of varying severity and expression which depend upon the precise area involved. A detailed description of potential disabilities cannot be undertaken here—the problems are covered in textbooks of neurology.

Some mention must be made of the generalized pathological conditions or symptoms that may properly be attributed to injury. Sepsis may be introduced through an open wound of the skull—especially one involving the nose. The origin of this may be obvious if the open fracture involves the vault of the skull. Fracture of the base of the skull, which may communicate with the outside through either the nose or ear, is less easy to detect and is certainly harder to repair. Generalized infection or overt abscess formation attributable to such injuries may be delayed for days or weeks. Even in the absence of infection, a distressing leak of cerebral spinal fluid may persist for some time.

Neuropsychiatric sequelae are considered in more detail in Chapter 28. After head injury many persons suffer from chronic headache, loss of concentration and unexplained attacks of giddiness. Post-traumatic epilepsy occurs after head injury without fracture in some 3 per cent of cases and follows 16 per cent of severe head injuries.

The prevention of head injury

The prevention of head injury is of major concern in mining, in the construction industries in general and, of greatest general importance, in vehicular transportation.

Different forms of head protection have been developed for these various situations. Because it has to protect against impacts of very varying intensity and direction, the helmet used in transportation is the most sophisticated and merits a short consideration.

The prototype helmet on which nearly all models now in use are based was developed by the Royal Air Force, the major design feature being the separation of the skull from the hard shell by the use of a suspension harness. The importance of good fit was apparent at an early stage of development and the need for ear flaps was emphasized by the number of head injuries that were found to originate in the temporal region. The introduction of head protection in military aviation coincided with the emergence of very high-performance aircraft; the forces involved in crashes of such aircraft generally exceed by far the protective capacity of any reasonable helmet and, currently, the main safety function of the military aviator's helmet is to protect against the buffeting associated with low-altitude, high-performance flight and against the possibility of injury during in-flight escape. It is disheartening to see that helmets are seldom used in the one form of flying where they would provide maximum benefit—that is, in light private aviation; there are no regulations to compel civilian fliers to protect themselves in this way.

The use of helmets in motor-car racing is dictated by both domestic and international controlling organizations. It would be too much to expect the ordinary driver or front-seat passenger in a family motor car to wear protective headgear—although some lives would certainly be saved thereby—but there is undoubtedly a case for their use in open sports cars. This is because, in addition to windshield contact injuries—the prevention of which is largely a matter of shoulder harness (*see* Chapter 10)—preventable skull injury in road-traffic accidents stems from secondary impact with the roadway after ejection from the vehicle.

Of all the vehicles in which this type of injury occurs, the motor cycle stands supreme and it is now compulsory by law in the United Kingdom to wear a 'crash helmet' while driving or travelling on a powered vehicle of motor-cycle type[3]; such helmets must conform to designated standards[4]. The imposition of helmets on motor cyclists has met with far less opposition than has legislation compelling the use of seat belts in cars, despite the fact that arguments against both are based on the concept of individual liberty in regard to self-protection. This is just as well—the motor-cycling fatality rate rose by an average of 38 per cent in those States of the USA that repealed helmet laws on libertarian grounds[5,6].

[3] Motor Cycles (Protective Helmets) Regulations 1980 (SI 1980 No. 1279). But there is an exemption for Sikhs (Road Traffic Act 1972, s. 32 A, added by Motor Cycle Crash Helmets (Religious Exemption) Act 1976, s. 1).

[4] Road Traffic Act 1972, s. 33.

[5] A grim experiment. *British Medical Journal* (1980), **281**, 406.

[6] The Courts take a similar attitude to contributory negligence in relation to safety helmets as in relation to restraining harnesses—O'Connell v. Jackson [1971] 3 W.L.R. 463.C.A. This attitude to head protection applies also in industrial accidents.

12

Transplantation of organs and the Human Tissue Act

The processes involved

Mechanical organ substitutes are often bulky, they restrict the lifestyle of the user, they may break down, and ultimately some form of incompatibility arises between patient and machine—e.g. there is thrombosis of the vessels, infection and the like. The concept of transplantation of biological organs is, therefore, extremely attractive both from therapeutic and from economic aspects.

The major difficulty in the procedure, apart from the required technical expertise, lies in the rejection by the body of foreign substances (or antigens), a principle which has been discussed in Chapter 1. The more 'foreign' the substance, the more rapid and inevitable will be the body's resistance to the graft. In the present state of knowledge, transplantation of organs from, say, apes to man is impossible save as a 'stop-gap' measure; all organs for long-term human transplantation must be obtained from human donors. The closer the antigenic similarity between recipient and donor, the more likely is the acceptance of the transplant. Antigenic similarity is, however, by no means the simple matter described under paternity testing and blood transfusion (Chapters 18 and 31); far more subtle relationships are involved and, apart from identical twins, the chances of finding two persons completely 'graft compatible' are negligible; at best, some—for example, siblings—are less incompatible than others. It follows that:

1. Transplantation must be accompanied by efforts to reduce the instinct of the recipient to reject the donated organ (immunosuppression).
2. Immunosuppression in humans cannot, as yet, be selective. The defences of the body against invasion are, therefore, reduced overall—e.g. against bacterial infection.
3. The body may still reject the graft when, ultimately, its powers to do so exceed the available immunosuppressive methods.

But any transplant must be effective in its own right if it is to be useful. A donation from a living person is more likely to succeed than is one from a dead donor and, in the latter case, success will be inversely proportional to the length of time between death and donation. Two problems of ethical and medico-legal importance arise—the lesser one of consent to make a living donation[1], and the major issue of obtaining cadaver specimens.

---

[1] Fully argued by Skegg, P.D.G. [1974]. Medical procedures and the crime of battery. *Criminal Law Review*, 693.

The propriety of live donation of organs for transplantation depends on three main factors. First, there should be a reasonable prospect of the transplant being successful; it might be legal for a man to consent, but it would certainly be unethical for a physician to encourage him to do so unless the recipient were a close relation by consanguinity, or a very accurate matching had been achieved.

Secondly, the benefit to the recipient must far outweigh the likely detriment to the donor. Potential donations are of three types:

1. of tissues that are readily replaceable, blood being the most obvious example, which cause no difficulty;

2. at the other extreme, of organs that are essential to the life of the donor. Since consent is no defence to a charge of homicide, removal of such organs in life must clearly be illegal;

3. of one of paired organs, the remaining one of which would be capable of maintaining life so long as it were healthy; for all practical purposes, this limits consideration to a kidney. Consent to such a donation may well be properly obtained, but this can be only after a very full explanation has been given. One would feel that two doctors should be required to certify that the donor has fully considered the implications, though there is certainly no requirement in law for such a practice[2].

Finally, the donor must be capable of consent as described in Chapter 30. The major problem specific to the present discussion is whether parents or guardians can give consent for a minor to undergo a surgical procedure that can be of no benefit to him or her. Although Lord Kilbrandon appears to have given this his tacit approval[3], it is doubtful whether such a practice would be wholly desirable because it is unlikely that a child would fully understand a complex subject, and because the possibility of a child subsequently needing his own donated organ may be greater than is so in an adult.

The ultimate success of a transplantation rests on the quality of the donated organ; this, in turn, depends upon the 'warm anoxic' time to which it is subjected—i.e. the time between cessation of the arterial oxygen supply and refrigeration of the isolated organ. Living donation therefore offers two major advantages. First, time is available for a full appraisal of the case, and, secondly, the warm anoxic time can be reduced almost to zero. In the case of a cadaver donation, however, the kidneys must be removed from the dead body within 30–60 minutes of circulatory failure and, in general, can be stored for no longer than 12 hours. Simpson has described the moment of death as 'the starting pistol for a race to save life'. The dramatic improvement in the results of transplantation surgery that has developed in recent years has been largely due to the approximation of the cadaver to the living donor through the medium of the 'beating-heart donor'—a concept that is discussed later in this chapter.

The law

Under English, Scots and American common law, the deceased has very limited rights as to the disposal of his body and, in the event of conflict, the wishes of the next-of-kin

---

[2] The South African Union Anatomical Donations and Post-Mortem Examinations Act 1970 does require certification by two doctors in the case of donation of 'naturally irreplaceable tissue'. Conditions in France are even more exacting; see Farfor, J. A. (1977) Organs for transplant: Courageous legislation. *British Medical Journal*, i, 497.

[3] As quoted by Meyers, D. W. (1970). *The Human Body and the Law*, p. 123. Edinburgh; University Press.

would normally be supported rather than those of the dead person, irrespective of how the latter had expressed his intentions. The common law position appeared to be supported by the Secretary of State for Health and Social Security in 1973[4]. Statute law is, however, tending to replace common law. In America, the Uniform Anatomical Gift Act has done much to regularize and standardize the situation; the Human Tissue Act 1961 serves the same purpose in the United Kingdom.

Section 1 of the British Act deals first with the situation when the deceased has asked during his life that his body should be used for transplant donorship. Then, the 'person lawfully in possession of the body' after his death may authorize the removal of any part of his body for use as requested. In the absence of a specific request, subsection (2) empowers the 'person lawfully in possession' of the body to authorize removal of organs 'if, having made such reasonable enquiry as may be practicable, he has no reason to believe (a) that the deceased had expressed an objection to his body being so dealt with after his death and had not withdrawn it; or (b) that the surviving spouse or any surviving relative of the deceased objects to the body being so dealt with'.

Cadaver organs for transplantation must have been healthy in life and it follows that, apart from occasional cases of fatal natural cerebral disease, violent deaths will provide the major source of donations. Other than those professionally concerned with the transplant procedure, there are thus two groups of persons with a practical interest in the provision of cadaver organs—the medico-legal authorities, represented by the Coroner or the Procurator Fiscal, and those 'lawfully in possession' of the dead body.

Lawful possession

The main problem related to those 'in lawful possession of the body' lies in the definition of 'lawful possession' as now applied. The discussion involves three parties—the deceased, the authorities in charge of the place where the body died and the next-of-kin. It has first to be decided whether the Act is speaking of those 'in possession' of the body—who are clearly the hospital authorities—or of those 'with a right to possession'—who are the next-of-kin; obviously, there may be a saving in time, and possibly, an increase in available treatments, if the former interpretation is correct. There is still some doubt on this. The English Medical Defence Union adhere to their opinion that it is the executors or relatives of the dead person who must authorize the removal of any organ. On the other hand, Lord Kilbrandon in Scotland and Lord Edmund Davies in England clearly believe that, for the purposes of the Act, the Hospital Board are lawfully in possession of the body. In this they have the support of the British Medical Association. The Act itself infers the correctness of this view—in Section 1 (6), undertakers are specifically excluded as being in possession of the body for the purpose of authorizing organ donation while, in Section 1 (7), allowance is made for the delegation of authority within the hospital. If there is no authority how can this be delegated?

The legal significance of a living person's declared desire to dispose of his body after death has already been mentioned; the effect on such authorizations as 'kidney donor cards' is obviously a matter for concern. If the relatives are in 'lawful

---

[4] *British Medical Journal* (1973), **iii**, 360.

possession' of the body they may well be legally entitled to refuse to authorize organ donation even under Section 1 (1) of the Human Tissue Act[5]. One cannot help feeling that, if put to the test, modern opinion would approve the principle that so long as the instructions given are reasonable and not contrary to public health or decency, a person has a right to dispose of his body in the same way as anything else he controls in life.

The meaning of 'reasonable enquiry' must also be questioned. Authoritative opinion believes this must be interpreted in relation to the time available; it would appear to be *unreasonable* to carry enquiries beyond the point in time after which an effective transplant would be unlikely. In practice, most suitable donors will be maintained on a ventilator (*see below*) and timeous difficulties related to consultation now occur only rarely.

Medico-legal authorities

All of the above considerations are, of course, subject to the authority of the Coroner or the Fiscal. They will nearly always be responsible for disposal of the body, and it is axiomatic that there must be no interference with a body so constrained unless specific permission is granted—unauthorized removal of tissue is expressly prohibited under the Human Tissue Act s. 1(5). But since no authority wishes to obstruct unreasonably a potentially life-saving measure, most Coroners and Fiscals agree to prior discussion of cases and the consequent immediate granting of permission in the event of death[6]. Previous inquiry will dispose of the possibility that the removed organ may have been of importance to the medico-legal investigation—in practice, this will only be of major concern in heart transplantation. Although a successful plea of *novus actus interveniens* is now extremely unlikely[7], some medico-legal authorities may incline to the view that a patient whose death is likely to be the subject of criminal proceedings should not be used as a transplant donor.

Brain-stem death

It is now appreciated everywhere that persons dying in hospital as a result of brain damage may be sustained in a state of animation by machine. The damage may, among others, be due to violence, to poisoning or to natural causes, the common

---

[5] Although accompanied by the proviso that the matter can be finally determined only by the Courts, NHS Circular 1975 (Gen) 34, issued in May 1975, leaves no doubt that the person lawfully in possession of the body is the Health Board or Area Health Authority responsible for the hospital. Only if and when the deceased's executors or relatives ask for the body to be handed over to them do they take over lawful possession of the body from the Board. It is further stated that, if the relatives or executors ask that the body be handed over to them after an authorization under Section (1) has been given, this action goes not revoke the authorization which continues to be legally effective. The Circular states that if the deceased during his lifetime had recorded an appropriate request then it would, in these circumstances, be reasonable for the authorization to be acted upon.

[6] Such 'permission' is still confined by the interpretation of s. 1(1) and 1 (2) of the 1961 Act.

[7] In Re Potter (*Medico-Legal Journal* (1963), **31**, 195), a man was committed for trial by the Coroner on a charge of manslaughter. His victim was used as a 'beating heart donor'. At the subsequent trial he was convicted only of common assault. This case had many unusual features and has been overtaken by Finlayson v. H.M. Adv. and R. v. Malcherek and Steel (*see below*).

denominator being that the brain suffers anoxic—or more correctly hypoxic—damage. The treatment of anoxia is to give oxygen; the effect of cerebral anoxia can be measured in degrees rather than in stages—the brain cannot recover from such damage but the condition will not progress once oxygen is provided. It follows that, in practice, the great majority of patients in coma of this type are placed on ventilator support, at least for a period of assessment. Respiration, which normally depends on a functioning respiratory centre in the brain stem, is thereby taken over by the machine and the oxygenated heart continues to beat, thus perfusing the tissues with oxygen. By traditional standards, which relate death to cessation of the heart and respiration, the patient is alive. But life is artificially supported and, at *some* time, that support must be removed. The medical profession is thus faced with the double dilemma of 'what is death?' and 'who is responsible for death if "life" is dependent on a machine?'.

The standard methods of diagnosing death are inapplicable in the context of ventilator support. *Figure 12.1*, however, attempts to show that, in such circumstances, it is logical to use the brain, which controls the heart and lungs, as a

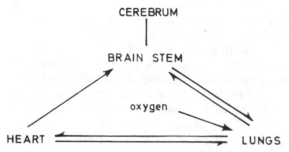

CEREBRUM

BRAIN STEM

oxygen

HEART   LUNGS

Figure 12.1 The process of dying. Both the heart and lungs are functionless without the other and both can be overridden mechanically. The brain will die without circulated oxygen, but the lungs cannot function without the brain stem. Since the brain stem is irreplaceable, it is reasonable to regard it as the seat of life and the measure of death.

measure of death—a practice that has led to the concept of 'brain death'. This term is capable of misinterpretation. Simplistically, one can speak of functional regions within the brain that vary in their resistance to oxygen deprivation (*see* Chapter 1). The most sensitive is the cortex, broadly responsible for the intellect or humanizing functions of the brain; this is followed by the thalamic region which is, in general, responsible for our animal behaviour; and, finally, there is the brain stem which regulates the basic functions of the body and, in particular, respiration. Thus, various degrees of oxygen lack will lead to varying degrees of 'brain death', and these may range from intellectual deterioration[8] to the suppression of all functions save the capacity to remain alive—this is known as the 'persistent vegetative state'. In any discussion of death, it is essential to appreciate that death is an absolute concept[9]; the body is not dead unless the whole brain is dead. The brain stem is not

[8] Despite being the least form of hypoxic damage, the results may be catastrophic. For a discussion of the complexities of awarding damages in such cases, *see* Lim Poh Choo v. Camden and Islington Area Health Authority [1979] 2 All E.R., 910.
[9] Skegg, P. D. G. (1974), Irreversibly comatosed individuals: alive or dead? *Cambridge Law Journal*, **33**, 130, discusses the problem in depth.

only the controller of 'life' but is also that part of the brain which is most resistant to hypoxia; for these reasons, it is strongly urged that the common expression 'brain death' is replaced by the unambiguous term 'brain-stem death'.

It is now firmly established that the diagnosis of brain-stem death can be made while the heart is still beating[10]. Stringent criteria are laid down. These include the exclusion of drug overdose, hypothermia or metabolic disorder as a cause of deep coma; establishing that the reason for the coma is irremediable structural brain damage; testing to establish that all brain-stem reflexes are absent; and in particular, establishing, under very standardized conditions, that no respiratory movements occur when the patient is disconnected from the mechanical ventilator. It is recommended that the tests be repeated, the interval between investigations depending upon the nature of the primary condition and the clinical course of the disease. It is now standard practice for the diagnosis to be made by two doctors[11], and it is axiomatic that they should be independent of any transplant team concerned with the case. More elaborate tests, including the use of the electro-encephalograph (EEG) are not considered necessary to establish a diagnosis of brain-stem death[12]. It has further been agreed in the United Kingdom that the establishment of brain-stem death means that the patient is dead[13], and there is growing evidence that the heart will cease to beat even with continued ventilator support within a few days of brain-stem death having occurred.

The answers to the problems concerning causation when ventilator support is removed are not quite definitive. Every patient must ultimately be withdrawn from the machine. In some, the criteria of brain-stem death may not have been met yet the patient's condition is such that further mechanical support is pointless, offensive or both. A proportion of such patients will then breathe spontaneously[14]. These cases pose no immediate legal or ethical problem; only the dilemma of what to do in the event of later respiratory failure remains to be faced. Others—and such cases must be rare—will be unable to maintain their respiration and will die. In either circumstance, the decision to withdraw support must be made by the physicians on the basis of clinical judgment. It would seem that, in doing so, the doctor does nothing to attract criminal sanction[15]. There is no problem if brain-stem death has been declared; the patient is dead and the decision as to whether to terminate or continue ventilation rests upon whether the corpse is to be used as an organ donor.

Since there are different indications for ventilator withdrawal, British judges have perhaps been ingenious, rather than evasive, in failing to define death in legal terms. First in Scotland[16] and then in England[17], appeals against conviction for

[10] Conference of Medical Royal Colleges and their Faculties in the UK (1976). Diagnosis of brain death. *British Medical Journal*, ii, 1187.

[11] Positively enacted in the Uniform Anatomical Gift Act of the USA.

[12] A lawyer's view of the validity of this diagnosis is given in Kennedy, I. M. (1981), *The Unmasking of Medicine*, p. 162; London; George Allen & Unwin.

[13] Conference of Medical Royal Colleges and their Faculties in the UK (1979). Diagnosis of Death. *British Medical Journal*, i, 332.

[14] Such was the much publicized case Re. Quinlan (1976) 70 N.J. 10 355A 2d 647. In the welter of legal argument surrounding her removal from ventilator support, it is important to appreciate that she was not dead.

[15] Kennedy, I. M. [1977], Switching off life support machines: the legal implications, *Criminal Law Review*, 443, makes the clear distinction between the doctor and others who could be charged with homicide or attempted homicide.

[16] Finlayson v. H.M. Adv. 1978 SLT (notes) 60.

[17] R. v. Malcherek, R. v. Steel [1981] 2 All E.R. 422 CA.

unlawful killing have been based on the argument that switching off the machine broke the chain of causation. In neither instance did the judges consider specifically the question of death; in both, the appeals were dismissed on the grounds that the doctors had followed good medical practice. The situation in the United States is less uniform but is, in some ways, more positive[18]. Whether there should be a law defining death is arguable[19]; what is certain is that legislation should not attempt to tell doctors *how* to make the diagnosis.

While many of the problems of criminality and brain-stem death seem to have been settled, civil litigation may demand greater legal precision, particularly as to the time of death. Brain-stem death may occur at a given point, but this is imperceptible; the time at which the actual diagnosis is made is to some extent arbitrary. One can thus conceive, for example, of problems arising in relation to the currency of life insurance policies. There is also the real dilemma in applying the criteria of brain-stem death to the solution of *commorientes*—a dilemma that seems to the author to be insoluble, save in a negative sense[20].

The 'beating-heart donor'

The retention of the patient on the ventilator after brain-stem death has been established opens the way to a fully oxygenated cadaver transplant—the so-called 'beating-heart donor'. The outcome of the transplantation is thereby greatly improved, and there is a medico-legal possibility—and perhaps reality in the United States[21]—that to transplant anything other than the 'best possible' organ could be construed as medical negligence. Unfortunately, there is still some public disquiet at the concept of the 'beating-heart' donor, which derives from a failure to understand the nature of brain-stem death; perhaps one of the most unsatisfactory aspects of the current position is the general failure to establish acceptable international criteria[22]. The public—and, indeed, the surgeon[23]—might also be reassured if a death certificate were always completed before the donor operation, but at present there is no such obligation. Although the majority of cases are likely to be the subject of a Coroner's or Fiscal's post-mortem examination, both authorities have the power to override the terms of a certificate should the need be indicated by their inquiries. Moreover, it is common practice for the medico-legal authority to regard the donor operation as part of the autopsy and to insist on the presence of the pathologist.

There is little doubt that the success or failure of the transplant programme is now dictated by public attitudes, and a major advance in statute law will probably only be achieved when kidney donation, which is now recognized as an established method of saving valuable lives, is separated from the more experimental and

[18] Reviewed by Smith, A. M. (1980), Brain death: A case for legislation?, *Journal of the Law Society of Scotland*, 113.

[19] *See* for example, the debate between Skegg, P. D. G. and Kennedy, I. in *Journal of Medical Ethics* (1976), **2**, 190; and (1977), **3**, 5.

[20] For example, if tests indicate that two persons are 'brain-stem dead', the time at which the tests were done cannot be used as evidence of relative survival.

[21] Brain death. *British Medical Journal* (1975), **i**, 356.

[22] The interested reader is referred to a most useful review by van Till, A. (1975), How dead can you be? *Medicine, Science and the Law*, **15**, 133.

[23] Particularly in relation to s. 1(4) of the Human Tissue Act 1961, which states that the operator must have verified by personal examination of the body that life is extinct.

flamboyant procedures, of which heart transplantation generates the most emotion. This probably stems from the fact that, in a cardiac transplant, one is removing an organ that is still supporting life no matter how imperfectly and is replacing it by something that must, in the present state of knowledge, fail sooner rather than later—at which point the situation is irretrievable. No such absolute limitations affect kidney transplants, which are usually performed only as a substitute for mechanical supports to which return can reasonably be made in the event of biological rejection.

The British Transplantation Society has put forward, as a matter for discussion, the suggestion that the Human Tissue Act 1961 should be amended so as to allow the person lawfully in possession of the body to authorize removal of organs without having to take positive steps to ascertain whether there were objections on the part of the next-of-kin[24]—in other words, the onus would be on individuals to 'contract out' of a cadaver donor system in the event of objection. The author's limited experience with public opinion on the matter suggests that the modification would be unacceptable; in practice, the very great majority of cases likely to provide organ donations are accompanied to hospital by relatives whose opinions must be sought and respected.

[24] British Transplantation Society (1975). The shortage of organs for clinical transplantation: Document for discussion. *British Medical Journal*, i, 251.

13

Asphyxia

Asphyxia is here defined as the result of interference with the oxygenation of the red blood cells. Tissue hypoxia due to anaemia, which is a deficiency of the red blood cells themselves, is therefore excluded from discussion.

Asphyxia is of five main types (*see Figure 2.2*):

1. *Mechanical*—in which the airways are blocked in an unnatural fashion.
2. *Pathological*—where the transfer of oxygen to the lungs is prevented by disease of the upper air passages or of the lungs themselves.
3. *Toxic*—whereby poisonous substances prevent the uptake of oxygen.
4. *Environmental*—or an insufficiency of oxygen in the inspired air.
5. *Iatrogenic*—or caused by the medical profession and mainly associated with anaesthesia.

Mechanical asphyxia

Atmospheric oxygen may be excluded from the lungs at various levels.

First, the nose and mouth may be obstructed—the process of *suffocation*[1]. Secondly, the glottis—or upper entry to the air passages—may be blocked as in *choking* due to impaction of food or of a gag. The most important level of occlusion in the context of forensic medicine is at the larynx, where the process is generally described as *strangulation*—if this is accomplished by hand alone it is manual strangulation or *throttling*; strangulation by ligature or cord may also be performed manually, the most specific example being *garrotting*, or it may result from suspension, i.e. *hanging*. Still lower in the air passages, the whole trachea or a main bronchus may be blocked after *inhalation* of foreign bodies or of stomach contents. Finally, the muscles of respiration may themselves be immobilized, for example, by crushing; the condition known as *traumatic asphyxia* results.

Suffocation

Unnatural suffocation in infancy presents one of the most difficult problems in

---

[1] Total occlusion of the nose and mouth by liquid—that is, drowning—is described separately in Chapter 14. Although suffocation also results from burial in trenches following land falls etc., the results are then very comparable with those described later under 'traumatic asphyxia'.

forensic pathology. It is a simple matter to place a pillow over a baby's face leaving, as likely as not, no evidence of external pressure. The only signs demonstrable at autopsy will then be those of anoxia in general, which can be summarized as:

1. *Cyanosis.* In the absence of oxygen, most of the oxyhaemoglobin will be converted to and remain in its reduced form; the colour of this is of dark plums which will be seen in the skin. This sign is of little medico-legal value because death itself is a matter of permanent tissue anoxia; some degree of cyanosis is therefore found in most natural deaths and may be very marked in those due to cardiac failure.

2. *Venous congestion.* Failure of the right side of the heart, with stagnation of blood in the veins, is an accompaniment of all asphyxial deaths save those that terminate suddenly. Congestion of the lungs is most common but, as this is a frequent finding in natural heart failure, its significance is slight; major diagnostic importance is confined to systemic congestion—that is, congestion of the skin and of the organs other than the lungs. A main result of venous congestion is capillary rupture and consequent formation of *petechial haemorrhages* which are often found in asphyxial deaths[2]. The distribution of these haemorrhages is of diagnostic importance and is greatly influenced by:

    (i)   impairment of the venous exit from the capillaries. Thus, pressure on the veins of the neck while the heart continues to beat, as in strangulation, will cause local pressure in the capillaries of the head—petechiae will, therefore, be pronounced in the eyes and on the face;

    (ii)   the nature of the tissue. The capillaries will give way more readily where they are least supported—thus petechiae will appear to be more concentrated in fatty fibrous tissue such as the eyelids;

    (iii) general visibility. Other than on the skin, petechiae will be most readily visible when confined by a transparent membrane. Internally, therefore, they are seen most often on the lungs beneath the pleura or on the heart beneath the pericardium. In infancy, they are often obvious beneath the covering of the thymus gland and, in severe asphyxia, they will be seen underneath the inner covering (mucosa) of the pharynx, larynx and other hollow organs;

    (iv)   intensity of congestion. The intensity of congestion may cause the petechiae to coalesce into larger haemorrhage; if the pressure builds up still further, the covering material may rupture and frank bleeding will occur.

Although back pressure is a major factor causing the petechiae, a deficiency of oxygen alone will damage the capillaries; since such a deficiency must occur during any process of dying, the question arises as to whether petechiae can be found following natural death. There is certainly no shortage of written authority to the effect that they *can* be[3]. In these circumstances, the 'spots' are usually confined to the pleural surface of the lungs, most often between the lobes. The distinction between 'natural' petechiae found in this condition and those resulting from asphyxia is essentially a matter of quantitation; the former are generally few in number and must be sought with determination.

---

[2] This evidence of asphyxia was first described in infant suffocation by a French police surgeon; as a result, the haemorrhages are often referred to as 'Tardieu spots'.

[3] *See*, for example, Polson, C. J., Gee, D. J. and Knight, B. (1985) *Essentials of Forensic Medicine*, 4th edn., p. 354; Oxford; Pergamon; and Gordon, I. and Shapiro, H. A. (1982), *Forensic Medicine* 2nd edn., p. 83; Edinburgh; Churchill Livingstone.

3. *Oedema.* Hypoxic damage to the capillaries will result in increased permeability of their walls which will allow the passage of fluid plasma rather than of particulate red blood cells; oedema (or 'water in the tissues') will accompany asphyxia provided the hypoxic stimulus is relatively long lasting. The process is generally best demonstrated in the lungs. Again, the distribution of oedema may be important as its production will be exaggerated by intravascular pressure—thus, oedema of the face, tongue and pharynx is a feature of strangulation.

The suffocated infant, therefore, may well show no more than generalized congestion with the formation of petechial haemorrhage on the surface of the lungs, heart and thymus; the changes are non-specific and their interpretation must depend largely on the circumstantial evidence. Suffocation with the hand may leave identifiable evidence because the generalized congestion of asphyxia will not develop at the points of pressure; there may be similar findings on the back of the head if the baby's face has been forced into a pillow. Such appearances must be distinguished from the normal effects of hypostasis which are present in 'cot deaths' (*see* page 212); in these cases, the baby has often been dead for some time before discovery and pressure areas of pallor will have formed—since the child is invariably moved by distraught parents, the consequent anomalous position of these areas may cause some confusion.

Can suffocation of accidental type occur in infancy? Most authorities would agree that it is an improbable occurrence because a baby suffocating with its face into a pillow will move reflexly so as to breathe; but there may be cases when, because of entanglement in a harness or bedclothes, movement is impossible and true accidental suffocation can result. Suffocation by overlaying, essentially a matter of overcrowding, is now rare; occasional instances are associated with drugs and drunkenness (Chapter 20). The condition may never have been as common as tradition supposes; many deaths so diagnosed must have been unrecognized 'cot deaths'.

Accidental asphyxia in older children focuses attention on the specific hazards of 'plastic bags'. Numerous tragedies have occurred due to such activities as 'playing spacemen' when a 'helmet' of polythene, attracted to the nose and mouth by respiration, becomes moulded firmly to the shape of the face; if the airway occlusion is sudden, rapid death may result with the classic signs of asphyxia. The great majority of plastic bags are now marked as 'dangerous' and others are perforated when their intended use permits[4].

The sexual asphyxias

Plastic bags also play a part in the interesting group of conditions known as sexual asphyxias; these may also include features of strangulation.

These deaths are characterized by a strongly male distribution and by an equally common association with transvestism together with the use of some asphyxial mechanism, such as a plastic or other bag; a masochistic tendency is often shown by tying the hands or binding the torso and by the superimposition of some form of suspension by a neck ligature. The sexual nature of the condition may be emphasized by a display of pornographic literature.

[4] *See* Toy (Safety) Regulations (S.I. 1974 No. 1367) arising from the Consumer Protection Act 1961.

These features taken together virtually eliminate the involvement of another party, particularly when, as is usual, the victim has taken precautions to preserve his solitude. Occasionally, however, the possibility that the dead man was the victim of a sadomasochistic partnership needs to be excluded—death may be very rapid in any highly emotional state, particularly when the neck is involved, and should it occur, any others involved are likely to leave the scene. The common problem in the classic sexual asphyxial death is, however, to distinguish between accident and suicide; unless there is specific evidence to the contrary, such deaths should generally be regarded as accidental, caused either by unexpectedly rapid loss of consciousness or by failure to escape from the manufactured conditions. It is less easy to be so certain in cases involving females.

Obstruction at the laryngeal opening

Gagging is seldom intentionally homicidal. More commonly, death occurs accidentally when the mouth has been stuffed with material to stifle calls for help—this may have been premeditated as when immobilizing a night watchman or done on impulse, say, during the course of a sexual assault. Suicidal gagging must be very rare. I have personal experience of one case in which a depressed hospital patient forced his handkerchief down his throat. Death may be of an asphyxial type but sudden death due to reflex vagal inhibition of the heart is a strong possibility.

Accidental gagging—or choking—can also follow impaction of a bolus of food in the larynx. This may be associated with drunkenness but is most commonly seen in elderly persons who bolt their food as a symptom of senile dementia—the process of mental ageing—or who cannot masticate efficiently without teeth. Death is almost always sudden and is due to stimulation of the vagus nerve. An asphyxial type of death may follow if the food passes the larynx and lodges in the trachea; impaction of something smaller—for example, a nut—in a main bronchus may result in death of almost any degree of suddenness ranging from vagal stimulation to death far removed in time due to bronchopneumonia or lung abscess. This type of death needs to be distinguished from that due to aspiration of regurgitated stomach contents—discussed later in the chapter—which is far less satisfactorily defined.

Strangulation

Strangulation is that aspect of asphyxia that most often results in serious criminal charges. It is, therefore, considered here in some detail.

Manual Strangulation

Except in unusual circumstances—for example, in retributive gang warfare—it is doubtful if throttling is often the result of deep premeditation; far more frequently, exasperation or fear provokes a murderous impulse which, in the absence of any weapon, is satisfied by 'wringing his or her neck'. The circumstances surrounding the crime and the precise type of a strangling are, therefore, of great importance in assessing the mind of the assailant at the time. Much may be reflected in the mode of death, and the pathological evidence may be of particular significance in the final evaluation.

Throttling can be accomplished single-handedly, in which case the thumb of a right-handed assailant is pressed into the right-hand side of the victim's neck close to the angle of the jaw, or bimanually, when each thumb is used to exert pressure; in an attack from behind, the fingers of each hand act as the main constricting agent.

The local signs of throttling may consist, therefore, of bruising or superficial abrasion of the neck corresponding to a number of thumb or finger-pads. Both structures involved—the neck and the fingers—are relatively soft and bruises, although often obvious, may have indefinite edges; the appearances may well be clearer some hours after death when the process of blood stasis has produced a general pallor of the area. The edges of the bruises may show elliptical abrasions caused by the finger-nails of the assailant.

The signs of death from throttling depend upon the precise mode of death; this also applies in other types of violence to the neck. There are, essentially, four mechanisms:

1. The windpipe is occluded. In this case, the changes will be those of generalized oxygen deficiency and, because of the associated struggling, petechial haemorrhages are likely to be prominent. Pulmonary oedema will have been provoked if the anoxia has been prolonged and may show itself as froth at the nose and mouth if the pressure has been intermittent. This finding is not specific and occurs in prolonged hypoxia of many other types.
2. The venous return is obstructed. Anoxia in the brain results from stagnation of the blood and, because this is a gradual process, the cumulative effects of local oxygen lack will be prominent—thus, suffusion of the face with many petechial haemorrhages will be found; but generalized signs of asphyxia will be slight because the rest of the body is adequately oxygenated. There is some division of opinion amongst authorities as to how long is the agonal period in such cases. Some believe that, in throttling with the hands, the pressure must be applied for 2 minutes or more to cause death[5]. Such estimates cannot be based on experiment and there is no doubt that 2 minutes is a lengthy period for sustained activity. Others[6] hold that most stranglings are over within half a minute—irrespective of the intervention of factors discussed below in (3) and (4). This latter estimate has been borne out in studies of accidental strangling and would seem to be the more reasonable.
3. The blood supply to the brain is cut off by pressure on the carotid vessels. Except in strangulation by suspension (*see below*) this can be little more than a theoretical possibility as, first, it is mechanically difficult to achieve the necessary compression through the tissues and, secondly, an alternative blood supply to the brain is available through the arteries of the vertebral column. Pressure on the carotid arteries is far more likely to cause:
4. Death from vagal inhibition of the heart. As described in Chapter 1, a sudden unexpected and, particularly, abnormal sensory stimulation may result in an equally sudden and abnormal reflex through the motor component of the vagus nerve; the heart is arrested and death occurs with great suddenness. The carotid plexus in the neck is particularly sensitive and pressure at this point may well be the predominant cause of this type of sudden death: alternatively, fracture of the laryngeal cartilages may provide the main reflex stimulus.

As discussed in deaths associated with anaesthesia (Chapter 31), autonomic reflexes are likely to be less inhibited when the higher control centres are functionally

[5] *See*, for example, Camps, F. E., Robinson, A. E. and Lucas, B. G. B. (eds) (1976), *Gradwohl's Legal Medicine*, 3rd edn., p. 333; Bristol; Wright.
[6] I am indebted to the late Professor C. K. Simpson for a personal communication on this point.

depressed and it is certainly my impression that vagal activity is more common in death due to strangulation when the victim is moderately to severely affected by alcohol—often of the order of 200 mg per 100 ml blood; there is support for this observation in the literature[7].

Injuries to the tissues of the throat and larynx provide the most important findings in the post-mortem dissection after manual strangulation. Bruising is the most constant of these and is found at all depths corresponding, in the main, to the pressure marks under the fingers; posterior bruising of the larynx may be caused by pressure against the spine and the base of the tongue may be affected by traction as much as by direct pressure. The thyroid gland may, itself, show bruising.

Fracture of the laryngeal cartilages is another diagnostic finding. The most frequent fracture involves the superior cornu of the thyroid cartilage, since the natural position of the thumb in manual strangulation is to rest on the ligament that joins the thyroid cartilage to the hyoid bone. The hyoid is, therefore, also often involved, due either to upward displacement by the thumb or to downward traction as the point of attachment to the thyroid is broken. Associated haemorrhage is a most important post-mortem observation; this is the acid test of injury in life. It is, however, well established that bruising can occur as a result of the dissection itself—particularly around the neck structures. For this reason it has been suggested that the cranial cavity should be dissected first in any case of suspected throttling; the potential for artefact is thus reduced by releasing the pressure in the engorged veins. The laryngeal cartilages can be broken during removal of the neck organs but this should not occur other than in unskilled hands. Finally, the possibility that an injury discovered derived from a previous episode far removed in time cannot always be entirely discounted; such a fracture will, of course, be bloodless.

The pathologist is almost always asked for his opinion on the force required to cause a fracture of the larynx. Such an assessment is bound to be to some extent subjective. However, damage to the larynx beyond fracture of the cornua of the thyroid and hyoid—for example, fracture of the main wings of the thyroid—will imply 'considerable force'; this type of fracture may result from the karate-blow type of assault rather than from simple throttling. Cartilages that are calcified are certainly easier to fracture than are those that are young and supple—but this is a comparative estimate only, which still fails to answer the question of how much force was applied in the individual case. In order to improve the objectivity of the assessment, it is advised that the larynx be X-rayed in every case in which fracture is discovered. But it must be remembered that the muscles and ligaments will tend to realign any broken ossicles; a fracture may well be present but may not be visible in the X-ray because of this tendency to a normal position and because of variable calcification in the area.

Strangulation by Ligature

Strangulation by ligature without suspension is not uncommon as a form of homicide. Apart from the classic premeditated crime of garrotting—in which the

[7] *See*, for example, Simpson, K. (ed.) (1965), *Taylor's Principles and Practice of Medical Jurisprudence*, 12th edn., p. 359; London; Churchill—'States of narcosis and drunkenness may considerably shorten the period [of time taken to die from asphyxiation]'.

Gonzales, T. A., *et al.* (1954). *Legal Medicine*, 2nd edn., p. 472; New York; Appeleton-Century-Crofts—'Alcoholic individuals may be asphyxiated easily by manual compression of the neck and succumb without revealing any demonstrable signs of violence at autopsy'.

assailants used their own prepared form of ligature—the material used to strangle is usually that which happens to be near at hand; because of the close association with sexual assaults and of the rarity of an original intention to strangle, nylon stockings or pantihose are most frequently found in adult cases; the victim's own scarf is also often used.

The ligature may or may not be knotted in homicidal strangling; although the former is more common, the assailant sometimes depends upon his own strength to maintain the pressure on the neck. This is usually sufficient to cause actual obstruction of the windpipe and must involve pressure on the veins. The usual post-mortem appearances are those of generalized anoxia with exaggerated appearances in the head; rapid death from vagal inhibition of the heart can, however, occur. The ligature causes a mark which is characteristically horizontal and of regular depth; it nearly always passes in front of the neck across the membrane connecting the hyoid and thyroid cartilages which are fractured far less commonly than in manual strangulation. Very little external evidence of the presence of a ligature may remain if it is composed of soft material and is removed immediately after death. Cord or rope may, however, leave a distinctive pattern while irregular finger-nail scratches, inflicted by the victim in an attempt to loosen the constriction, are highly suggestive of homicidal strangling.

Suicidal strangulation by ligature is uncommon but certainly occurs. It is generally associated either with an intricate system of tourniquet application or with the use of elastic material which will spring back to give powerful constriction after having been knotted—nylon stockings behave effectively in this way. At the same time, this effect may be accidental rather than suicidal—self-strangulation is used as a form of exhibitionism. Accidental strangulation either by self or by another in horseplay may occur in the absence of a tied knot; death is of a reflex type.

The umbilical cord is occasionally used to strangle a newborn infant—the question then arises as to whether the cord can encircle the neck so as to cause fatal accidental strangulation either *in utero* or during the act of birth. Few would dogmatize that either cannot happen and, in cases of precipitate labour, the cord may be markedly tightened. Such cases must arouse suspicion but, no matter how great this may be, the onus is still with the prosecution to prove the *fact* of a separate existence before a charge can be upheld. A separate existence will scarcely ever be possible in accidental strangulation by the cord, but proof *may* be forthcoming in cases of infanticide or child murder; the problem is discussed in Chapter 19.

Strangulation by Suspension

Death from hanging may be judicial or quasi-judicial. Judicial hanging in the United Kingdom[8] gave rise not to an asphyxial death but to disruption of the cervical spinal cord due to a separation fracture of the neck induced by the massive jolt following a drop of some 2.2 m (7 ft); the common fracture site was at the level C2–3. Asphyxial hangings of the 'Western' film type were resurrected in the quasi-judicial circumstances of partisan warfare but, nowadays, death by hanging is almost entirely suicidal with a small accidental element.

The suicidal nature of the case is nearly always apparent from the circum-

[8] Abolished under the Murder (Abolition of Death Penalty) Act 1965 apart from potential use in the event of treason or piracy with violence.

stances—although an attempt to disguise a homicide as a suicidal hanging is not unknown[9]. Arrangements involving some elaboration are often made and steps are usually taken to offset the possibility of detection before death; consequently, it is not unusual for suicidal hangings to have been dead for some days before discovery.

The main post-mortem findings are those of facial congestion coupled with severe hypostatic changes in the legs and forearms; the former may, however, be absent if the carotid arteries have been compressed. The ligature mark in the neck is deep and is maximal opposite the point of suspension; it often passes between hyoid and thyroid cartilages in front, rising to the point of an inverted V, corresponding to the knot of the noose, either in the midline posteriorly or behind one ear. The internal appearances will be those of generalized anoxia but, even if death has resulted rapidly from vagal stimulation, the effects of blood pooling will still result in severe changes which are visible externally; anomalies of lividity may indicate the possibility of simulation. Fractures of the laryngeal cartilages may occur in hanging but are by no means invariable; much depends upon the age of the subject. The ligature may be so firm and applied so rapidly that vital reaction is absent; a false impression of a post-mortem origin may be gained.

Accidental hanging is generally sexually orientated and is associated with the sexual asphyxias previously discussed; simple exhibitionism may, however, end disastrously. Death can be due to vagal inhibition of the heart even though steps have been taken to prevent a fatal outcome—for example, by having the point of suspension so low that the feet touch the ground. It is, in fact, surprising how many 'successful' suicides occur thus—the combination of motivation, nervous tension and mechanical cerebral hypoxia, which may be of great suddenness, combine to produce death in a situation that appears readily recoverable. Such deaths are well documented in conditions that eliminate the possibility of homicide.

Other forms of accidental hangings scarcely need special mention though many need careful differentiation from homicide—the baby strangled in its restraining harness is one example. Industrial accidents of many types can be imagined. A somewhat bizarre form of accidental hanging may occur in sport or military parachuting when the neck becomes entangled with the shroud lines; the severe jolt often imparted gives rise to intimal laceration of the carotid arteries—a minor sign at post-mortem dissection that strongly indicates a sudden stretching of the neck in hanging incidents of all types.

Obstruction in the lower air passages

Drowning, discussed in Chapter 14, is an obvious form of obstruction involving the lower respiratory tract. But it is also possible effectively to 'drown' in one's own body fluids—the accumulation of fluid in the lungs is known as pulmonary oedema, which forms part of the syndrome of hypoxia described above.

The condition is not specific to mechanical asphyxia. It occurs in all forms of hypoxic death, including those of central origin such as barbiturate poisoning. It is also a natural result of heart failure—an ineffective left ventricle is unable to clear the blood returning from the lungs; very severe oedema is commonly present in death due to coronary insufficiency. A similar manifestation of 'heart failure' is

[9] R. v. Emmett-Dunne, General Court Martial, Dusseldorf, 1954.

seen when the volume of the circulating blood is increased beyond the capacity of the left ventricle; this occurs when fluids are transfused over-liberally into the body and is a form of iatrogenic asphyxia which is discussed in Chapter 31.

Pulmonary oedema commences within the alveoli but it may be so intense that the bronchioles and bronchi are filled with fluid. Irritant gases produce extremes of the condition—the early war gases chlorine and phosgene are examples of such direct-acting substances but even tear gas may produce severe pulmonary reaction in high concentration.

The interpretation of obstruction of the lower airways by inhaled stomach contents presents a practical problem in forensic pathology. This is certainly a common post-mortem finding which is particularly frequent in hypoxic deaths. Although it is easy to presume a cause-and-effect relationship, a diagnosis of asphyxia due to inhalation of stomach contents may well be a misconception; it is widely held that vomitus in the air passages is usually there because of, rather than as the cause of, tissue anoxia[10] and this may be especially pertinent to 'cot deaths' (see page 212). To complicate matters further, the act of vomiting itself may cause the appearance of petechiae by suddenly raising the venous pressure. In practical terms, the presence of inhaled material from the stomach should not be accepted as the precise cause of death unless products of digestion can be demonstrated microscopically in the small air passages; a valid diagnosis is often associated with conditions that depress the reflex ability to expel foreign material from the lungs—head injury and intoxication due to drugs or alcohol are frequent causes.

Restriction of chest movement

Pressure on the chest sufficient to inhibit respiratory movement will cause asphyxia—the condition must be unnatural and is known as traumatic asphyxia. Circumstances likely to produce this effect are self-evident—crushing under rock falls, pinning in a vehicular accident and crushing in a crowd—particularly if the crowd collapses—are common accidental causes of traumatic asphyxia. The pathological findings are characteristic—there is intense congestion with widespread formation of petechiae in the tissues, especially in those of the upper thorax and neck; occasionally, there is little or nothing to be seen externally. The mechanism of traumatic asphyxia could just possibly be used homicidally by the assailant sitting on the victim's chest—some such method, coupled with manual suffocation, was admitted by Burke and Hare, hence the descriptive title of 'burking'.

Pathological conditions

Any pathological condition of the lungs that interferes with the free interchange of gases across the alveolar capillary membrane will cause some degree of tissue hypoxia. Bronchitis, emphysema and pulmonary fibrosis are the main conditions but, although they are a major cause of mortality in the general population, they have only limited medico-legal significance.

Many pathological pulmonary conditions are intimately associated with work

[10] See Knight, B. (1982) Legal Aspects of Medical Practice, 3rd edn., p. 179; Edinburgh; Churchill Livingstone.

and are likely to be the subject of compensation for industrial injury. They are discussed in some detail in Chapter 15.

The presence of lung disease may result in severe strain on the right side of the heart—that side which is responsible for pumping blood into and through the lungs; a failing heart in this situation is known as *cor pulmonale*. While most sufferers exist in a state of chronic ill health, an acute exacerbation may be a cause of sudden death resulting in a Coroner's or Fiscal's Inquiry.

The presence of a condition predisposing to tissue anoxia will compound the effects of any other asphyxial mechanism; the pre-existing condition of the victim's lungs may, therefore, have considerable bearing on the evaluation of a case of, say, manual strangulation. This concept of synergism holds for all the main categories of asphyxia discussed.

Paralysis of the respiratory muscles may result from disease—the most well-known example being acute anterior poliomyelitis or 'infantile paralysis'.

Toxic asphyxia

Toxic asphyxia is of two main types. Either the capacity of the haemoglobin to bind oxygen is impaired, or the enzymatic processes whereby the oxygen in the blood is utilized by the tissues are blocked.

Conversion of haemoglobin to the compound methaemoglobin is effected by many industrial poisons (*see* Chapter 22). This change produces more frightening signs than genuine pathological effects and the only haemoglobin derivative that is of major practical medico-legal importance is carboxyhaemoglobin—formed by the combination of haemoglobin with inspired carbon monoxide. Cyanides are outstanding examples of enzymatic poisons. These two substances will, therefore, be treated individually.

Carbon monoxide poisoning

Until a few years ago the most readily available source of this asphyxiant was the domestic gas supply which contained some 5–15 per cent of carbon monoxide (CO); this supply is now widely provided by natural gas which, although asphyxiant in that it is irrespirable, has no positive toxic qualities. Consequently, the number of cases of suicidal poisoning due to domestic gases in England and Wales fell from 988 in 1968 to 11 in 1978. Most CO with which the public comes in contact nowadays derives from the combustion of carbon-containing material; carbon dioxide (CO_2) is the end product of ideal combustion but, since very few flames are totally efficient, all gas produced by fire contains some carbon monoxide. CO_2 is relatively unimportant as its physiological effects can be compensated save in an enclosed environment (*see* page 137); the affinity of haemoglobin for CO is, however, some 300 times that of its affinity for oxygen. The formation of carboxyhaemoglobin (COHb) is, therefore, cumulative and a potentially fatal proportion of respirably inert COHb in the blood can derive from only a small concentration of CO in the inspired air.

In practice, therefore, two factors are needed to endanger life through carbon monoxide poisoning—first, there must be combustion and, secondly, the removal of the products of combustion must be inefficient.

The most common sources of poisoning include:

1. Solid-fuel, gas or oil fires fitted with inadequate flues or used in rooms without sufficient ventilation. Oil heaters in bedrooms (including caravans) or geysers in bathrooms are obvious examples.
2. Internal combustion engines having defective exhaust systems—or operating within closed garages.
3. Mines—where the perpetual minor fires leave pockets of contamination.

Death from CO poisoning may be homicidal, suicidal or accidental.

Homicidal poisoning must be extremely rare because of its uncertainty of success, although one could conceive of a town-gas supply being deliberately opened in the presence of a sleeping or otherwise unconscious victim; infanticide attempts combined with suicide are probably less uncommon. The use of CO during murder, presumably as a sexual stimulant, has been recorded but would not constitute the prime weapon in such an instance[11].

Suicidal poisoning was most often associated with the gas oven in the past; the motor-car exhaust is now the most frequent source of the poison for this purpose. The true nature of a suicidal CO poisoning is likely to be shown by the intricate arrangements made—not only to ensure a concentrated delivery of the gas but, often, for the comfort of the subject. Additional suicidal agents—such as drugs—may well have been used. Death ensues in some five minutes in an oven; car exhaust gas, which contains about six per cent CO, can also kill in a matter of minutes but this time will be greatly influenced by variations in the efficiency of delivery and ventilation[12].

Several other factors affect the individual's susceptibility to CO. As with all poisons, the elderly are likely to be killed more easily than the young and the presence of disease that, of itself, contributes to or kills through tissue hypoxia must be taken into account—coronary insufficiency is an obvious example. Similarly, an anaemic person will succumb more quickly than will the normal, as it is the sum of hypoxic factors that matters. It follows that the symptoms of CO poisoning will also depend on the physical state of the individual. Thus, it is generally stated that conversion of 30 per cent of the haemoglobin to COHb results in dizziness and headache, inco-ordination appears at 50 per cent saturation, unconsciousness at 60 per cent and death at 70–80 per cent; but these are proportions relative to the total oxyhaemoglobin available and it is this total that conditions symptoms. Moreover, the more rapid and deep is the respiration, the more contaminated air will be inspired and the faster will be the accumulation of COHb. From the purely legal aspect all these factors will be relevant when problems of survival arise as they may well do if members of a family are found dead in a room or caravan; they also greatly influence the medical assessment of accidental CO poisoning.

Accidental intoxication by CO is of interest on two counts—first, it may of itself be the cause of death and, secondly, it may be the cause of a vehicular accident and, indirectly, of death from trauma.

All sources of CO are associated with accidental poisoning. These include space-heating appliances, water heaters of the geyser type and the exhausts of

[11] See Camps, F. E. (1953) *Medical and Scientific Investigations in the Christie Case*; London; Medical Publications.

[12] An extraordinary self-recorded case has been reported in which death occurred in 20 minutes; the critical point of poisoning appeared to be at 6–7 minutes (Flanagan, N. G., *et al.* (1978). *Medicine, Science and the Law*, **18**, 117).

stationary cars left with engines running. Fumes from the exhaust of stationary cars contaminate the passenger compartment either through a faulty exhaust or heater system or as a result of escape into the air of a closed garage. Leaking pipes or loose taps conducting town gas must also be considered; mining accidents can occur but, thanks to safety measures taken, are now rare. Death is almost invariably associated with a degree of unawareness—senility, sleep, alcoholism or pre-occupation with other matters are obvious examples. Accidents connected with senility are those of forgetfulness in turning off taps, failure to remember open taps when recharging coin-operated meters and the like. Accidents in sleep are usually associated with open-flame heating apparatus. It must be remembered that individuals may react differently, that CO tends to layer and that concentrations in a room will vary greatly according to the positions of draughty windows and doors. The maximum concentration of CO in the air of a room will not be very great and the effects are spread over a relatively long period; alterations in the environment will exaggerate differences in clinical response and, when there are several persons in a room, it may well be that some will wake up or be roused when others are already dead—such a result by no means rules out accident. Alcoholism may be a particular feature predisposing to death amongst down-and-outs who are huddled around inefficient braziers or boilers, especially if these have inadequate flues. Preoccupation may be a feature of deaths in garages while making car repairs. The combination of preoccupation and exercise leads to sudden deaths during sexual activity—often in cars in which the heater is left running. Perhaps the bathroom geyser is the only apparatus likely to be lethal to a person normally aware and occupied; the usual small size of the room exaggerates the danger of failing to turn off the flame before entering the bath.

CO is a potential—and actual—cause of death due to traumatic injury in motor cars and in aircraft; the problem is discussed in Chapter 10. For the present, it is necessary merely to emphasize that only low levels of COHb—sufficient to cause no more than distraction or disorientation—are needed to cause a vehicular accident and, further, that there will be a marked synergistic relationship with other adverse physiological factors such as fatigue. The forensic pathologist and toxicologist will, therefore, be dealing with concentrations of COHb that are only slightly raised and which must be interpreted with care and in relation to the accident as a whole.

Cyanide

Poisoning by cyanide is uncommon but has historical interest; it is also the most significant example of histotoxic asphyxia—tissue enzymes are blocked by the process known as molecular substitution and are unable to transfer the oxygen in the blood. Death is essentially due to poisoning of the respiratory centre which is especially sensitive to hypoxia. If death is not sudden, the high proportion of oxyhaemoglobin in the venous blood may show itself through the bright pink colour of the skin and internal organs; the colour must be distinguished from that of COHb and from the effects of cold, including post-mortem refrigeration. Delayed death only occurs in cases of ingestion of cyanide salts; hydrocyanic acid is one of the most rapidly fatal poisons known.

Hydrocyanic acid is used as a gaseous fungicide or, more commonly, rodenticide; its use is specifically controlled[13]. Cyanide salts are used in the steel industry and in

---

[13] Hydrogen Cyanide (Fumigation) Act 1937.

other industrial processes; they are common laboratory chemicals; they are widely used in photography. Natural sources of cyanide include bitter almonds, the kernels of many fruit-stones and the leaves and fruit of some plants.

Death from cyanide poisoning is now rare. Homicidal poisoning seems to be a matter of history only—although cyanides were used for the genocidal killings of the 1940s. Accidental poisoning occurs mainly in industry and in laboratories. The sale of cyanide salts is unlawful save as provided by s. 4 of the Poisons Act 1972; such suicides as are now reported occur, therefore, among subjects who require the poison for their trade or business—e.g. chemists and photographers.

Poisoning from natural sources of cyanide is very rare. A number of very old cases involving bitter almonds themselves, or the essential oil, have been reported. The significant quantities of cyanide contained in fruit-stones are only available after laborious extraction, and cyanide poisoning from plants is extremely unlikely. There are, however, general dangers for children eating berries with which they are unfamiliar and these are emphasized in Chapter 22.

Environmental asphyxia

Reduction in the available oxygen to a level inconsistent with life arises as a medico-legal problem most commonly in relation to enclosed spaces—too many people may be closeted in too small a space or the space may be too small to support a single human life. The former may be murderous in intent—the 'Black Hole of Calcutta' is history's most vivid example—or a matter of reckless indifference; occasionally, overcrowding in small, cold rooms may cause the accidental death of whole families living in ghetto conditions. The second category is commoner and is typified by a child being trapped inside a disused refrigerator or trunk; it is generally clear that such instances are accidental—although the precise nature of the accident, particularly of the part played by other children, may be in doubt—but the pathologist has to be aware of the possibility of the disposal of a child dead from other causes. Adults can also be locked in containers—e.g. safes—accidentally though such circumstances would almost always be highly suspicious. Accidents of industrial type may also result in anoxic deaths—mining and submarine disasters are obvious examples.

There is often some difficulty in deciding whether to attribute a death of this type to oxygen deficiency or to poisoning by excess CO_2; I believe that the former is correct unless CO_2 is introduced into the environment in some way other than as a product of normal respiration. However, both physiological mechanisms operate and the process of asphyxiation in an enclosed environment is self-accelerating. As oxygen is utilized the concentration of CO_2 builds up; an increase in CO_2 reflexly increases the respiratory activity which, in turn, accelerates the depletion of oxygen; a rapidly fatal vicious circle is established, gross biochemical changes being added to lack of oxygen.

Environmental asphyxia due to altitude must be mentioned although, as it is virtually confined to aviation, it has only slight medico-legal implications. Death truly due to high-altitude hypoxia is rare. Mountaineers and those living at heights are able to adapt to the conditions; balloonists were early historic casualties but are scarcely a large group now; emergency oxygen is available to airline passengers and, so far as is known, has never failed when required.

Hypoxia at altitude is of greater importance in two other respects. In the first place, a person who is particularly susceptible to oxygen lack is at increased risk as ascent is made. An altitude of the order of 1500–1800 m (5000–6000 ft), which is quite safe for normal fit persons, may precipitate fatal myocardial ischaemia in the presence of an already inadequate coronary circulation; similar altitudes could precipitate a crisis in a person with sickle-cell disease. The ability of hypoxia to cause an aircraft accident is even more significant. Precision performance falls off rapidly with decreasing oxygen pressure, and it is generally accepted that 3000 m (10 000 ft) is the effective upper limit at which a man can operate an intricate machine without supplemental oxygen; above 9000 m (30 000 ft) this supplement must be supplied under positive pressure. The effects of hypobaric hypoxia are quite insidious, the victim being wholly unaware of his decreasing efficiency; it follows that failure of the oxygen supply to a military aviator or undiscovered loss of pressure in cabin-type aircraft[14] are potential causes of accidents. Sudden loss of pressure ('explosive decompression') in a large aircraft—such as might be caused by the detonation of a bomb or by major structural failure—is a complex pathological problem; death and injury may result from turbulence in the cabin, anoxia, the effects of low pressure and of cold and, of course, from the likely crash.

Iatrogenic asphyxia

Some degree of hypoxia may occur whenever a general inhalation anaesthetic is administered, the relative avoidance of this being a measure of the anaesthetist's vigilance and skill. Since oxygen lack in these circumstances is often imposed upon patients who are particularly susceptible by reason of disease, there is a real possibility of death due to hypoxia under anaesthesia. The medico-legal importance of the subject is great and is treated separately in Chapter 31.

---

[14] This is, of course, an impossibility in major commercial aircraft which have multiple means of detection available.

14

Fire, water, heat, cold and neglect

This chapter deals with a number of conditions which, while being related mainly to asphyxia, have a wider interest than the simple production of tissue anoxia. Those that are not so associated are logically related through at least one line of interest.

Injury and death from burning

Legally, burns include the destruction of tissue through the application of any form of heat or of any chemical substance. There is no distinction in law as to the degree of burning—to burn someone in any way is a serious assault and the use of corrosive substances is a specific aggravation in Scots law.

Burns may be natural—as in exposure to non-ionizing solar radiation or due to lightning; they may be due to dry heat—generally from open fires but also from such articles as hot plates, hot-water bottles, etc.; burns due to moist heat are commonly known as scalds; corrosive substances have their own individual pathologies, and burns due to electricity and X-rays should be included in this classification.

The distribution of these types of burn varies with age. Under the age of 3 years, a high proportion are due to scalding; scalding also occurs in later childhood but accidental setting light to clothes is more important in this age group and is the most significant source of burning in old age; in normal adult life the great majority of accidental burns stem from industry which provides examples of dry, wet and corrosive burning. However, with the exception of those due to lightning and man-made electricity (*see* below), the local medical effects of all burns are similar; this section will deal with burns due to fire as being the most typical, the most common and, medico-legally, the most important form of thermal injuries.

Burning in the human varies from simple reddening and blistering of the skin to severe charring and destruction of deeper parts of the body; I was involved in the investigation of one aircraft disaster in which no less than 23 bodies remained unaccounted for—it could only be assumed that they had been effectively cremated. It was at one time customary to classify burns according to their appearance; it is more rational to speak in terms of depth. If there is loss of only partial thickness of the skin it should be self-healing, whereas full-thickness loss will require skin grafting; very deep burning will inevitably cause some loss of function or lead even to amputation. This classification, essentially related to treatment, is also helpful in assessing the hurt and inconvenience sustained. The immediate prognosis of a burn depends to a great extent on susceptibility to pain—which is mainly a matter of conditioning and of age. Once over the initial impact, the outcome of a burn involving loss of skin is largely dictated by the escape of body fluids, the severity of which correlates, within limits, with the area rather than the depth of burning. There is a massive loss of water, protein and electrolytes from the raw areas and severe surgical shock arises if treatment is inadequate. Subsequently, the results of a burn are related to the risk of overwhelming infection. Children and the elderly are more susceptible to secondary infection and septicaemia than are young adults. The general rule is that burning that destroys more than 70 per cent of the skin is likely to be fatal irrespective of the treatment; the elderly may not survive a 20 per cent burn[1].

Severe burns due to fire may be accidental, suicidal or homicidal. The first is by far the commonest and is a particular hazard of childhood and of old age; catching the clothes in an open or an electric fire is very liable to occur in both age groups[2]. Statutory protection is given to children both in England and Wales and in Scotland[3] where it is declared an offence for a person over the age of 16 to expose a child under the age of 12 (age 7 in Scotland) in his or her care to the dangers of contact with an open fire grate or any heating appliance without taking reasonable precautions and, by reason thereof, the child is killed or suffers serious injury. Children are also prone to scalding by boiling fat and similar things to which they are drawn by inquisitiveness. There is a clear association between infirmity and burning in the aged; frank illness may lead to a sequence of collapse, concussion and burning while in the unconscious state. Acute alcoholism also plays an important part in accidental burning; the combination of intoxication and smoking in bed is extremely dangerous and the latter practice is illegal in hotels in the USA.

Mass accidental burnings are a risk whenever large numbers of persons are congregated in an enclosed area. The likely situations are obvious and need no detailed discussion; tenements, hotels, dance halls, theatres, etc., provide the common examples. Prevention of disaster is a matter of rigid application of building regulations, of ensuring a competent fire-fighting capacity and of provision of adequate escape facilities[4].

Burning in transport accidents must be mentioned. It is far less common than might be expected in automobile accidents but it is by no means rare in aircraft accidents, although the latter do not constitute a numerically important cause of unnatural death; it is noteworthy that the more 'survivable' an aircraft accident is in terms of crash forces, the more likely is death, when it occurs, to be due to burning—there is clearly room for improvement in the design of seats, passenger restraints and emergency escape procedures.

Suicidal burning is not all that uncommon—there were at least 74 and probably as

---

[1] The calculation of the area is based on the 'Rule of Nine'. The head and neck represent 9 per cent of the body area; each arm 9 per cent; the front and back of the trunk each 18 per cent; and each leg 18 per cent.

[2] Current Regulations require that a guard be fitted to all domestic heating appliances whether they be coal, gas, electric or oil fires (Heating Appliances (Fireguards) Regulations 1973, S.I. 73/2106 made under the Consumer Protection Act 1961).

[3] Children and Young Persons Act 1933, s. 11 as amended; Children and Young Persons (Scotland) Act 1937, s. 22.

[4] Fire Precautions Act 1971.

many as 111 instances in England and Wales in 1979. It may be adopted when maximum publicity is sought—igniting one's own kerosene-drenched body has become something of an extreme form of political protest. Otherwise this form of suicide must generally be associated with severe mental derangement; I have experience of only one case, where the subject also drank over a pint of paraffin, presumably in the hope of dying by explosion. The practice of suttee—or ritual suicide by a Hindu widow on her husband's death—has long been abandoned.

Homicide by burning must also be very exceptional owing to the uncertainty of success. But murder by fire after having immobilized the subject—say by injury or by drugs—or, more probably, attempted concealment of a murder through post-mortem incineration are not at all unlikely; many of the classic examples of inspired forensic pathology have derived from such attempts[5]. The distinction of ante- mortem from post-mortem burning is, therefore, essential. The demonstration of 'vital reaction' (see Chapter 4) around a burn is of minimal value in this context, as the body will almost always be severely charred. Major importance attaches to the demonstration of products of combustion either in the form of soot in the air passages or upper gastrointestinal tract or as COHb in the blood—values of 20–50 per cent are common. For reasons that are sometimes unclear, the two parameters do not always follow one another logically[6], but it is virtually impossible to force soot deeply into the tissues of a cadaver while no more than traces of COHb would be likely to result from post-mortem diffusion of gas from the atmosphere. In the event of fractures having been found, the discovery of bone-marrow or fat emboli in the lungs (see Chapter 10) would strongly suggest that the bony injuries were sustained in life; it has been claimed that burning by itself will cause fat embolism but I have not been able to substantiate this observation. The most certain evidence of a cause of death other than burning would be a finding positively indicating that cause—such as the discovery of a bullet or of evidence of manual strangulation.

The disposal of bodies by burning is something of a vexed subject. Practices differ in crematoria, but a reasonable programme for the reduction of a body to ashes involves exposure to a temperature of 600 °C for 1 hour. Such a temperature would be unlikely to be achieved in normal domestic conditions. It might be possible to destroy portions of the cadaver after disarticulation—in itself, a fairly complex task—in a domestic stove or on a very efficient bonfire, but it would be a prolonged process. In practice, attempts to promote a more spectacular fire are thwarted by neighbours reporting the matter to the fire brigade.

Burning of itself causes artefacts that should be distinguished from ante-mortem injury; the lawyer should have some knowledge of them as they may appear as unqualified factual statements in post-mortem reports. The most common of these artefacts are muscle contractures which often result in the so-called 'pugilistic attitude'; this is simply due to heat coagulation of protein and is not evidence of a defence reaction. Contraction of the skin may lead to splits which are very like incised wounds. Boiling of body fluids in enclosed spaces may lead to apparent intravital haemorrhage; the most common type presents as a false extradural haemorrhage. Burning may of itself cause bony fractures; these are common in the bones of the arms and legs but are also seen in the skull where they may result in

[5] For example, R. v. Rouse, 1931, Northampton Assizes; R. v. Dobkin, 1943, C.C.C.
[6] This problem is discussed in detail by Blackmore, D. J. (1973), in *Aerospace Pathology*, Ed. by J. K. Mason and W. J. Reals, p. 196; Chicago; College of American Pathologists Foundation.

severe loss of bone. The combination of artefactual haemorrhage and fracture can pose a most difficult pathological problem.

Death from burning may be immediate—the intense pain may cause reflex inhibition of the heart or the thermal injury may simply be so severe as to be incompatible with life. Alternatively, death may be asphyxial in type; fire victims do not die from carbon monoxide poisoning *per se*—the discovery of COHb is rather a measure of survival in a fire environment. Early stupefaction can occur but this is probably due to the inhalation of other poisonous substances—e.g. cyanides—which are combustion products of many man-made materials. The distinction of the mode of death is of more than academic interest; it may be important evidence in the application of the laws of succession (*see* Chapter 10). Delayed death from burning is commonly due either to traumatic shock, or to infection spreading from the damaged areas; even if the problems of fluid loss and toxaemia are overcome, acute renal failure may have occurred and the response to dialysis is universally bad when this condition follows burning. Death more remote in time may result from pneumonia due to enforced and prolonged immobilization, and it is possible—though not everywhere agreed—that the effects of prolonged stress may exhaust the capacity of the adrenal glands to sustain life.

It scarcely needs emphasis that the long-term results of survival from severe burning may be disfiguring and disabling and that such features must be considered in assessing damages. Some effects may not be immediately apparent—blindness, for example, may be threatened not only by the immediate fire but by an increasing inability to close the eyes or blink as the injured tissues contract. Overall, accidental burning results in a substantial reduction in the efficiency of the young and active population.

Death from electricity

Electricity is used on a vast scale even by persons with negligible understanding of its behaviour. The fact that it causes so few deaths is a tribute to the safety engineering that has accompanied the development of the electrical industry.

The outcome of an electric shock depends upon physical factors in the discharge and on the physiological state of the subject.

The determinants in the discharge are the current (measured in amperes), the voltage (or electromotive force of the current, measured in volts), the time over which the discharge is passed (amperes × seconds = coulombs) and the type of current—whether direct or alternating. The major factors in the subject include his resistance to an electrical discharge, his body weight—children are more susceptible than are adults—his earthing and his degree of preparedness.

The relative importance of the discharge factors depends significantly upon the period of application. Ultra-short exposures are unpredictable in their effects, which depend upon the precise state of excitability of the heart when the shock is received. If the electric current is passed for less than 3 seconds, the danger is related both to the magnitude of the current and to the duration of the shock. Applications of longer than 3 seconds depend almost entirely on the amperage for their lethal effect; amperage to some extent dictates duration, as a high current initiates muscle spasm—the subject is unable to release the conductor and long exposure results. Direct current is less hazardous to life than is alternating. The danger of the latter increases with the frequency and probably reaches its peak at the frequency of the public supply—50 hertz (cycles per second) in Britain and Europe and 60 Hz in the USA. Alternating current becomes less dangerous once the power frequency range of 1 kHz is passed, ultra-high frequencies being only a source of intense heat.

The voltage of the discharge is important when related to the resistance of the subject. The latter is almost entirely a matter of skin moisture; a completely dry person would have an exceptionally high resistance and might well tolerate voltages of the order of those used in supply systems. The skin is generally of such conductivity that voltages above 200 V are likely to be fatal due to the limb-to-limb passage of a current of over 50 mA. Efficient movement of current depends, in ordinary circumstances, on the efficiency of earthing—a subject standing on wet ground is at far greater risk than is one on a dry surface. In the worst conditions, an alternating current at 25 V and 50 Hz has been fatal. Short-duration impulse shocks are used in agricultural electric fences; pulses of the order one tenth of a second in each second are usually considered non-lethal, but children of small body weight have been killed in exceptional circuit conditions. All workers with electricity will testify to the protective effect of preparedness for a shock; this is scarcely surprising since death from electric shock involves a considerable element of reflex nervous activity.

As to the relationship between electricity and accident, suicide and homicide, the last can be virtually dismissed save, perhaps, in the context of the 'battered baby' (*see* Chapter 20). Even judicial electrocution—which involved the passage of a current of very high voltage followed by one of great intensity—is now extremely rare. Suicidal electrocution has been reported but is now very uncommon despite the ready availability of the methods; the diagnosis can seldom be in doubt owing to the complexity of the arrangements made—a factor that also serves to eliminate homicide.

Accidents are overwhelmingly responsible for death due to electricity and are of several types.

Industrial accidents are kept to a minimum by stringent safety precautions but nevertheless continue to occur as a result of genuine mishap or flouting of the regulations due to overconfidence. Direct contact may not be necessary if very high tension cables are involved as arcing may occur at a distance of a few millimetres. *Domiciliary accidents* are more common and are of three main types: the apparatus may be defective, due often to fraying of insulation; attempts may be made to repair equipment without disconnecting it from the mains supply while using makeshift tools, a particular hazard for housewives; or apparatus may be dangerously used—the most common example involves the use of electric equipment in the bathroom, where conditions for electrical conduction are optimal. Neutral fusing, which can give a false indication that the apparatus is 'dead', is a hazard peculiar to older apparatus of British manufacture. *Iatrogenic accidents* are of much medico-legal importance as they will almost invariably lead to actions for negligence. Electroconvulsive therapy, in which convulsions are deliberately precipitated by electrical stimulation of the brain, is occasionally used in the treatment of mental disorder; traumatic injury may be sustained during the convulsion and deaths have been reported due to the electric shock itself. Polson *et al.*[7] have drawn attention to the hazards of electricity used with 'invasive'

---

[7] In *Essentials of Forensic Medicine* (1985), 4th edn., p.302. Oxford; Pergamon.

diagnostic or therapeutic techniques—i.e. those that involve penetration of the skin or of a mucous membrane; since the resistance of the skin is eliminated and blood is an excellent conductor, death may be caused by misapplication of very low intensity currents. The same authors (at page 304) have also reported on the use of electricity as an *autoerotic stimulant*. I have seen one case in which a penile vibrator was connected to a mains plug; when the dead body was discovered the plug was not in the socket and no marks were found on the penis—the cause of death could not, therefore, be attributed to electricity with certainty.

The diagnosis of death due to electric shock may, in fact, be difficult—electric marking is not always present. Characteristically, however, there is a mark which may correspond to the shape of the electrode and shows a central area of necrosis surrounded by a white zone which is, in turn, encircled by a blush of dilated vessels. A true burn of parchmented or charred type may result if the current has been prolonged. An 'exit' mark may also be present and may take on the shape of the exit contact.

Death is predominantly physiological when due to the electric shock itself; the post-mortem findings are, accordingly, often slight and generally non-specific. Three modes of death are described. In the least common, the respiratory centre of the brain is directly affected if the current passes through the head; a variant hypothesis is that vagal stimulation causes cardiac arrest. Alternatively, the entire musculature may be involved in the spasmodic contracture described above; death is then akin to that in traumatic asphyxia (*see* page 133) and accounts for those cases of electrocution that show the post-mortem changes usually associated with mechanical hypoxia. The most common cause of death is said to be ventricular fibrillation—that state in which the ventricles of the heart beat so rapidly as to be ineffective pumps. Interestingly, the current passing must be of fairly critical intensity to produce this effect—the deliberate application of a high-intensity current is used medically as a *treatment* of ventricular fibrillation, and this may account for some remarkable survivals that are reported after very high intensity electric shocks (any counter-shock, including painful injury, can act as a defibrillator). There are two major points of medico-legal interest associated with death from fibrillation. First, it has been reported that death may not be immediate and can be preceded by volitional movement. Secondly, and of far greater importance, cardiac function may be restored; prompt resuscitative measures are therefore essential and artificial respiration can be successful even after having been applied for very long periods.

Finally, death may be caused by, but not be due to, electrocution. Thus the fatal outcome may be due to burning if the clothes are set alight; alternatively, death may result from traumatic injury if a high-intensity shock precipitates the subject, for example, from a high ladder.

Lightning as a source of electrocution

A lightning flash incorporates several physical features. These include the application of an electric current of extremely high intensity, the effects of primary 'flash' and secondary thermal burning and the pressure effects of a high-intensity blast wave (*see* page 92). The subject struck may, therefore, sustain injuries of traumatic type—including fractures—which must be distinguished from those due to homicide. Superficial skin burns of a leafy or arborescent type are characteristic, when present, of lightning strike. Beyond this aspect of differential diagnosis, lightning strikes are of no medico-legal importance since they are always occurrences of unpredictable, accidental type. Despite the apparent ferocity of a lightning strike, it is noteworthy that death occurs in less than half the subjects who are treated promptly.

Death from hyperthermia

Although it has little medico-legal significance, a note on hyperthermic death is added for the sake of completeness. The human body is fairly well adapted to hot climates; sweating is the main protective mechanism and severe effects may follow abnormalities of this function.

Direct effects of heat on the brain may lead to heat stroke. The thermoregulating mechanism of the body is affected and the body temperature rises precipitously in association with a failure to sweat. The condition is essentially due to exposure of the head to direct heat, usually in an arid climate. This type of death could be criminally associated with deliberate exposure of soldiers or prisoners; some cases were the subject of war crimes.

Heat exhaustion is, medically, a different condition and arises in two forms. Anhidrotic heat exhaustion—that is, heat exhaustion due to failure of sweating—is secondary to a form of skin disease that occurs in hot, damp climates and is of no concern in the present context. Hyperhidrotic heat exhaustion, due to excessive sweating, could well form the subject of a medico-legal inquiry. In this condition, sweat flows so freely that enough sodium chloride is lost to provoke severe physiological effects unless it is purposefully replaced. This is the characteristic exhaustion of the long-distance runner or of the soldier on forced march, but the pure condition is not often seen in outdoor activity—a highly dangerous situation arises when heat stroke is superimposed. Heat exhaustion has considerable importance in industry and is a hazard to stokers in ships, etc., where the effects have been declared industrial accidents[8].

Death due to drowning

Although closely related to asphyxia, death from drowning is not a simple matter of oxygen lack. This certainly occurs but an additional, and perhaps main, effect of water inhaled in the lungs is to alter the biochemical balance of the blood; how this occurs depends upon the medium of immersion.

Drowning in salt water is closest to a true asphyxial death and, generally, there is ample evidence of a struggle to breathe; petechiae, however, rarely form in the lungs due, possibly, to the mechanical pressure of the inhaled water upon the capillaries. During the death throes, water not only passes into the lungs but is gulped into the stomach and is forced into the middle ear. Death may result from total immersion for some 2–3 minutes.

---

[8] For example, Maskery v. Lancashire Shipping Co. Ltd. (1914) 7 B.W.C.C. 428; Ismay, Imrie & Co. v. Williamson [1908] A.C. 437; but see Pyper v. Manchester Liners Ltd [1916] 2 K.B. 691 when death due to heat stroke was not considered the result of injury by accident—in fact, this appears to have been more probably a case of heat exhaustion.

The mechanism differs in fresh water which is removed from the lungs and transferred to the bloodstream far more quickly than is sea water. During this process, which, by raising the blood volume, is dangerous in itself, the protective covering of the alveoli—so-called 'surfactant'—is removed and this, among other results, causes the classic frothing at the mouth. Such frothing is not specific to drowning—it occurs in burning and in virtually any condition associated with pulmonary oedema—but it is very good evidence of death having been due to drowning when found in a body removed from the water. The fresh water passing into the pulmonary capillaries dilutes the plasma and an osmotic differential is built up between the plasma and the interior of the red blood cells. Water then passes into the cells which burst, liberating large quantities of intracellular potassium; a state of *hyperkalaemia* results which poisons the heart. Death from drowning in fresh water is, therefore, predominantly cardiac rather than asphyxial in nature and, consequently, is more rapid. It is fair to add that not all authorities are convinced that this sequence occurs in the human.

The nasopharynx and larynx are particularly sensitive to unusual stimuli; the sudden impact of cold fresh or salt water on the back of the throat is a classic potential cause of vagal inhibition of the heart (reflex cardiac arrest). Those who have fallen out of boats, slipped into canals and the like may, therefore, show none of the standard signs of drowning and often present a difficult pathological problem. Persons who slip in the bath, particularly children, may die in this way; indeed, a *normal* type of drowning in the bath would, in itself, be a suspicious circumstance[9].

Death from drowning may, again, be accidental, suicidal or homicidal. Accidental drowning is commonly associated with steep-sided, unnatural water courses or containers. Thus, children tend to drown in water tanks and the domestic swimming pool takes a severe toll, particularly in the USA; brewery workers may drown in the vats and adults falling into canals are less able to extricate themselves than are those who fall into rivers. Alcohol is a very important factor in the last example and ill health may also contribute to accidental drowning; something of the order of 4 per cent of drownings are epileptic in origin, and epileptics may drown face down in only inches of water. Unconsciousness from any cause will produce the same effect and a person falling into a dock may sustain concussive head injury in the process; the importance—and difficulty—of distinguishing such an injury from one due to an assault needs no emphasis.

Suicidal drowning is surprisingly common—even by walking out to sea, a method that must give ample scope for reconsideration. The placing of weights in the pockets or the tying of legs may be indications of suicide but such methods will also be adopted in criminal activity. The distinction of suicide from either homicide or accident must depend largely on the circumstantial evidence. In this connection, Simpson[10] stresses the importance of the location of the hat; the handbag in the case of a woman is, perhaps, an even better distinguishing feature.

There are many variations in homicidal drowning. The possibility of immersion in the bath has already been discussed. Pushing a non-swimmer into inshore water would scarcely be an elective method of murder due to the likelihood of rescue;

---

[9] George Smith, who drowned his 'brides in the bath' is, nevertheless, thought to have done so through the medium of vagal stimulation—the method being suddenly to immerse the woman's head by lifting her feet.
[10] In *Forensic Medicine* (1979), 8th edn., p. 103. London; Edward Arnold.

such cases are' more likely to be in the nature of manslaughter—the drowning resulting from a brawl on land. On the other hand, even the best of swimmers will die if thrown from a boat on the open sea; a conclusive distinction between murder and accident might well be impossible on pathological grounds and, indeed, a charge of murder may be brought in the absence of a cadaver. However, the most likely association between criminality and 'drowning' is the disposal in the water of a body already dead; as in incineration, the pathological problem is to distinguish between ante-mortem and post-mortem immersion.

This is often complicated by severe putrefaction following failure to recover bodies from the water for relatively long periods. Not only do the pathological findings change—fluid, for example, passes from the lungs into the pleural spaces—but, during the period of immersion, there is opportunity for destruction of tissue by fish and crustaceans. Additionally, artefacts simulating ante-mortem injury can be produced by contact with rocks, ships' propellers and the like. The rare condition of cadaveric spasm is probably most often found in drowning; almost certainly the casualty was alive on entering the water if weeds or flotsam are discovered firmly clenched in the hands. However, the finding of mud or weeds in the upper air passages has been criticized as good evidence of respiratory movements while under water. It has been stated that such foreign bodies can enter a dead body; it is difficult to generalize on this—the interpretation depends on the amount of foreign material and the depth of its penetration. Two further approaches to the diagnosis of inhalation of water are theoretically available. First, there is the biochemical concept that a high concentration of electrolytes entering the lungs from sea water will be reflected in a higher chloride content in the blood of the left side of the heart than in that of the right; the converse should hold if the pulmonary blood is diluted by fresh water. The test is, however, relatively insensitive—a difference of at least 25 mg chloride/100 ml blood must be demonstrated—and becomes non-specific with the onset of putrefaction. It generally gives a good result when the diagnosis of death from drowning is obvious; it fails in just those instances where help is needed. The demonstration of other sea-water constituents—for example, magnesium—may be of more value, while others have drawn attention to the low specific gravity of the blood in the left side of the heart that is found in deaths from drowning irrespective of the type of water. The second test of inhalation depends on the demonstration of diatoms within the body. These are silica-covered organisms of minute size which are found to a varying extent in both salt and fresh water—the precise type of diatoms discovered in the cadaver has been used as an indication of the exact place of death. Most diatoms will be found in the lungs but it is generally held that organisms must be discovered in the systemic circulation—for example, in the bone marrow—to give proof of inhalation *intra vitam*. This is to guard against the possibility of passive entry of water into the lungs after death; the test has also been criticized on the grounds that airborne diatoms are widespread in some districts. The problem seems to be simply one of quantification—the finding of many diatoms is good evidence of drowning, but if only a few are discovered the result must be considered equivocal. The extreme resistance of the organisms to all forms of digestion makes the test especially valuable in the face of severe putrefaction.

Drowning is associated with one specific form of delayed death—post-immersion pneumonitis. This inflammatory condition is the result of the structural damage inflicted on the lungs by inhaled water. It may come on only hours after an apparently successful rescue and has a high mortality.

Death from hypothermia

Hypothermic deaths of medico-legal importance fall into two major groups—first, those associated with fit persons exposed to the cold, as an example of which immersion in water forms a logical link with the preceding section; secondly, there are the cases involving elderly, unfit persons who die in conditions associated with subnutrition.

In contrast to its relatively good defences against a hot environment, the human body adapts very poorly to cold; the protective mechanism of shivering operates only when the body temperature has actually fallen. The warmest clothing compatible with function, and not artificially heated, will fail to protect a man at rest from a fall in body temperature when that of the ambient temperature is $-20°C$; it will not keep him in comfort at an ambient temperature of $0°C$ or less. The subject is at grave risk when the body temperature falls to $30°C$, evidence of life is difficult to detect at $27°C$ and recovery from a fall in temperature to $24°C$ is unlikely. Shivering ceases when the body temperature has fallen to $33°C$ and, after that, the only defence open to the body is one involving shifts of blood from the periphery to the deep core. This causes profound physiological changes to which the body may be unable to adapt. Concurrent alcoholism accelerates death probably by interfering with these protective vascular responses.

The body temperature falls with surprising speed. It is doubtful if many persons could survive for more than 15 minutes in the North Sea in winter. Clothing may postpone the end and fat persons will survive longer than thin. I have seen one case in which three partially clothed children equipped with life-jackets were precipitated into the Bristol Channel in very cold weather; there was no evidence of drowning and death was estimated to have occurred in about 10 minutes. A moribund condition of persons removed from the water may be due either to drowning or to hypothermia but the treatment of the one condition is likely to be lethal in the other. The diagnostic dilemma confronting the the attending physician may be one of great complexity.

As metabolism approaches zero, so do the body's requirements for oxygen; sufficient quantities of the gas may, in fact, be dissolved in the plasma. States of 'suspended animation' can, therefore, occur. The most outstanding example reported is that of a young boy who travelled for 9 hours in the unpressurized nosewheel compartment of an aircraft at 8800 m (29 000 ft). Death in these circumstances would be expected either from hypoxia or from hypothermia; occurring together, they resulted in unconsciousness which was rapidly reversed in hospital. Any condition greatly reducing the body's need for oxygen—for example, narcotic poisoning—coupled, perhaps, with a low atmospheric temperature as in extreme poverty, might simulate death so closely as to deceive the examining physician; conditions in the mortuary refrigerator might conceivably perpetuate the simulation and cases have occurred when life has been discovered on the autopsy table. Hypothermic deaths do, therefore, require very careful certification and this applies particularly to the classic case of the elderly person living alone in poor conditions.

The post-mortem diagnosis of death due to hypothermia is largely circumstantial and a matter of exclusion. The circulation of blood is affected and leads to the development of a type of surgical shock; characteristically, the inefficient circulation results in the presence of microthrombi—or widespread clotting of the blood in the small vessels. Haemorrhage into the bowel and acute inflammation without bacterial invasion of the pancreas also occur in a high proportion of cases, the underlying mechanism being the same. Very likely, however, nothing specific will be found. Deaths of this type are unlikely to be anything more than a sociological problem although, occasionally, the management of an old people's home might be called into question.

Death due to neglect

Neglect is, in practice, divisible into two categories—self-neglect and the neglect of children; occasional cases of deliberate neglect of old persons occur but these must be rare[11]. While skin ulcers, parasitic infestation and the like are an integral part of neglect, it is the accompanying starvation that is the most important factor contributing to death. 'Starvation' consists of subnutrition—which is the intake of an insufficient quantity of food—and malnutrition—which is feeding of inadequate quality. Malnutrition can and does occur as a separate entity; subnutrition must always include some degree of malnutrition.

The usual case of neglect, therefore, presents as an emaciated body that shows multiple trophic ulcers, is verminous and shows evidence of severe vitamin deficiency. The inevitable weakening of the body may open the way to wide dissemination of natural disease but disease may, of course, be the primary cause of the marasmic state; this distinction between cause and effect is of great importance in the event of criminal charges being pressed. In the typical case of neglect the person must have been taking or been provided with *some* sustenance to have survived a sufficient time for the other changes to develop; total starvation is fatal in some 2 weeks, but life may be prolonged for up to 10 weeks so long as fluid is available.

Self-neglect commonly represents a failure of society itself, often abetted by the individual's ignorance or fault—alcoholism being a frequent precipitating factor. Other cases of self-neglect have a psychiatric background; certainly not all elderly persons suffering from malnutrition are impoverished although the fear of impending poverty may motivate the condition. Neglect in the well-to-do may be not so much true self-neglect as the result of an incapacity to get about: the possibility that the condition derives, effectively, from neglect by family or society must be considered. If a death is to be the subject of criminal charges there has to be more than simple neglect—there must be evidence of deliberate intent to cause harm or of a reckless indifference to the well-being of a person in the charge of the accused. Nevertheless, all cases of apparent self-neglect deserve intensive forensic study because, irrespective of the elimination of criminality, this is an area of community preventive medicine in which the medico-legal services can be properly involved.

The hunger strike is one aspect of self-neglect—virtually suicidal in nature—that has recently returned to public interest. This situation raises fascinating problems in criminological and medical ethics; the point at which a doctor should actively engage in saving life against the wishes of the subject, thereby committing an assault and often apparently associating himself with a political bias, is one that needs careful assessment—it is fortunate that the great majority of cases are

[11] There is an interesting discussion of manslaughter by neglect in the *British Medical Journal* (1977), i, 722, which notes, in particular, R. v. Stone [1977] 2 W.L.R. 169.

resolved by the politicians themselves, and current policy is that the doctor's role is to advise the prisoner of the dangers of starvation, to have treatment and hospital space available but, otherwise, to refrain from interference[12]. While this policy accords with the Declaration of Tokyo[13], the physician must at times be concerned as to whether the prisoner can, in truth, form an 'unimpaired and rational judgment'.

Child neglect is by far the most important aspect of the subject. Undoubtedly, some parents are so ignorant as to be incapable of adequately caring for their children but, in many cases, child neglect must have criminal undertones. The obligation placed upon a parent, or other person legally liable to maintain a child, to provide adequate food and clothing, to obtain medical care and to provide housing—or, in the event of these being impossible, to take steps to procure such advantages—is statutory throughout the United Kingdom[14]. The pathologist has often a difficult task in the interpretation of a death due apparently to child neglect. The mere discovery of subnutrition or malnutrition is not evidence of criminal neglect, while the role of intercurrent disease may be very difficult to assess; much will depend upon the ancillary evidence—often this will be in the form of unusually severe skin disease. Death due to neglect should be a rarity as efficient social services are widely available to arrange for adequate care and protection while recovery is still possible. The subject of child maltreatment is discussed further in Chapter 20.

Child neglect includes abandonment or exposure which, in the event of death, could amount to infanticide (or child murder), manslaughter (or culpable homicide) or even murder. The pathological contribution will be likely, in these cases, to be equivocal as the findings will not be those of neglect but rather those of simple hypothermia. Infants are more susceptible to the cold than are adults, but the post-mortem diagnosis can seldom be made other than on the basis of exclusion.

In a very different context, the concept of what might be termed *iatrogenic neglect* has recently attracted public attention. In certain circumstances, and particularly at each end of the natural lifespan, doctors may, as a clinical decision, withhold treatment from patients and authorize, for example, 'nursing care only'. The subject is considered further in Chapter 30.

[12] The controversial judgment in Leigh v. Gladstone (1909) 26 T.L.R. 139 is thus overturned. The subject is extensively discussed by Zellick, G. (1976), The forcible feeding of prisoners: an examination of the legality of enforced therapy, *Public Law*, 153–87.

[13] (1975). Guidelines concerning torture and other cruel, inhuman or degrading treatment or punishment in relation to detention and imprisonment. The complete text is reproduced in Mason, J. K. and McCall Smith, R. A. (1983) *Law and Medical Ethics*, App. D, London; Butterworths.

[14] Children and Young Persons Act 1933, s. 1(2); Children and Young Persons (Scotland) Act 1937, s. 12(2). But the offence is not one of strict liability (*see* R v Sheppard and Another [1980] 3 All E.R. 899).

15

Industrial injury and disease

Definitions and administration

It is axiomatic in a developed society that persons should be compensated for disability attributable to their working conditions. Ideally, such compensation should be payable irrespective of contributory fault and, while not excluding the possibility, should be free from the uncertainties of litigation on the bases of negligence or of contributory negligence. Such a system has been in operation in the United Kingdom since 1948 when the original National Insurance (Industrial Injuries) Act became operative. The relevant legislation is now consolidated in the Social Security Act 1975[1].

All persons employed in an insurable occupation are automatically insured—through contributions from employees, employers and the Exchequer—against disablement, incapacity or death resulting from an injury by accident arising out of and in the course of employment. The definition of injury is wide, including any physiological injury or change for the worse, and that of accident is equally embracing, being 'an unlooked-for-mishap or an untoward event which is not expected or designed'. The course of work need not be the proper course—for example, failure to take such safety measures as have been ordered has no effect on the payment of benefits (s. 52). Accidents due to skylarking or misconduct by another also attract benefit (s. 55).

There are, however, limits to which an insurance fund can stretch and disputes as to definition[2] are bound to occur; nor is industrial disease an entirely straight-forward subject.

Injuries that are self-evident—that is, those that involve external mutilation—will not be discussed here; not only are these beyond dispute but they are so various that a detailed description would be impossible. But the term 'accident' also includes injuries sustained in circumstances that are accidental merely by virtue of being unexpected. These circumstances need not be exceptional; an unexpected

---

[1] Previous legislation is repealed in Social Security (Consequential Provisions) Act 1975. Northern Ireland has its own Act (Social Security (Northern Ireland) Act 1975).

[2] Examples being the definition of 'place of work' in relation to transport and physical boundaries. A person is generally held to be at his place of work if he is in transport provided by his employers (positively enacted, s. 53) but not when in his own; an accident occurring in the grounds of a factory would also probably qualify for compensation.

event may be brought about by the routine engagement in work and it is immaterial that the work did no more than exacerbate known pre-existing disease[3]. A person more prone to accident than normal is still covered by the Act; thus, a known epileptic who has a fit at work and, as a result, suffers injury still sustains an industrial injury[4].

Disease contracted at work is dealt with in two main categories. There is first a disease that results from a single occurrence at work—and this is clearly an accident. The precise moment of injury need not be defined in all circumstances; a nurse contracting tuberculosis was clearly infected at a certain time although the precise exposure that was responsible for infection cannot be ascertained. In certain circumstances, however, there is continuing exposure to a work hazard and a disease contracted as a result is a matter of process rather than of accident. To qualify for insurance benefits, the second category of disease must be prescribed by regulations (s. 76). These diseases are loosely defined as those that can be attributed with reasonable certainty to the occupation and that do not constitute a risk to the whole population; sufferers from such diseases are treated for insurance purposes exactly as if they had sustained an accidental injury. A list of prescribed diseases is given in Appendix I.

Benefits for industrial injuries are available as:

1. *Injury Benefit*—payable as an allowance during the period in which the insured is unable to work through injury. It is not payable in respect of pneumoconiosis, when it is replaced by special benefit. Injury benefit is given for 156 days disregarding Sundays and is then replaced by:
2. *Disablement Benefit*—payable according to the disability (including disfigurement) sustained expressed as a percentage of total disablement. Less than 20 per cent disability is paid in gratuity form; otherwise it is distributed weekly. The disablement pension can be increased by an unemployability supplement and, *inter alia*, in respect of special hardship or exceptionally severe disablement.
3. *Death Benefit*—payable as a pension to a widow until remarriage at which time a gratuity is paid. The amount payable is modified according to the number of dependants of the dead person.

Problems as to whether an injury is to be regarded as industrial are decided by an Insurance Officer; referral or appeal is to a local tribunal consisting of a chairman and a representative each of employers and employees. There is a further right of appeal to a National Insurance Commissioner. Cases of special difficulty may be heard by a tribunal of three Commissioners. The degree of disablement is, however, decided by Medical Boards consisting of two or more medical practitioners. Appeals from their decisions are made to Medical Appeal Tribunals consisting of a chairman and two consultant medical practitioners; both the board and the tribunal may reverse their assessments if there are reasonable grounds. They cannot, however, reverse the Insurance Officer's decision that a condition did result from industrial injury[5]. Final appeal against the decision of a Medical Tribunal is to a Commissioner, such appeal being permissible only on a point of law.

Specific regulations are made as to prescribed diseases—in particular, the

---

[3] Clover, Clayton & Co. Ltd. v. Hughes [1910] A.C. 242; Oates v. Earl Fitzwilliam's Collieries Co. [1939] 2 All E.R. 498.
[4] Tankard v. Stone-Platt Engineering Co. Ltd. (1946) 174 L.T. 277.
[5] Jones v. Secretary of State for Social Services [1972] 1 All E.R. 145.

establishment of special medical boards and the appointment of special medical officers—and provisions are made in regard to the pneumoconioses that cover initial and periodic medical examinations and also allow for suspension or non-employment of persons found to be suffering from pneumoconiosis. Attendance at, and provision of facilities for, such examinations are compulsory. Byssinosis, or dust disease following inhalation of cotton dust, was once considered separately but is now benefited in the same way as any other occupational dust disease. A list of prescribed occupations is given in Appendix J.

The role of the lawyer in industrial compensation

A worker seeking industrial benefit may be represented—and, indeed, need not be present—at hearings of the local tribunal and before the National Insurance Commissioner. The main function of these appeal bodies is to decide whether or not the ruling of the Insurance Officer as to the definition of an industrial accident is valid[6].

Decisions, unless setting a precedent, will largely depend upon previous rulings which can be studied under the heading of 'Commissioners' Decisions'; these are published individually or bound under categories of benefit in the continuing 'Index and Digest of Decisions'. The list of conditions that have been held to be industrial accidents is steadily lengthening—some of the more extreme examples including a nervous shock resulting from watching a fatal accident that involved a workmate; a 'drop foot' sustained as a result of continual kneeling (this being something of an extension of accident as opposed to process) and coronary thrombosis arising during the act of tightening a nut.

It follows that not only must the lawyer be aware of these decisions but that, in the case of death, these should have been founded on sound medical evidence. Ideally, all deaths occurring at the place of work should be reported to the Coroner or the Fiscal irrespective of the certifying doctor's opinion as to the causative association with the deceased's occupation[7], and the cause of death should be certified as a result of post-mortem dissection; such a procedure would at least narrow the fields of dispute as to fact. It has been noted that appeal from the decisions of the Medical Appeal Tribunal can be made only on points of law; the role of the lawyer is then self-evident.

Both the solicitor and the advocate may be further involved in industrial litigation in so far as there is an ultimate appeal from a decision of the Commissioner to the High Court or the Court of Session on a point of law. Much civil litigation is initiated by employed persons against their employers based on negligence resulting in loss, injury and damage; in a proportion of these, the provisions of the Law Reform (Contributory Negligence) Act 1945 are invoked when the damages fail to be reduced on account of the contributory negligence of the injured party himself. There have recently been a significant number of successful actions for negligence against employers by workers who have contracted prescribed diseases. All such cases appear to have been settled out of court and are therefore unreported, but damages of £7500 have been awarded to a man with coal miners' pneumoconiosis[8].

[6] It is the Secretary of State who is charged with the duty of deciding whether the *occupation* was insurable under the Act (s. 93).
[7] See the Brodrick Report, para. 6.33 (*Report of the Committee on Death Certification and Coroners*. 1971, Cmnd. 4810. London; HMSO).
[8] *Sunday Times*, 1 February, 1970.

The medical nature of conventional 'accidents' at work is generally readily understandable and the logical sequence implied in disease contracted as a result of an accident is also normally clear. The nature—and rationale—of the prescribed diseases may not, however, be common knowledge in legal circles and a brief description is apposite.

The pneumoconioses

Pneumoconiosis is defined as fibrosis of the lung due to silica dust, asbestos dust or other dust and includes the condition of the lungs known as 'dust-reticulation'; a list of such conditions is given in Appendix J.

Fibrogenic dust may be mineral or vegetable in nature. The former is by far the more important and, while all occupations associated with mineral dust carry some risk, three conditions are outstanding—coal miners' pneumoconiosis because of its incidence in the United Kingdom, silicosis because it is, perhaps, the underlying basis for the clinical manifestations of the majority of mineral dust diseases, and asbestosis because of its severe effects and because it is a particularly good example of how workers other than miners—perhaps even the general population—may be affected by dust.

Coal miners' pneumoconiosis

Some 35000 certified cases of coal workers' pneumoconiosis are on record in the United Kingdom. About 500 new cases are still certified each year although the average age at which the different stages of the disease present has increased[9].

Pulmonary changes are often originally symptomless and are gauged radiologically; but this may not necessarily be so and the interrelationship of pneumoconiosis with other lung disease poses a considerable clinical problem which may result in differences of expert opinion when litigation or problems of compensation arise. The disease is divided into simple and complicated forms and, in view of the difficulties of clinical assessment, the former is empirically quantified on the radiological appearances. The lesions seen in the X-ray are known as nodules and these are classified according to size (Group p nodules are up to 1.5mm in diameter, Group m from 1.5 to 3.0mm and Group n between 3.0 and 10.0mm). The severity of the disease is further classified by its distribution, Category 1 diseases being limited to defined portions of the lungs while Category 3 denotes affection of the whole of both lungs; Category 2 is intermediate.

Complicated pneumoconiosis is alternatively known as progressive massive fibrosis (PMF). Nodules larger than 10mm in diameter appear and coalesce to produce extensive destruction of the lung with severe symptoms of respiratory distress. The incidence of PMF rises with the extent of the simple disease but, while the two must be in some way connected, the relationship is by no means a simple one. The effects of any coincident tuberculosis are treated as though they were the effects of pneumoconiosis.

It is officially stated[10] that simple pneumoconiosis is not itself a cause of disability

---

[9] The approximate comparable figures for pneumoconiosis as a whole are 40000 and 800.
[10] Ministry of Social Security (1967). *Pneumoconiosis and Allied Occupational Chest Diseases.* London; HMSO.

and does not reduce the expectation of life. Certainly other respiratory diseases are often present as no more than coincidentals, but the total validity of this pragmatic view is, at least, open to challenge[11].

The main conditions that are agreed as complicating simple pneumoconiosis are chronic bronchitis and emphysema; provided the primary disability is not less than 50 per cent, any disability due to these is added to the assessment of the dust disease for the purposes of benefit.

Because of the clinical difficulties involved, compensation is largely based on 'rule of thumb' observations. The suspected case is examined by two members of the Pneumoconiosis Panel and the subject is certified as suffering from pneumo-coniosis if they agree that Category 2 disease is present—Category 1 disease is sometimes accepted if the subject is young. The degree of disability is assessed on the basis of the vital capacity of the lungs—which is a measure of the amount of oxygen the lungs can make available to the body—and on the forced expiratory volume of the breath—which is a measure of the effectiveness or impairment of the elasticity and, hence, efficient function of the lungs. No appeal is normally available against the decision of the Pneumoconiosis Medical Panel save, in special circumstances, to the central Pneumoconiosis Medical Board; rejection of a claim does not prohibit repeated applications.

This valiant attempt to ensure a uniform procedure, the rationale of which is readily demonstrable, causes some problems which are particularly related to the difficulties of correlating clinical symptoms—which may have several different origins—with the radiological appearances, which are related to a single causative factor. It is often difficult for a legal adviser to understand how one man with apparently appreciable respiratory distress can be denied benefit while a much fitter colleague is a certified pneumoconiotic; yet it can and does occur.

Further causes of confusion may attend the result of post-mortem dissection. The Registrar of Deaths is obliged to report to the Procurator Fiscal or to the Coroner any deaths due to or arising from industrial disease or poisoning (*see* Chapter 2)[12]. The Coroner must also notify the Pneumoconiosis Panel of the date and place of the post-mortem examination and the Panel may be represented there; no such obligation rests on either the Procurator Fiscal or the Registrar in Scotland. While the Rules prevent a Coroner asking a member of the Pneumoconiosis Medical Panel to carry out the dissection[13], there is an informal arrangement whereby the thoracic organs are later made available to the Panel[14]. Thus the Coroner's certificate of death—whether it be by virtue of his own Form B or of a Certificate after Inquest—may include pneumoconiosis as relevant to death, whereas the Pneumoconiosis Medical Panel may decide that there is no entitlement to industrial death benefit; the converse may also hold. The important fact is that the report of the Coroner's pathologist is only indirectly associated with death benefit, in so far as the Pneumoconiosis Medical Panel will usually take into account the results of the Coroner's inquiries and these may also be used as evidence on appeal against the decision of the Insurance Officer; in the final analysis, however, it is the

[11] *See*, for example, Davies, D. (1974), Disability and coal workers' pneumoconiosis, *British Medical Journal*, **ii**, 652.

[12] In neither case is there a requirement for a doctor, who is willing to provide a certificate to the cause of death, to draw attention to any occupational condition that, in his opinion, has no association with that cause. The effect of the Industrial Diseases (Notification) Act 1981 on this generalization has yet to be seen.

[13] Coroners' Rules 1984 (S.I. 1984/552), Rule 6(1)(d).

[14] Home Office Circular 79/69.

opinion of the Pneumoconiosis Panel that exerts the main influence on the Insurance Officer. The importance of post-mortem dissection and of the availability of the evidence to the equitable settling of cases is obvious.

Silicosis

Silica in its large particulate form causes no more than a harmless reaction to a foreign body. But when the size of particles is small, a fibrotic reaction is set up which has profound effects on the lungs. Silica is, in essence, the primary source of the pneumoconioses, and is likely to be dispersed whenever rock is drilled or sand is particularized as in the cleaning of blast furnaces, building in sandstone, grinding and the like. Coal dust as such is relatively innocuous in the absence of silica; true silicosis in coal miners generally occurs only in those confronted with the harder seams—that is, in anthracite miners and in the 'hard headers' who drive the tunnels to reach the face. Gold mining is particularly dangerous as a source of the disease.

The lesion in silicosis is that of formation of fibrotic nodules due to the locally poisonous properties of silica when dissolved—possibly in the form of silicic acid. The process is self-perpetuating, the amount of fibrosis is disproportionate to the quantity of dust and the end result is massive destruction of lung tissue with death from a combination of cardiac and respiratory failure. In the process, the original isolated nodules coalesce to form what is known as massive conglomerate nodular silicosis; alternatively, a form of progressive massive fibrosis, not unlike that seen in coal miners' pneumoconiosis, may arise.

Silicosis is clearly associated with tuberculosis and potentiates the virulence of the organism causing the latter disease. There is, however, no fully acceptable evidence that silica stimulates the formation of cancer[15]. Thus, silicosis differs markedly from the third of the most important dust diseases—asbestosis.

Asbestosis

Asbestos occurs in two main types—chrysotile and amphiboles. There are three varieties of amphiboles: crocidolite, amosite and anthophyllite. The fibres of chrysotile are long and are used mainly for the preparation of asbestos clothing; those of amphiboles are shaped like needles and are used to make roofing, tiles and insulating material.

As with all dust disease, asbestosis consists of fibrosis of the lung tissue which can be finely nodular or dense and massive. Since asbestos is virtually indestructible, its effects on the lung are progressive even after removal from the dusty environment. Fibrosis of the lung does occur in asbestos miners but, because the main offending condition is the 'asbestos cloud', those who are exposed to asbestos in its purified—or purifying—form are at greatest risk. Asbestos is used in very many industrial processes but maximum exposure outside the factories concerned with preparation occurs in the building trade; in shipbuilding, where it is used mainly as a thermal insulator; and in the manufacture of brakes, clutches and the like. The danger is particularly great during the destruction of asbestos products when

[15] Two haematite mines in Cumbria, separated by only 48 km (30 miles), showed a marked difference in the incidence of lung cancer. In the mine associated with soft clay substrate, cancer was not an occupational hazard; the incidence of cancer among workers in the hard-rock mines was some 70 per cent above the general level. The difference, however, might well have been due to radioactivity—cf. the iron-ore miners in Czechoslovakia.

masses of very dry dust are dispersed in relatively uncontrolled conditions. There is, therefore, a potential hazard to the public in the vicinity of large reconstruction projects, which are now limited by very strict controls[16].

Although simple asbestosis may cause lethal dysfunction of the lungs, it is distinguished from almost all other forms of pneumoconiosis by its incontrovertible association with malignant tumours of the lungs—at least 60 per cent of workers who are accepted as disabled by pneumoconiosis due to asbestos subsequently develop lung cancer; the death rate in asbestos workers from the common form of lung cancer, bronchogenic carcinoma, is some ten times that of the general population. The increase is largely taken up with an association with smoking although the risks are also substantial for a heavily exposed non-smoker. Bronchogenic carcinoma is probably associated with all types of asbestos and with a relatively long exposure, but one particular form of cancer—mesothelioma—is particularly associated with exposure to crocidolite or 'blue asbestos'[17]. It is very rarely associated with chrysotile and never with anthophyllite. There is some evidence that mesothelioma occurring in miners results from exposure to an asbestos/manganese complex, but it is workers in an atmosphere laden with the dust from prepared asbestos products who are at greatest risk; the exposure to blue asbestos need only be short and, of major medico-legal significance, there is always a long incubation period—the condition may not manifest itself for some 20–40 years after exposure. A cause-and-effect association may be difficult to prove—or defend—at such a distance in time particularly as mesothelioma may occur without any other features of asbestosis; the provisions of the Limitation Act 1980, which extend the period in which an action for personal damages can be brought in the event of there being no symptoms for some time after an untoward event, must be invoked in any suit for negligence.

Other prescribed diseases

The pneumoconioses are so distinct and of such importance that they have been given particular prominence. Other prescribed diseases are less common and are of such diversity as to preclude a full description outside a work confined to industrial medicine. The reader will be able to understand the great majority from a simple view of Appendix I; some specific aspects of poisoning are, however, considered in Chapter 22.

Safety at work

The subject of safety at work is now dominated by the Health and Safety at Work, etc. Act 1974, which attempts to provide a comprehensive system of law designed to integrate the safety and health of work people and of the public. In the words of s. 1(2) 'the making of health and safety regulations and agricultural health and

---

[16] Asbestos Regulations 1969 (S.I. 1969/690). The Commission of the European Communities (*Public Health Risks of Exposure to Asbestos* (1977). London; Pergamon Press) has argued that simple ambient exposure to asbestos carries no definite risk but that too many uncertainties exist to deny such a risk. The *British Medical Journal* contains a number of important leading articles relating to the subject (1976), i, 1361; (1978), i, 1164; (1981), 283, 457).

[17] Mesothelioma may be greatly reduced in future due to the banning of crocidolite under the Asbestos (Prohibition) Regulations 1985 (S.I. 1985/910).

safety regulations and the preparation and approval of codes of practice shall in particular have effect with a view to enabling specified enactments and the regulations . . . in force under those enactments to be progressively replaced by a system [operating under this Act] and designed to improve the standards . . . established under those enactments.' Thus, the 1974 Act does not repeal but rather integrates all previous legislation devoted to specific industries or aspects of working conditions[18].

Part 1 of the Act imposes strict obligations on employers—in particular, the duty to establish 'safety committees'[19]—and sets up a Health and Safety Commission and Health and Safety Executive. The Commission, consisting of representatives of employers, employees and local authorities, is charged with effecting the purposes of the Act and with arranging research, training and provision of information relevant to safety at work. The Executive, a triumvirate, gives effect to the decisions of the Commission, enforcing these through appointed inspectors who are given wide powers of entry, investigation, interrogation and discovery, although answers given to the inspector carrying out his duties cannot be used in evidence in any proceedings taken against the person answering.

Inspectors may serve 'improvement' or 'prohibition' notices on persons in control of activities who then have the right of appeal to an industrial tribunal at which they may be represented by legal advisers. A number of offences concerned with obstructing or disobeying the Executive are specified, and proceedings may be taken against the person as a result of a Coroner's inquest or a public inquiry under the Fatal Accidents and Sudden Deaths Inquiry (Scotland) Act 1976. No public inquiry under this Act is held if an investigation is being undertaken by the Health and Safety Executive.

A very large number of consequential regulations have been issued under the Act which have had a profound effect on those areas of employment not covered by the previous essentially 'industrial' legislation, including hospitals and laboratories[20]. Many of the regulations are of a consolidating type, an important example being the Notification of Accidents and Dangerous Occurrences Regulations 1980 (S.I. 1980/84). An accident is notifiable to the Executive if it involves the death of any person or injury to an employee resulting in more than 3 days absence from work—in the latter case, a consequent death occurring within 1 year must also be notified. Fourteen examples of dangerous occurrences that are notifiable wherever they occur are specified, and there are additional notifications in the cases of mines, quarries and railways[21].

Certain industrial diseases must also be notified by a doctor to the Chief Inspector of Factories[22]—these include poisoning by lead, phosphorus, arsenic and mercury when contracted in a factory. Subsequent to the original Act, poisoning by beryllium and cadmium have been added to the list together with a number of other diseases which are listed in Appendix K.

The Employment Medical Advisory Service Act 1972 amends the Factories Act

[18] The relevant Schedule specifies 31 statutes of which the following are representative and especially important: The Alkali, &c. Works Regulation Act 1906; Employment of Women, Young Persons and Children Act 1920; Petroleum (Consolidation) Act 1928; Mines and Quarries Act 1954; Agriculture (Safety, Health and Welfare Provisions) Act 1956; Factories Act 1961; Offices, Shops and Railway Premises Act 1963; Nuclear Installations Act 1965; Employment Medical Advisory Service Act 1972.
[19] Safety Representatives and Safety Committees Regulations 1977 (S.I. 1977/500).
[20] See, for example, the Dangerous Pathogens Regulations 1981 (S.I. 1981/1011) and the Health and Safety (Genetic Manipulation) Regulations 1978 (S.I. 1978/752).
[21] The list is not exhaustive as other accidents or occurrences must be notified under other regulations—e.g. the Civil Aviation (Investigation of Accidents) Regulations 1983 (S.I. 1983/551).
[22] Factories Act 1961, s. 82.

1961 in relation to the carrying out of statutory medical examinations and examinations of young persons. Official Appointed Factory doctors have been replaced by Employment Medical Advisers. The Employment Medical Advisory Service Act 1972 was incorporated *in toto* into the Health and Safety at Work etc. Act 1974 and the Employment Medical Advisers form the medical wing of the Health and Safety Executive; the medical advisers are granted the full powers of an Inspector and they may investigate the cause of death, injury, disease or poisoning resulting from employment.

In England and Wales and in Scotland, the Minister may direct that a full investigation be held into the causes and circumstances of any accident occurring or of any disease acquired in a factory—it is not uncommon for a legal man to be appointed as the Assessor and lawyers will be involved on behalf of the parties concerned.

Deaths resulting from a notifiable disease or accident must be reported to the Coroner or to the Procurator Fiscal. The former is obliged to hold an Inquest with a jury at which any interested party may be legally represented. In Scotland, the same situation is covered by the inquiry that is held under the Fatal Accidents and Sudden Deaths Inquiry (Scotland) Act 1976 but such an inquiry will not normally be held if a Ministerial Public Inquiry has been ordered.

16

Medico-legal aspects of sport

Generally speaking, medico-legal aspects of sport are governed by the doctrine of *volenti non fit injuria*. However, this cannot always hold. There are several interests involved in organized sport—including those of the participants, the promoters and the public—and while the Roman crowds no doubt felt themselves well entertained, it is unlikely that the early Christians were happy with their representation. So much is now materially at stake in what once were games that the law must become involved; injury and death at sport are now integral parts of forensic medicine.

It is not intended to consider all potential injuries that can arise in risk sports; most are relatively obvious and few—other than accidental gunshot wounds which are discussed in Chapter 9—have particular medico-legal significance other than in relation to standards of professional medical care—negligence in treatment of a knee injury occurring in a man who made his living from football would be likely to attract greater damages than would be the case in similar circumstances involving an elderly bank clerk. But those sports that are, in effect, legalized assaults require separate consideration, and there are other more general aspects of forensic medicine that can conveniently be discussed under this chapter heading.

Boxing and wrestling

Springing from its roots in illegal prize-fighting and being most obviously associated with 'intent to inflict bodily injury', boxing has inevitably attracted the greatest forensic attention among sports.

Attitudes to boxing have altered dramatically in a lifetime. In the amateur sphere, the annual school boxing tournament has fallen so far from its position as the event of the year that the Royal College of Physicians has concluded 'it must be generally questioned whether there is any justification for including boxing as a school sport'[1]. It is fair to point out that, against this view, there are many who regard organized boxing as a controlled method of unleashing normal violence and, consequently, as a positive contribution to the reduction of violent crime. On the

[1] Royal College of Physicians (1969). *Report on the Medical Aspects of Boxing*. London; Royal College of Physicians.

professional side, there is no doubt that stricter controls introduced since the Second World War have transformed the image of boxing. Perhaps the administrative changes have been accelerated by the campaign against the sport which has been based to some extent on its mortality and, more importantly, on the associated long-term morbidity.

There are, in fact, surprisingly few acute fatalities in boxing. Between 1955 and 1958, only one death was attributed to boxing in the United Kingdom out of 50 deaths occurring during sport—astonishingly, during the same period, 14 persons were killed playing cricket[2]. It is claimed that there have been less than 20 deaths from boxing since 1945. When it occurs, death is most commonly due to intracranial haemorrhage; intracerebral bleeding into the midbrain is the injury said to be most specific to boxing, but subdural bleeding with its attendant latent period, is, in practice, less uncommon and may be cumulative as a result of repeated sheering forces being applied to the brain (see Chapter 11); abnormal stimulation of the autonomic nervous system, as by blows to the neck or to the solar plexus, are occasional causes of sudden death.

Far greater interest centres on the long-term effects of boxing—traumatic encephalopathy or 'punch drunkenness'. There is no doubt as to the reality of this syndrome although its prevalence may have been exaggerated. The precise mechanism is unknown but it probably results from a succession of attacks of 'diffuse neuronal injury' described in Chapter 11 as the cause of concussion. The condition, which is characterized by defects of memory, slurring of speech, unsteadiness of gait and clumsy movements, appears related to persistent repetition of severe injury to the head—it is, therefore, one that occurs in poor-quality boxers forced by economic necessity into frequent bouts beyond their capability and who consequently receive more than average punishment; there is also some evidence that punch drunkenness is associated with the length of each bout—while the brain can recover from five contests of three rounds each, it has no interval in which to do so during 15 consecutive rounds. The Report on the Medical Aspects of Boxing concluded that, while the likelihood of severe disablement due to brain damage was rare in boxers, there was evidence of a lesser degree of damage in a high proportion of persons who had boxed professionally for over 10 years.

This being so, the effects of boxing should be preventable by regulation and, certainly, much effort is put into this aspect of the spectacle. A strict medical code has been enforced in British professional boxing since 1953 and includes general annual examinations of licensed boxers as well as immediate pre-fight medical check-ups. The number of bouts is controlled by the Medical Commission of the British Board of Boxing Control, who also have the power to withdraw a man's licence on the grounds of ill health. Appointed doctors are present at the ringside to advise on fitness to continue the fight and to assess the injury in the event of a knock-out; an injured boxer must be suspended until he is declared fit for another bout. Moreover, an investigation is mounted if a boxer loses four fights in succession.

In view of all these precautions, a death in the ring can scarcely be regarded as anything other than accidental; this, however, depends upon the regulations being observed[2a]. Death resulting from a deliberate mismatch could certainly attract a charge of culpable homicide as would one that could be attributed to premeditated

[2] Parliamentary Debates, House of Lords, 1962, **240**, col. 366.
[2a] See Attorney General's Reference (No. 6 of 1980) [1981] Q.B. 715.

failure to stop a fight that was clearly leading to severe injury. Disability sustained because of inadequate pre-fight medical examination could be, and has been, construed as being attributable to medical negligence[3].

It may seem inequitable that the *voluntary* provision of medical care can lead to litigation when such care is seen to fall short of acceptable standards; there are, for example, no comparable controls in professional wrestling, yet this causes no adverse comment. There would, however, be a popular demand for medical supervision of wrestling should the need become apparent; the fact that death or severe injury is virtually unknown in professional 'all-in' wrestling in the United Kingdom can probably be left to speak for itself—interestingly enough, there is a considerable morbidity in Eastern Europe. It is doubtful if boxing would have survived the political attacks of the early 1960s had it not set its own house in order; public opinion, having forced a standard, requires that standard to be maintained.

Sudden death in non-contact sports

Occasional deaths occur in apparently healthy young adults engaged in strenuous exercise such as long-distance running, protracted swimming or severe marching. Sometimes the environmental conditions are obviously extreme and can be held responsible for the death—e.g. in severe heat, death may be due to heat stroke or heat exhaustion (*see* Chapter 14) or, at the other end of the spectrum, an enforced stop may lead to death from exposure; many deaths of this type result from ignoring authoritative advice or from inadequate planning.

Very often, however, the cause of death is obscure and may only be assumed after a diligent search has revealed some unusual abnormality; equally, no cause may be demonstrable and the death is, in effect, physiological (*see* Chapter 7 for a fuller discussion). Any abnormal conditions discovered are generally those that might be expected to leave the heart dangerously short of oxygen during excessive demand—in particular, anatomical abnormalities of the coronary circulation or an unusual degree of atheroma. The importance of these conditions in a medico-legal context is twofold—first, they would not have been recognizable by routine medical tests for fitness and, as a corollary, no blame for the death can reasonably be attached to the organizers of the activity. A number of such deaths have been attributed to blood disorders that are sensitive to hypoxia; sickle-cell disease has been cited and other unusual conditions[4] may cause collapse and dangerous sequelae if not sudden death. Selection both for employment and for recreation on the basis of sickle-cell trait is seldom practicable in the absence of symptoms; nevertheless, persons known to have the trait should be warned of the possible dangers and doctors responsible for certifying fitness should obtain written acknowledgement that appropriate advice has been given. Some form of abnormal reflex nervous stimulation—or, equally nebulously, an acute failure of an essential endocrine gland such as the adrenal—must be supposed in those cases in which no cause of death can be discovered; I have been impressed by the number of these

---

[3] Polson, C. J. and Gee, D. J., in *The Essentials of Forensic Medicine*, 3rd edn., p. 184 (Oxford; Pergamon), quote a case of retinal detachment in which a claim against the Medical Officer of the boxing club was settled for £4600. There was an element of contributory negligence in this case.

[4] For example, the condition known as 'march haemoglobinuria' in which the red blood cells break down in the particular circumstances of strenuous exercise. The main danger lies in associated acute renal failure.

deaths that appear to be associated with very full stomachs—this suggests the former possibility, but such diagnoses are rarely satisfying.

Sport and steroids

Competition in any walk of life leads to the search for advantages of doubtful morality. International sport is no exception and, in the last decade, much attention has focused on the use of a group of hormones known as *anabolic steroids* as intended aids to the improvement of physical performance.

The total muscle mass is undoubtedly increased by their use but it may well be that this is achieved through water retention rather than by an increase in the size and number of fibres[5]; much of the physical result attributed to steroids has been ascribed to psychological effects, including a euphoric attitude to hard training. The balance of evidence would seem, however, to be that, provided the subjects are already highly trained, steroids can significantly improve performance—and this applies particularly in power events. It has been pointed out that standards in women's field sports improved very rapidly from 1968 and it could well be that this coincided with the general introduction of steroids—there is little doubt that the habit of steroid medication is now fairly widespread among high-grade athletes.

Against their probable benefits must be balanced the ill effects of steroids, particularly as there is a strong probability that some self-medicators will inevitably overprescribe, especially if there has been a good response to small doses. The side effects involve hirsutism, spotty skin (acne), prostatic enlargement and, of greater importance, some degree of liver damage. There is loss of libido and, perhaps, loss of fertility. Many of these effects are due to the associated androgen (or 'maleness-producing') effects of the steroids. More serious effects on growth, etc., may, therefore, result from the use of these hormones in high dosage in prepubertal subjects. As with any substance used essentially to alter the physiology of the body, withdrawal should be gradual lest a sudden imbalance be precipitated.

Laboratory tests for anabolic steroids are available, but are expensive and require considerable expertise; control of their abuse in sport is, therefore, difficult—prohibition without detection is an unsatisfactory state of affairs. The Technical Commission of the International Federation of Sports Medicine has condemned the use of steroids by healthy sportsmen, but the onus of discovery and elimination rests on the governing bodies of the sports concerned[6].

Other forms of 'doping' have been—and may well still be—used in competitive sports; the amphetamines, for example, had a vogue as stimulants. The amphetamines, in particular, are unlikely to pose any problem in British athletics, since they are now Class B controlled drugs[7]—they are also readily demonstrable in body fluids. The difficulties in screening for known drugs that are excreted in the urine or saliva are not, in fact, so much technical as emotional and political; very adequate control can be exercised over racehorses.

---

[5] A distinction that is of no consequence in 'body building' competitions; steroid adjuvants are permitted by the organizers of these events.
[6] *British Journal of Sports Medicine* (1975), **9**, 111.
[7] Misuse of Drugs Act 1971 (*see* Chapter 23).

Sex and sport

Problems in the differentiation of sex are discussed in relation to marriage in Chapter 17. In recent years, comparable problems have arisen in competitive international sport where intimate medical examinations of competitors as a routine would be unacceptable. This is, therefore, an appropriate place to draw attention to some of the unexceptional methods available for the determination of the genetic sex on a screening basis; such methods depend upon the positive demonstration of either the Y chromosome or of what may be the XX agglomerate.

The latter process is that most commonly used and depends upon the fact that a high proportion of female cell nuclei show one or two dots of chromatin, easily visible under the microscope, beneath the nuclear membrane—the so-called 'Barr bodies'. These bodies are well seen in the skin or smooth muscle when a surgical biopsy is taken but this is, of course, impossible for routine use. Screening on a large scale is facilitated by the fact that the surface cells of the mucosa of the mouth are a good source of diagnostic Barr bodies. It is quite practical to rub the inside of the cheek with a blunt edge, to transfer the cells removed to a slide and to stain them. The proportion of cells showing Barr bodies is not high. One must find them in at least two nuclei out of every 100 cells examined to make a firm diagnosis of femininity.

A variation on this theme is the demonstration of sex chromatin or 'Davidson' bodies in the polymorphonuclear white cells of the blood. These appear as drumstick appendages to the multilobular nuclei. They are not easy to distinguish with certainty from other nuclear excrescences which occur independently of XX chromosomes and they are, again, by no means universal in the cells. The classic test for femininity involves discovery of six drumsticks. If these are found in less than 300 consecutive polymorph cells then the subject is regarded as 'chromatin positive'—this being a properly purist way of expressing 'femininity' through the finding of chromatin bodies.

The only advantage to be gained in sport from a sex transfer is for a chromosomal male to masquerade as a female—the deception need not be deliberate and may be due to genuine error. The tests described above therefore suffer from being of a negative nature. It is the *failure* to demonstrate chromatin bodies that indicates a deception. It would be preferable to demonstrate the Y chromosome positively and this can be done using, again, either desquamated cells from the inside of the mouth or white blood corpuscles; a positive result depends on the ability of the Y chromosome to fluoresce when treated with the dye quinacrine. The technique is considerably more complex than is that involved in searching for female chromatin masses. The portion of cells that are clearly 'Y positive' varies from 15 per cent to 80 per cent with different observers; a very occasional cell that is apparently male may be found in normal females. The technique is now sufficiently perfected to be regarded as being beyond the stage of mere development.

Problems of false sex are of decreasing importance in sport largely due to their increasing ease of discovery. Sexing by cells is, however, widely used in population studies and in the investigation of infants of doubtful genital sex—the chromatin bodies are developed *in utero* and much psychological difficulty can be avoided by an early diagnosis.

Death and injury in the crowd

The extent of violence in a crowd depends on two main characteristics—the quality of the crowd and its quantity as related to available space.

As to quality, it is a matter of common observation that the corporate nature of crowds at sporting events has changed dramatically in the last 20 years, so much so that a proportion of spectators at some events appear to attend with the express intention of being violent and others must take steps to defend themselves. Despite intensive police action, offensive weapons find their way into stadiums and injuries ranging from those due to kicking, through bottle injuries, to those involving the use of razors and knives are sustained each week. Violence may, of course, be continued after the event itself. Inevitably, there is a close association between fighting and alcohol; Scotland has taken the lead with legislation to prevent drunkenness at major sporting events[8]. Apart from the unusual environment in which they are inflicted, the injuries do not differ materialy from those that are described elsewhere and they need no further consideration here. Some forms of traumatic injury and death that are related to the number and density of persons are, however, typified by sports crowds and can conveniently be discussed in this section.

A human being can tolerate considerable crowding in normal circumstances and in a normal atmosphere. Minor physiological disturbances such as fainting or collapse due to heat exhaustion occur frequently but, provided the subject can be removed from the crowd, no lasting injury results. Danger is associated with loss of 'herd' control which may be accidental or impulsive. The former is exemplified by the collapse of a stand or of crowd-control barriers and the latter by a crowd's reaction when attempting to move in difficulty or under threat of danger.

In the event of crowd collapse, death may result from traumatic asphyxia. This has already been mentioned in Chapter 13. The sheer weight of bodies—the condition is very rare except on inclined terraces or when the subjects are supine—prevents the use of the thoracic and abdominal muscles of respiration. An element of suffocation by occlusion of the nose and mouth may be added. A feature of this type of death is that the blood vessels are also compressed; the classic appearances of asphyxia—congestion and petechial haemorrhage—are characteristically exaggerated in traumatic asphyxia.

Similar deaths will occur if the crowd piles up at an exit, particularly when the route funnels downwards. The conditions are self-generating as those who find themselves obstructed by others in front attempt to escape the crush of those behind. Panic ensues and injuries due to trampling may well predominate; the extreme of such a situation is seen when a pressing danger such as fire is propelling the crowd forward. A remarkable example of a human 'stampede' occurred in the London underground in 1942 when 173 persons died while taking shelter from an air raid. The disaster was precipitated by one or a few persons stumbling and obstructing the free flow of people.

The responsibility of the owners of a stadium for the safety of spectators was, until recently, governed only by liability in tort or delict; heavy damages were, for example, awarded to the estates of those killed at Ibrox Park, Glasgow in 1971 when a crush barrier collapsed following an unexpected goal-score. Safety standards are, however, now also regulated by statute[9]. Safety certificates are required for stadiums accommodating more than 10 000 persons, stipulating the number who can be admitted to various parts of the ground, the number of entrances and exits and the number of crush barriers required. Records of attendance and maintenance must be kept. Before issuing a certificate, the local authority must confer with the local police, fire and community health officers.

[8] Criminal Justice (Scotland) Act 1980, Part V. See, now, the Sporting Events (Control of Alcohol etc.) Act 1985.
[9] Safety of Sports Grounds Act 1975. The inadequacy of the controls was demonstrated at Bradford, where 56 persons died from fire in a stand in 1985.

In the event of a person being crushed, death may be delayed for some days and be ultimately due to the 'crush syndrome'. This condition, which is certainly not confined to crowds[10], results essentially from the crushing of the muscle masses and release of degeneration products. Death is due to acute renal failure but, in practice, recovery is the rule in those who survive the initial trauma.

The hazards of diving

An appreciable number of recreational divers die each year and the exploitation of North Sea oil has recently focused attention on the hazards of professional diving. The diver is essentially at risk on three counts—the effect of pressure, the need for an artificial respiratory environment and the dangers from marine predators. To these should be added the hazards of the external environment, whether they are natural or arising out of the type of work being done.

The pressure increases by 101 kPa (1 atmosphere) with every 10 m (33 ft) of depth. A great excess of air is therefore needed to fill the lungs and this expands during ascent; the same principles apply to gases dissolved in the body fluids.

While breathing air at depth, the diver may suffer from either nitrogen narcosis—a condition that has been likened to acute alcoholism—or acute oxygen poisoning which can occur when this essential gas is inhaled under pressure (over 300 kPa) and causes convulsions of central cerebral origin. In either case, the diver may die from the direct effects, he may become incoordinated and mismanage his task or his apparatus, he may drown or he may ascend precipitously.

Rapid ascent leads to massive expansion of the lungs and to release of bubbles of gas—nitrogen being especially significant—from the body fluids. Pulmonary distension is of no consequence provided that the airways are opened; rupture of the alveoli and blood vessels may occur if the glottis is closed and, in severe cases, death may result from air embolism—or blocking of the circulation by bubbles of gas (*see also* page 198). Release of gas into the tissues causes severe pain in the joints ('the bends'), difficulty in breathing ('the chokes'), pain in the air-containing ear or skull sinuses (barotrauma) or death due to widespread air embolism. The greater the number of exposures, the greater the risk of developing cavitation of, and permanent damage to, the central nervous system and the bones. Decompression sickness is a hazard of all work undertaken at pressure and is prescribed (Appendix I, A3). Both commercial and sports divers are at risk from serious neurological complications; good monitoring may compensate for the greater risks undertaken by the more severely exposed professional.

The hazards of diving may be increased by anxiety (overbreathing) or by hypothermia (*see* page 148), either of which may be fatal in their own right. Overbreathing endangers life by reducing the respiratory centre's sensitivity to oxygen lack; the diver may simply lapse into hypoxic unconsciousness and drown. Fatalities of this type have been recorded even during underwater exercise in swimming pools. The prevention of diving fatalities rests on good training, maintenance of apparatus, adjustment of the artificial atmosphere—for example,

---

[10] It is seen mainly in persons buried under falling rocks or masonry and is common in garage accidents when the subject is impacted between two vehicles. Train accidents provide a number of cases due to the often lengthy process of extricating survivors (cf. the accident at Moorgate underground station in 1975).

by the substitution of helium for nitrogen, the correlation of depth of dive with the apparatus available[11] and on the rigid application of decompression schedules—the deeper the dive, the longer the time that must be allowed for ascent[12]. Sports divers should always conform to the advice of a body such as the British Sub-aqua Club.

Somewhat similar, though generally far less severe, exposures to the hazards of decompression result from ascent in unpressurized high-altitude machines. Serious effects, which include some unique and baffling deaths due to post-descent shock, are limited to professional aviators and astronauts; prevention rests on pressuriz-ation either of the cabin environment or of the man by a pressure suit. The effects of high and low pressure may, however, be summative; occasional holidays have ended tragically through taking a 'last quick scuba dive' before the aircraft, the cabin pressure of which is equivalent to a height of some 1800m (5500ft), leaves for home—diving should not be practised within 24 hours of an intended flight.

The sea has its share of dangerous animals. Many have poison apparatus in tentacles, gills or fins and are most dangerous at spawning time. Marine venoms are generally toxic to the central nervous system and, while most 'stings' cause little more than local pain, others may be rapidly fatal. As with all poisons, the effect is to some extent dependent upon body weight and children are, therefore, more susceptible; highly poisonous fish are virtually limited to tropical waters.

Fish are carnivores and some may attack man; of these, the shark is pre-eminent—but, even so, is probably unfairly maligned. The size and aggressiveness of sharks, of which there are many varieties, is very roughly proportional to water temperature. Their teeth cause extensive laceration and death from shark-bite can result rapidly from haemorrhage; occasionally, drowning may be precipitated by panic. The moods of sharks are unpredictable; adults have died from shark-bite sustained while paddling. Shark netting or shark patrols are essential where bathing occurs in infested tropical or subtropical waters.

[11] A mixed-gas breathing mixture is now obligatory at depths exceeding 50m (Diving Operations at Work Regulations 1981, S.I. 1981/399, r. 5).

[12] While companies and clubs may devise their own criteria, the Royal Naval Diving Tables form a useful basis.

17

Medico-legal aspects of marriage and pregnancy

A number of legal problems that are of immediate concern to the medical profession, or that can be resolved only on the basis of medical opinion, surround the state of matrimony. The subject is fundamental to forensic medicine though cases for decision are relatively rare.

Disputed sex

Marriage is defined as the union of a man and a woman, and on occasion, the definition of sex may be difficult. A declaration of nullity could properly follow if it were shown that the sex of one spouse was not that supposed[1].

The sex of a person can be judged on various criteria. First, there is the chromosomal or genetic make-up. As has been discussed elsewhere (*see* page 3), the possession of a Y chromosome in the cell nucleus determines maleness. If a Y chromosome is discovered on testing, it is reasonable to assume that the person is a male, save in very rare circumstances when, as a result of abnormal division of the sex chromosomes, there is effectively a preponderance of X chromosomes and the subject is bisexual to a varied extent. Mosaicism, or the presence in one body of both male and female cell populations, may produce even more bizarre anatomic anomalies. Such cases usually become apparent at puberty and are of no concern in relation to marriage.

Secondly, the sex may be indicated by the gonads—basically, whether there are testes or ovaries. Again, there are instances in which the testes fail to develop normally and, as a result, the Y chromosome does not exert its influence on the general sex characteristics. In the extreme of the condition (the testicular feminization syndrome), the subject may have clearly female appearances yet have XY chromosomes.

Thirdly, there is the appearance of the external genitalia and here there may be very great difficulties. The commonest abnormalities are failures of the development of the normal male genitalia when a gross condition of *hypospadias* may leave the genitalia closely resembling those of a female. Alternatively, there may be

---

[1] Matrimonial Causes Act 1973 (s. 11(c)); but this Act does not apply in Scotland where the same situation would be covered by common law.

excessive secretion by the adrenal gland in a female which leads to great hypertrophy of the female genitalia and to a spurious appearances of maleness (the adreno-genital syndrome). Cases of either type may easily be mistaken at birth[2] but are usually discovered during childhood and puberty; again, these cases are of little significance in the context of marriage but they may be of considerable psychiatric importance as the subject may have been reared incorrectly for some years.

Fourthly, there is the person's own psychological assessment of his or her sex which may be contrary to all the other evidence; in its most advanced form, this state is known as transsexualism[3]. The importance of this abnormal state is that it may lead to surgical intervention—generally to remove the male genitalia and to fashion others simulating those of the female; femaleness is maintained by treatment with female sex hormone (oestrogen)[4]. In very unusual circumstances, a person who had been so treated might 'marry' another of the same genetic and gonadal sex. Such a marriage has been declared void in England on the grounds that both persons were male, the respondent having at all times been a biological male notwithstanding operative intervention; it was held that, even if the marriage had been valid, normal intercourse—which means intercourse *per vaginam* and not through an artificial vaginal passage—could not occur[5].

Other reasons for nullity of marriage

Sexual intercourse is a most important factor in a functioning marriage and, as discussed above, must be of normal type and must be potentially satisfying to be acceptable in civil law as true intercourse[5a]. Incapacity on the part of either spouse to consummate the marriage in this way enables the Court, on the appropriate proceedings being taken, to declare a marriage null and void provided that the incapacity is incurable. The incapacity is still so regarded if the spouse refuses a remedial operation and the same is true if the proposed operation is likely to be dangerous or is unlikely to succeed. Consummation of marriage depends on successful coitus; sterility or failure of emission is immaterial[6]. The procreation of children is not, in law, a principal intention of marriage and, therefore, neither the use of contraceptives nor the practice of coitus interruptus constitute grounds for a declaration of nullity[7].

[2] There is provision in both the relevant English and Scottish Acts for the correction of registration as to sex; the name may also be changed. In Scotland, a Register of Corrections is maintained. This does not, however, apply in cases of 'sex change'—whether surgically assisted or accomplished by natural anatomic changes (X Petitioner 1957 S.L.T. (Sh. Ct.) 61).

[3] This should not be confused with transvestism which is the wearing of clothes of the opposite sex; transvestism may, of course, be a prominent sign of transsexualism.

[4] Meyers, D. W. (1970), *The Human Body and the Law*, p. 52, Edinburgh University Press, has argued that such surgery is of doubtful legality in England, consent to a severe and unlawful physical invasion not being possible. The modern view, however, is that the large number of operations now undertaken are clearly legal by virtue of their therapeutic value (for an extensive review of comparative law see Petit, P. (1976), L'ambiguité de droit face au syndrome transsexuel, *Rev. Dr. Civ.*, **74**, 263).

[5] Corbett v. Corbett [1971] P. 83. The importance of biological sex is emphasized by comparison with S. Y. v. S. Y. (orse. W.) [1963] P. 37 where it was held that vaginal atresia in a *woman* could be corrected by operation and *vera copula* completed.

[5a] W. (orse. K.) v. W. [1967] 1 W.L.R. 1554.

[6] R. v. R. [1952] 1 All E.R. 1194.

[7] Baxter v. Baxter [1948] A.C. 274; White v. White [1948] P. 330—but they could result in a divorce decree being granted since such behaviour might be held to be unendurable; irretrievable breakdown of marriage would be proved thereby.

The Court must, in practice, base its decision on medical evidence and, in England, appoints its own medical examiners to whom both parties must submit for examination. In Scotland, however, it is for the pursuer to lead what evidence he or she can; the Courts will not normally order a defender to undergo an examination. Obvious defects may be apparent externally, the extreme being sufficient to induce a geniune error as to sex although, as described above, such cases are unlikley to persist until marriage. Even so, a true penis may be of such small size as to be incapable of penetration and a vagina may be so rudimentary as to inhibit entry of a normal male organ.

Most often, however, the allegation will be based on impotence in the male. Statutory impotence exists in England in boys under the age of 14 but, since marriage below the age of 16 is unlawful, this has no present relevance. In neither English nor Scots law is there an upper age limit beyond which there is a presumption of impotence.

Impotence may be physical in origin—it is a frequent, though not invariable, accompaniment of paraplegia—or it may have apparently no more than a psychological basis. Demonstration of the former may be easy for the doctor but, in the presence of normal genitalia, the latter may be hard to prove in the face of a resolute defence.

Impotence in the female in the sense of failure to have orgasm is clearly not grounds for annulment but frigidity—or hatred of intercourse—to the extent that the vagina was thereby stimulated to a state of persistent spasm would be competent grounds, were it possible to prove its existence. Occasional women reach the same condition by reason of the pain experienced in sexual intercourse. Physical disease other than malformation in women is an uncommon cause of impotence.

Impotence arising from any cause after the marriage has been consummated cannot be grounds for a declaration of nullity. There is, however, a famous case in which a declaration was made despite the fact that there was a child who was the undisputed offspring of the couple concerned[8]. It was held that entry of the sperm and fertilization of the ovum could occur without legal penetration; medically speaking this is so, though it must be a fortunately rare occurrence.

There are other bases for nullity which are, in the main, statutory but as to which medical evidence may occasionally be called. A bigamous marriage is one obvious example but, medico-legally, perhaps the most important are that a marriage is null if one of the parties was aged less than 16[9]; certain degrees of consanguinity and affinity are a lawful impediment whether the relationships exist in the legitimate or illegitimate state[10]; a marriage can be annulled if, at the time of the marriage, one party was suffering from mental disorder of such a kind or to such an extent as to render him or her unfitted to marriage; there are grounds for annulment in England

[8] Clarke v. Clarke [1943] 2 All E.R. 540.

[9] Matrimonial Causes Act 1973 (s. 11), but see page 220 as to sexual offences in such a circumstance.

[10] Twenty-three prohibited relationships are listed (Marriage Act 1949, Sch. 1). A man cannot marry (and the reverse applies for women) his mother, daughter, grandmother, granddaughter, sister, mother-in-law, stepdaughter, stepmother, daughter-in-law, aunt, niece and a number of more distant relations by affinity. The list in Scotland is even longer (Marriage (Scotland) Act 1977, Sch. 1) where, as in the case of incest, the possibility of an association between more distant generations is taken into account. Marriage between a man and his adoptive mother or adopted daughter is prohibited (Marriage Act 1949 as amended by Children Act 1975, Sch. 3; Marriage (Scotland) Act 1977) but marriage between cousins is permissible as is marriage to a former wife's sister, aunt or niece (Marriage (Enabling) Act 1960).

and Wales when one partner was suffering from venereal disease at the time of marriage—provided that the petitioner was unaware of the situation when the marriage took place. Pregnancy by another man at the time of marriage unsuspected by the petitioner is grounds for annulment in England and Wales but not in Scotland—contrariwise, a false threat of pregnancy as a spur to wedlock does not constitute grounds for nullity.

Pregnancy

Aside from these considerations, and the criminal connotations that are discussed in Chapter 19, pregnancy is of obvious medico-legal importance in civil litigation involving problems such as divorce and succession. The question of paternity will loom large in these issues and Chapter 18 is devoted to the scientific basis of its settlement. For present purposes, it is intended only to recapitulate the circumstantial evidence that bears on the probability of conception being as averred by one or other party.

Certain presumptions as to age and pregnancy are made—at least in relation to perpetuity law. These include, first, that a young woman is capable of conceiving a child in her 13th year and, secondly, that an old woman is past childbearing in her 56th year[11]. As to the lower age limit, it has been pointed out that many very youthful pregnancies result from incest and such an instance has been recorded in a girl aged 12½ years. The most extreme cases reported are those of a Peruvian girl who is said to have given birth at the age of 5¾ and of another pregnancy that occurred in a child 6½ years old. These, however, must be regarded as freak occurrences and it would be reasonable to accept the 13th year as the practical lower limit for young birth with the 12th year as the earliest at which conception is possible. At the upper end, it is generally agreed that impregnation is unusual after the age of 45 but that exceptions here are more numerous and more acceptable; each case must be considered individually as to probability. It has certainly been held that inability to bear children after the age of 53 was a rebuttable presumption[12].

The duration of pregnancy is of greater medico-legal significance. The normal average gestation period is regarded as 280 days, but this depends on numerous factors, including the length of the menstrual cycle which may vary quite markedly from the norm of 28 days. Additionally, allowance must be made for the possibility that fertilization of the ovum does not occur immediately after coitus; although spermatozoa lose their viability rapidly in the vagina (*see* Chapter 21), they can survive for some 48 hours in the receptive environment of the uterus and, exceptionally, have been demonstrated as fecund 5 days after injection—natural fertilization probably occurs most commonly in the Fallopian tube.

Such physiological variations will account for divergences from the normal of at most 10 days; there is no doubt, however, that less explicable cases do occur, and the Courts are prepared to accept wider limits in reaching decisions as to paternity when the length of a pregnancy is the main or only evidence. What is, perhaps, the extreme decision held that a husband was not entitled to a divorce on the grounds of adultery simply because a child was born 349 days after the last intramarital

[11] Perpetuities and Accumulations Act 1964, s. 2. (subject to a medical opinion in the case of the living). There are no general presumptions in Scots law.
[12] These cases are reported in *Glaister's Medical Jurisprudence and Toxicology*, (1973), 13th edn., pp. 360, 371; Edinburgh; Churchill Livingstone.

coitus[13]. A similar claim involving a gestation of 360 days was, however, upheld[14]. Medical investigations have also indicated that a period of 354 days from coitus to live birth is not impossible[15], while a newspaper report described the birth of a normal child to a woman who believed herself to have been pregnant for 13 months[16]. This case is unreported in the medical press and may have been an example of superfetation. This condition arises from the fertilization of ova liberated from the ovaries at different monthly ovulations. It is generally believed that, even if it is accepted that a second ovulation can occur in the presence of a normal fetus, it must be incredibly rare; it is possible, however, that a fetus could die *in utero* and a second impregnation occur before the onset of a menstrual period—the appearances would therefore be of a grossly prolonged gestation period. Superfecundation is a different and well-accepted concept whereby two ova released at the same ovulation are fertilized by two different acts of coitus; such an event would be distinguishable from the bearing of binovular twins only in exceptional circumstances.

Problems as to the minimum length of a pregnancy are complicated by the fact that short pregnancies may terminate either as miscarriages, stillbirths of premature births—medical viability in the last category depending largely on the efficiency of the obstetric services available. Legal viability (*see* Chapter 19) is, however, a different matter and refers only to a fetus of 28 weeks' gestation. It has been held that the fact that a premature child lived when the notional history of marital intercourse indicated that it could only have been of less than 28 weeks' gestation was not proof of illegitimacy[17]. The precise age of a newborn infant, whether alive or dead, may, therefore, be of very considerable medico-legal importance, and the process whereby it is assessed is discussed in Chapter 19.

Artificial insemination

Artificial insemination of an otherwise healthy woman who is unable to conceive a child through coitus with her husband may be chosen as an alternative to adoption. It is practised in two forms—insemination by the husband (AIH) or by an unrelated donor (AID); occasionally, in an attempt to side-step the issues, the husband's ejaculate may be mixed with that of the donor (AIHD). In any case, the seed is introduced into the cervical canal by means of a syringe.

Artificial insemination with the semen of the husband poses no problems other than its possible effect on a plea of nullity on the grounds of incapacity to consummate. The Departmental Committee on Human Artificial Insemination[18] recommended that the birth of a live child through the medium of AIH should be a bar to subsequent proceedings for nullity by either party; the Courts are, however, unlikely to agree to this in the present state of the law[19].

[13] Hadlum v. Hadlum [1948] 2 All E.R. 412.
[14] Preston-Jones v. Preston-Jones [1951] 1 All E.R. 124.
[15] McKeown, T. and Gibson, J. R. (1952). The period of gestation. *British Medical Journal*, i, 938.
[16] *The Scotsman*, 9th June, 1975.
[17] Clark v. Clark [1939] P. 228. The medical evidence in this case vividly demonstrates the advances made in medical technology since the war.
[18] *Report of the Departmental Committee on Human Artificial Insemination* (1960). Cmnd. 1105, para. 108. London; HMSO.
[19] L. v. L. [1949] 1 All E.R. 141. The main question in this case was whether the wife had accepted the conditions of an abnormal marriage having become pregnant by AIH. By implication, the Court did not consider the marriage to have been consummated thereby. *See* also the Scottish case of G. v. G. 1961 S.L.T. 324.

Artificial insemination by donor is loaded with forensic problems for all concerned—including the medical practitioner who may be called to advise on or to complete the procedure.

From the doctor's point of view, the most important feature is the consent of both husband and wife to the process. A doctor who became involved without the consent of the husband might be guilty of serious professional misconduct (*see* Chapter 30); when obtained, such consent can only be valid after the most complete explanation of the procedure and of the associated complexities. It is certain that the doctor must take a responsible attitude to the selection of the donor including a positive attempt to exclude communicable disease or an unsatisfactory genetic history[20]. He must also be responsible for the assessment of the recipient and her husband. The physical fitness of the intended mother is well within his compass, but it is less easy to avoid subjectivity when considering the psychological and social circumstances. Who can, or should, adjudge the suitability of a couple for parentage in what is, at best, an abnormal situation? There is the further problem that the presence of a single donor in a district could lead to consanguineous marriages in the future; this is one reason why records of donations should be kept. On the other hand, the availability of medical records could lead to considerable difficulties not only for the doctor but also for the donor (*see below*). It is an area in which the ethics of professional confidentiality are currently ill defined.

The position of the donor is by no means trouble free. Speller[21] has suggested that the donor's spouse might have grounds for divorce if it were known he were the father of other women's children; it is doubtful if this could constitute grounds for 'irretrievable breakdown of marriage' by virtue of intolerable behaviour, but it is reasonable to expect that consent to his role should be obtained from the donor's wife. In times of difficulty, the child might have a legal right to maintenance from its biological father and it is mainly for this reason that donors demand, and obtain, absolute secrecy. On the other hand, it is conceivable that a man might want to trace his progeny at some time in the future. Moreover, it is difficult to see why an AID child should not have the same right as to discovery of its biological parenthood as has one who is adopted. In practical terms, however, there would probably be no sperm donation if the guarantee of secrecy were removed[22].

The relationships between husband and wife in the AID situation are becoming clearer. The Departmental Committee already cited has urged that the birth of a child as a result of AID should be a bar to proceedings for nullity (at para. 156); but if it is not so in the case of AIH, there is even less reason why it should be so in AID. It seems now certain that AID, even without the consent of the husband, does not constitute adultery—this being on the grounds that adultery involves coitus[23]. Nevertheless, to attempt to conceive in this way without the husband's

[20] It has been recommended in *Glaister's Medical Jurisprudence and Toxicology* (1973), 13th edn., p. 367, (Edinburgh, Churchill Livingstone) that the criteria for a choice of donor additional to those described in the text should include that he is not a relative of either spouse, he should be potent, should be of age, his age should not exceed 40, he should have children of his own and his race and characteristics should resemble as closely as possible those of the husband of the woman to be inseminated. There seems, however, to be little uniformity in practice even in the USA where AID is practised on a large scale (Curie-Cohen, M., *et al.* (1979). Current practise of artificial insemination by donor in the United States. *New England Journal of Medicine*, **300**, 585–90.

[21] In *Law of Doctor and Patient* (1973), p. 42; London; H. K. Lewis.

[22] The whole arena of reproductive biology has recently been the subject of the *Report of the Committee of Inquiry into Human Fertilisation and Embryology* (1968) (Warnock, M., Chairman) (Cmnd. 9314) (hereafter cited as the Warnock Report).

[23] MacLennan v. MacLennan 1958. SC 105.

consent would almost certainly be considered conduct such as to cause breakdown of a marriage and the Departmental Committee (at para. 117) recommended that such behaviour should constitute grounds for divorce. Once having consented, however, and having accepted the child into the family, the wife's husband would be treated as the natural breadwinner and would be responsible for the child in the event of family disunity[24]. There is important law on this point in the United States[25].

Nevertheless, as the law now stands, a couple must be advised that a child conceived by AID is illegitimate and, strictly speaking, should be registered as such at birth. In practice, parents must do this very rarely and the law is, to this extent, being flouted. It is quite unreasonable to stigmatize a child as a result of something done essentially for the benefit of the parents, and this alone indicates the need for a change in the legal stance.

It has been suggested that the decision in *MacLennan* solves the problem in that there can be no illegitimacy if there is no adultery; this cannot hold as it confuses the two quite separate items of adultery and biological parenthood. A positive step would be to alter the heading on the relevant column of the birth certificate to some such formula of 'father or accepting husband'; this, however, would solve only the dilemma of registration—it would still leave doubt and would disturb the great majority who are certain of their fatherhood. The legal strategem of adopting the baby after true registration has been advocated but this is solely to the benefit of the parents; the effect on a child of discovering it was not only adopted but also conceived by AID could be very bad. Most would agree that, with the increasing public acceptability of AID, there is a need for positive legislation to place the consenting husband of a woman and her AID offspring in the same position as a natural father and a legitimate child[26]. The need for this is demonstrated by the unsatisfactory condition of case law[27], and 18 of the United States have now enacted legislation implying a presumption of legitimacy of the AID child conceived with the consent of both the mother and her husband. The Uniform Parentage Act 1974, s. 5(a) states that a husband who consents to his wife being artificially inseminated by a donor is treated in law as if he were the natural father of the child thereby conceived. Similar legislation has been enacted in New South Wales and in Victoria.

It could be argued that legislation is unnecessary in that the possible disadvantages to the child born as a result of AID have, in common with all illegitimate children, been very largely removed by the provisions of the Family Law Reform Act 1969, ss. 14–19 and of the Law Reform (Miscellaneous Provisions) (Scotland) Act 1968, ss. 1–4. There are, however, sufficient difficulties associated with the practice of AID to make it a separate case. 'The law has got to consider AID not in a prohibitory way and perhaps in a regulatory way to make the technique acceptable to society'[28].

Artificial insemination is essentially a remedy for a procreative defect in the male partner. The common abnormalities leading to sterility in the female result in failure of the ovum to reach the uterus. Many such cases can be treated successfully

[24] Matrimonial Causes Act 1965, s. 34 (4); Matrimonial Proceedings (Children) Act 1958, s. 7.

[25] People v. Sorensen (1968) 68 Cal. 2d 280.

[26] The unanimous view of the Report of Panel on Human Artificial Insemination (1973) (Peel, J., Chairman) *British Medical Journal*, iii, Suppl. 3, and of the Warnock Committee (n. 22).

[27] The Court in Australia in Roberts v. Roberts (1971) V.R. 160 refused to rule on legitimacy but said 'the plain fact is that the husband is not the father'; early US decisions were conflicting—e.g. Strnad v. Strnad (1948) 78 NYS 2d 390 upheld the legitimate state of the child while the contrary view was taken in Doornbos v. Doornbos (1954) 12 Ill. App. 2d 473.

[28] Leading article (1975). Artificial insemination (donor). *British Medical Journal*, iv, 2.

by surgery but there are still women who remain sterile. The technique of reimplantation of a fertilized ovum may offer a chance of childbearing to some of these.

In essence, the process consists of removing a mature ovum from the abdomen, fertilizing it with the husband's sperm in the laboratory and implanting the resultant zygote in the uterine cavity. The techniques have advanced rapidly in the last few years and, although they are expensive and confined to specialized units, something in the region of 20 per cent of *in vitro* fertilizations result in a continuing pregnancy; the miscarriage rate is, however, higher than normal. While the great majority of embryo transfers involve ova from a wife whose husband's semen is used—in which case, the result is comparable to AIH—donated ova may be used. An entirely new range of problems as to maternity are, thereby, introduced.

A further ethical dilemma relates rather to the experimentation that is essential to the perfection of the technique and to the status of the human embryo[29]—in effect, an extension of the abortion issue which is considered in Chapter 19. The practical problem lies in the possibility that the manipulations necessary to achieve successful implantation could damage the embryo and lead to disability in the infant; liability would then become a major issue. In the event, such a hazard is relatively unlikely as an embryo damaged so early in life would be more likely to abort spontaneously than to reach full term.

Surrogate motherhood

Surrogate motherhood offers a bizarre alternative to both reimplantation and adoption. It has thus far attracted more attention in the news media[30] than in medicine or the law. It is apparently practised to an extent in the USA[31] and advertisements appear in the less widely read journals of Britain. The technique involves artificial insemination of another woman with the sperm of the barren woman's husband; the infant is passed to its biological father and his wife at birth. Inevitably, such a method or parenting is based on a commercial transaction and is wide open to abuse, the most important from the would-be parents' points of view being that the biological mother could recant and fail to surrender the baby—although the instigators themselves might also have a change of heart; in either case it is unlikely that any Court would enforce such an unnatural contract—*ex turpi causa non oritur actio*. Otherwise, the legal problems of surrogate motherhood are those of AID, only more so—particularly as it would seem that most would-be 'womb-leasers' are married. It is worth noting that, money having changed hands, the option of adoption may not be open to the 'parents', although the purposes of the payment are not strictly those that the Adoption Act 1976, s. 57, was designed to avert. Anticipatory legislation has already been expedited[31a].

Objections become even stronger if the logical development of this practise—the implantation of a fertilized ovum into another woman's womb—is considered. The possible permutations and legal complexities then become bewildering.

[29] The problems as seen in the USA are neatly summarized in Culliton, B. J. and Waterfall, W. K. (1978), Flowering of American bioethics, *British Medical Journal*, **ii**, 127. The situation polarized in the United Kingdom with the introduction of the Unborn Children (Protection) Bill 1985 which failed only on technical grounds.
[30] *See*, for example, a remarkable article by Disney, A. (1981), Surrogate mothers, *Sunday Telegraph*, Magazine, No. 265, p. 80.
[31] Even there, its legality is suspect; *see* Erickson, E. A. (1978), Contracts to bear a baby, *Cal. L.R.*, **66**, 611.
[31a] Surrogacy Arrangements Act 1985. In Re a Baby (1985) Times, 15 January, the 'parents' were awarded custody in the interests of the infant.

Sterilization

A woman may be surgically sterilized—that is, rendered incapable of bearing children—by removal of the ovaries, by section, ligation or diathermy of the Fallopian tubes or by removal of the uterus. Similarly, a man may be made unable to procreate by removal of the testes or by section of the vas deferens on each side. Removal of the ovaries or testes, which is castration, may cause considerable hormonal upset and is undertaken only in exceptional circumstances.

Sterilization may be the primary object of, or merely incidental to, the operation. A man may have both testes removed because they contain tumours; but by far the most common form of unavoidable sterilization is associated with the removal of the female uterus—either for the eradication of a tumour or as a relief of problems in menstruation.

There is no serious medico-legal difficulty associated with sterilization which is imposed as a price for treatment of a medical condition. A woman—one can, for practical purposes, exclude a man in this context—is entitled to consent to or dissent from medical treatment for herself whether she is married or not; it seems perfectly clear that a husband has no right of veto nor has he any redress against the surgeon who operates on his wife without his consent so long as the decision was reached in non-negligent fashion. This implies fully informed consent by the wife; ideally this should include consent by the husband after the patient has given permission for him to be brought into discussion. But Speller[32] has also pointed out that a doctor who refrained from necessary gynaecological treatment *because* of lack of consent on the part of the husband might find himself in a difficult professional position.

Primary sterilization is a different matter. It poses a basic problem of ethics as to whether a surgical procedure not designed for treatment of a medical condition is sufficiently 'against the public interest' as to constitute criminal assault and, therefore, to be beyond the protection of consent[33]. Sterilization may be performed, among other reasons, as a punitive measure, on eugenic grounds or as a form of birth control. The first, although permissible in some states of the USA, is so foreign to British thought as to need no consideration. The second is rather different. There can be no question but that eugenic sterilization without consent must be an assault. But, with consent, sterilization was at least advocated some time ago by a Departmental Committee on Sterilization[34] in certain cases of mental defect and of hereditary disease; the risks are, however, formidable and no legislation to this end has been passed. The nature of consent in such cases poses an inherent problem—if a person is suffering from disease of the mind to the extent that he ought to be sterilized, can he give a valid consent? It would also seem that parents ought not to be able to consent to a non-therapeutic operation on behalf of a minor; there can rarely be any compelling reason why sterilization should not be postponed until the subject is aged 18[35].

---

[32] In *Law of Doctor and Patient* (1973), p. 37 by S. R. Speller. London; H. K. Lewis.

[33] *See* Denning, L.J.'s minority opinion in an early case (Bravery v. Bravery [1954] 1 W.L.R. 1169 at p. 1180).

[34] *Sterilization*. Report of Departmental Committee (1934). Cmnd. 4485. London; HMSO.

[35] In Re D (a minor) [1976] 1 All E.R. 326, the mother of a girl who was aged 11 and suffering from severe behaviour problems attributed to Sotos syndrome gave permission for her to be sterilized to avoid the possibility of bearing an abnormal fetus. Despite challenge from other professionals, the gynaecologist concerned refused to defer the operation. An application to make her a ward of court and to continue that wardship was upheld on the grounds that the proposed operation was one that deprived a woman of her basic human right to reproduce; an operation without her valid consent would be a violation of that human right and not solely within the clinical judgment of a doctor. The subject is well discussed in 'Sterilization of minors', *British Medical Journal* (1975), **iii**, 775.

The ethical issues relating to sterilization as a form of birth control have been settled. Both the English and Scottish Medical Defence Unions have long ago advised their members to the effect that it is a legitimate undertaking[36]. It is doubtful if it would ever have been criminal in Scotland owing to a lack of evil intent. Vasectomy has now been specifically authorized under the National Health Service (Family Planning) Amendment Act 1972. Abortions performed under the Abortion Act 1967 are combined with sterilization in some 16 per cent of cases and there may also be good psychiatric indications for the operation in many sterilizations which are apparently of 'convenience' type. Myers[37], however, draws a distinction between sterilization (e.g. by tying the tubes) and castration; although limiting his argument to the operation in the male, he believes that the latter is an offence that consent cannot legalize.

The secondary problem of the *nature* of the consent is far more important. One would have thought that, in the absence of medical grounds, sterilization of a normal person ought to be validated by consent of both the subject and the spouse; it was unanimously held in *Bravery v. Bravery* (n. 33) that an operation in the absence of such agreement would be grounds for divorce. Recently, however, that view has been challenged because an adult is entitled to confidentiality in his or her own right[38]. The older view is, however, to be preferred and, rather than lay himself open to a possible action for tort or delict for performing an operation without bilateral consent, the doctor would be better advised to dissociate himself from the case if disclosure to the spouse were refused. It should be noted that sterilization before marriage is not grounds for a declaration of nullity.

There remains the problem of civil liability in the event of failure of sterilization; this is probably the main medico-legal hazard associated with sterilization as a method of contraception.

It is often insufficiently understood that sterilizing operations cannot always guarantee infertility. Some techniques are more efficient than others but, in general, the certainty of success is related proportionately to the extent of mutilation. The ethical problem thus resolves itself into balancing the immediate effect against the possibility of a later wish to reverse the procedure—say, on remarriage or on the death of an existing child.

This poses a real dilemma. The success rate for reversal of sterilization by vasectomy in the male is unlikely to be better than 25 per cent and many surgeons would decline to perform an operation that was specifically limited by the patient to one that could be undone. Reversal in the female is likely to be more successful— up to about 70 per cent—but the original operation must have been of limited extent and the risks of an ectopic pregnancy (*see* page 73) are definitely increased following a reparative operation; sterilization techniques that eliminate the possibility of failure must be regarded as irreversible.

With a sound technique competently performed, the risk of pregnancy after female sterilization is very small indeed—but it would be a brave surgeon who averred that it was non-existent without removal of the uterus. Sterilization in the male is not so straightforward. When the subjects are tested for the presence of sperm in the ejaculate, it is found that a small number of motile organisms are still present 6 months after the operation in some 40 per cent of the men treated. Very

[36] Legality of sterilisation: a new outlook, *British Medical Journal* (1960), **ii**, 1516.
[37] In *The Human Body and the Law* (1970), p. 18, by D. W. Meyers. Edinburgh University Press.
[38] Samuels, A. (1980). The duty of the doctor to respect the confidence of the patient. *Medicine, Science and the Law*, **20**, 58.

occasionally, sperm are found later in those who were apparently sterile 3 months after the operation but, in these instances, the organisms are generally immobile and probably dead. The most serious complication is spontaneous recanalization of the ducts which may occur in up to 1 per cent of cases; instances have been reported even after surgery of moderately severe type.

All these considerations must be explained to the patient and to the spouse before consent can be valid. Having done so, the usual rules covering medical negligence apply—if the patient fully understood the risks, if the operation was properly performed and if the procedure was one that was accepted by competent colleagues in the profession, then the mere fact of pregnancy would not be proof of negligence[38a]. The proper procedure must, however, include adequate follow-up: this consists of routine examination of the ejaculate[39] and pathological proof by microscopy that the correct tissue was removed. It scarcely needs pointing out that if a husband who had been sterilized brought an action on account of an unexpected pregnancy in his wife, it would be quite reasonable for the surgeon to question the paternity of the child.

Divorce

Divorce in England and Wales can only be granted on the basis of an irretrievable breakdown of marriage[40]. There are a number of specific conditions that are taken either together or individually to show that this situation exists. One or more of the following must be proved—the fact that the respondent has committed adultery and the petitioner finds it intolerable to live with him or her[41]; that the respondent has behaved in such a way that the petitioner cannot reasonably be expected to live with the respondent; that the respondent has been in desertion for 2 years; that the spouses have lived apart for 2 years and the respondent consents to a divorce; and that the parties have lived apart for 5 years—in which case, the respondent's consent to divorce is not required.

The position is now very similar in Scotland. The common law ground of adultery and the several other possible bases for divorce detailed in the Divorce (Scotland) Act 1938 are now consolidated under the general heading of irretrievable breakdown of marriage in the Divorce (Scotland) Act 1976. Behaviour on the part of the defender can be regarded as unendurable irrespective of his or her mental state. Both the English and the Scots legislation contain provisions designed to encourage reconciliation; in particular, the continuation or resumption of cohabitation for a limited period—for example, after the discovery of adultery—does not bar a petition and, hence, spouses are not deterred from an attempt to make up.

There is, therefore, surprisingly little forensic medicine associated with divorce. The greater part will involve proof or disproof of adultery and this, in turn, is mainly a matter of paternity. Occasionally, however, the length of pregnancy will be decisive as may be evidence of venereal disease that could not have been contracted from the spouse. Forensic departments are often presented with bed

[38a] The terms of the contract, and the warnings given, are all important. *See* the contrast between Thake and another v. Maurice [1986] 1 All E.R. 497 and Eyre v. Measday [1986] 1 All E.R. 488.

[39] An acceptable regimen would be to require two negative specimens 2 weeks apart taken 2 months after the operation followed by a third negative specimen 1 month later before pronouncing the subject sterile.

[40] Matrimonial Causes Act 1973 (s. 1).

[41] But the two phrases are independent—Cleary v. Cleary [1974] 1 All E.R. 498.

linen, cushions and the like to establish the presence or absence of seminal stains; while these are usually presented in the hopes of proving adultery, such evidence can rarely be more than indicative of unseemly conduct on the part of the wife even if the stains are positively seminal and proven to be of a different secretor group (*see* page 191) from the husband's.

There remains unendurable behaviour, for proof of which there need be no evidence of physical injury. Nevertheless, such evidence, if present, would carry much weight and the medical practitioner may have an important part to play here if a woman seeks his advice and assistance; this must include an assessment of injury to health other than by physical means.

Non-accidental injury to married women

Medical evidence must play an important part in the application of the Domestic Violence and Matrimonial Proceedings Act 1976 when a wife is seeking an injunction against molestation[41a]. But what if the doctor notices evidence of physical ill treatment in a female patient when she has consulted him for other reasons? There is strong evidence that non-accidental injury in married women is a problem comparable in extent with that in children (*see* Chapter 20).

There is far less medical literature on the subject of 'wife-battering', probably because there are essential differences in the aetiology and management of these two types of household violence[42]. The wife who is being ill treated is adult and capable of taking her complaint to the appropriate authorities. There is no need for the doctor to protect a helpless patient, as applies to babies, and if there is no need there may be no justification for disclosure of confidential information; indeed, there is evidence that many women, whether because of genuine choice or of fear, would themselves resent such an intrusion[43]. The role of the doctor is perhaps limited to counselling not only as to his women patients' course of action but also as to the advisability of the husband being induced to seek medical help; in contrast to fathers who injure their children, many of those who seriously assault their wives are older and suffer from psychiatric disease—in the event of trial, a higher proportion of hospital orders are made than in cases of child abuse. The keeping of accurate records by the doctor, particularly including an assessment of the mental state of the women and of injuries noted in examination but of which no complaint is made, is of equal importance; such evidence might be invaluable in subsequent criminal[44] or civil proceedings.

[41a] Protection of varying type is also available, among others, under the Matrimonial Homes Act 1983, the Matrimonial and Family Proceedings Act 1984 and the Matrimonial Homes (Family Protection) (Scotland) Act 1981.

[42] The most useful reference is the *Report from the Select Committee on Violence in Marriage* (1975), Vol. **1,** H-C.533-i; London; HMSO.

[43] But many wives do seek help, especially from voluntary organizations. *See* Gayford, J. J. (1975), Wife battering: a preliminary survey of 100 cases, *British Medical Journal,* **i,** 194.

[44] Gordon, G. H. (1978), *The Criminal Law of Scotland,* 2nd edn., p. 821; Edinburgh; W. Green & Sons, holds that, in Scots law, an assault may be aggravated by being committed by a husband on his wife. Nevertheless, police involvement in domestic affrays is relatively infrequent.

18

Elementary genetics and testing for parentage

General principles

The normal human nucleus, which defines the 'personality' of the cell, contains 46 chromosomes arranged in two sets of 23 pairs, one set being derived from each parent. The sex cells, ova or spermatozoa, are therefore unique in containing only a single series of 23 chromosomes, but this series is formed from a random choice between one of two paired chromosomes present in each parent. Certain severe abnormalities are the direct result of an abnormal number of chromosomes being present—mongolism is, perhaps, the classic example.

Chromosomes consist of large numbers of genes. These are formed from deoxyribonucleic acid (DNA) and function as templates from which further identical genes can be formed at will through the medium of ribonucleic acid (RNA) which acts as a 'messenger' or carrier of a carbon copy. The original genetic pattern of the fertilized ovum is thereby maintained as the fetus and free-living body are developed.

Save in abnormal circumstances, each paired chromosome will contain one of a pair of genes that refer to the same genetic characteristic; each gene is derived from either the father or the mother but both cannot come from a single parent. These paired genes are known as *alleles*. The allelic genes may be the same, in which case the individual is said to be *homozygous* for that particular factor, or they may be different, resulting in the *heterozygous* state.

In the simplest heterozygous state, one of the pair of genes will express itself—or demonstrate its presence—and is therefore said to be *dominant*; the other member of the pair is known as *recessive*—it is still present and available for transmission to the offspring but is overshadowed or obscured by its dominant partner. This can be illustrated in simple fashion by hair colour for which characteristic the 'black hair' gene is dominant over the 'red hair' gene. *Figure 18.1* shows that, if a man (or woman) homozygous for black hair mates with a woman (or man) homozygous for red hair, all the offspring will be heterozygotes but all will be black-haired because the gene for red is recessive. But if two such heterozygotes mate, one of four offspring will be red-haired and three will be black-haired; two of the latter will, however, be 'carriers' of a recessive gene for red hair. It is pointed out in passing that this is a theoretical reason for prohibiting certain degrees of consanguineous marriage. Many harmful genes are recessive—it is scarcely possible for a truly disadvantageous gene to be dominant and for the strain to survive—and normal random mating leads to their natural suppression; 'in-breeding' must, however, increase the possibility of such recessive genes meeting as alleles—the harmful gene is then free to express itself with increasing frequency.

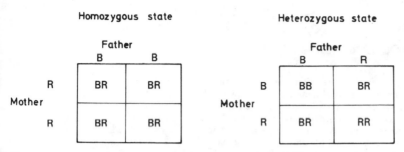

Figure 18.1 Homozygous and heterozygous matings. Either of the genes present in one parent may be paired with either of the genes present in the other; see text for explanation.

Reverting to the example of hair colour, ordinary observation will show that the position has been oversimplified since only a few people in whom it is not a racial characteristic have jet-black hair. In other words, dominance, save in some well-defined all-or-nothing situations, is relative; the capacity of a dominant gene to express itself is described as its degree of *penetration*—a gene of weak penetration may express itself only rarely when all the circumstances are in its favour. This is the justification for genetic counselling and for some legal abortions (*see* Chapters 19 and 20); if a very weakly penetrating harmful gene expresses itself once in a family, the conditions that encouraged its expression are likely to recur though, of course, they may not necessarily do so. Diseases or conditions that are thus dependent on the total genetic environment are called *multifactorial*; those that can be related to a single allele are known as *monogenetic*.

Some genetic variations are *sex-linked* or, better, *X-linked*. The sex chromosomes are designated X and Y; a normal female possesses the homozygous alleles XX while the male is XY. The combination YY is biologically impossible since Y is available only in a spermatozoon. Sex linkage is illustrated in *Figure 18.2* on the simple premise that a recessive gene is positioned in that area of the X chromosome that is absent in the male. A dominant 'unaffected' X arm suppresses the abnormal gene in the female; expression of the abnormality can only occur in the male while the female remains a 'carrier'—the only way for a female to express a sex-linked gene is for her to possess two abnormal X chromosomes, a possibility that is unlikely in the absence of 'in-breeding'.

If genetic studies are to be useful, the genes must be demonstrable. Some genes express themselves as *antigens* and can, therefore, cause the formation of *antibodies*; either may be used to demonstrate the other in the laboratory. Antibodies that are stimulated in a person who does not possess the corresponding antigens are described as immune—they arise in response to the presence of a foreign antigen and repeated exposures result in increasingly active antibody formation. Antigens may, however, be shared by many unrelated types of cell and antibodies can be formed in response to exposure to an antigen derived from a source unrelated to the form in which it occurs in the body. 'Naturally occurring' antibodies—of which

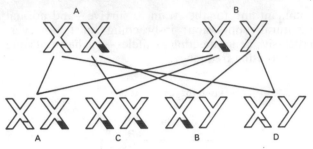

Figure 18.2 Sex linkage. In the illustration, the normal gene
absent from the Y chromosome is designated in black, while the
abnormal variant is white. A is a female carrier of the abnormal
gene which is suppressed by the normal; B is a normal male. Their
possible progeny are as follows: A, a normal 'carrier' female
similar to her mother; C, a normal female—the disease has been
eliminated from that strain; B, a normal male; D, a diseased
male—there is no normal X-linked gene available to suppress
the abnormal.

those reacting with the ABO blood cell antigens are the prime example—are
probably made in this way.

In the ideal situation, a gene should be demonstrable in both its dominant and
recessive forms. Suppose a gene Z has an allele z. If we can demonstrate both Z
and z by means of antisera (that is, blood sera containing antibodies) we can
distinguish the *genotypes*—or full genetic profiles—ZZ, Zz and zz; if, on the
other hand, we can only show the presence of the dominant Z we are limited to
describing a person as Z + ve or Z − ve and this inadequate genetic portrait is
known as a *phenotype* (although, Z − ve is, in fact, a genotype as, by a process
of elimination, it must represent zz). The genotype ZZ or Zz can be derived
from the phenotype either on the basis of probability—that is, by knowing the
proportional distribution in the population—or by a knowledge of the phenotypes of parents, siblings or children, the reverse process of paternity
testing.

Diagnostic antigens must be stable—they must not be affected by disease, age
and the like and they must not *mutate*, which is to alter their structure and their
expression. If a gene is to be useful in genetic studies—particularly if these are to be
used in a medico-legal context—natural mutation must be so rare as to be
unaccountable. The general mutation rate in humans is of the order of 1 in 1 million
gene generations; no proven example of a blood-group gene mutating between two
generations has ever been found[1].

The ideal genetic test substance should be readily available and it should contain
a number of systems that *segregate* independently thus increasing the number of
variable and recognizable characteristics.

The red blood cells meet almost all these requirements and, as a result, testing
for parentage, which forms the major part of medico-legal genetics, is virtually a
matter of blood testing.

[1] The principle that mutation can be accepted as excessively rare seems to have been agreed—*see
Halsbury's Statutes of England*, 3rd edn., Vol. **40**, p. 617. Excluded from paternity means excluded
subject to the occurrence of mutation (Family Law Reform Act 1969, s. 25).

Testing for parentage

Very occasionally, an allegation may be made that a child has been wrongly identified in the maternity crèche, while extraordinary instances of fabricated pregnancy followed by appropriation of an infant have been reported; there can be few other occasions in which the identity of a mother is in doubt and, for practical purposes, testing for parentage is a matter of paternity testing; it is in this context that the subject will be discussed[2]. The principal circumstances in which paternity tests are called for are in divorce proceedings and in the adjudication of affiliation orders.

In either case, the putative father is denying responsibility for a child and it is emphasized that standard genetic studies cannot prove paternity *conclusively*; although a very strong probability may be established (*see* page 188), the main function of the blood-testing laboratory is to exclude paternity in a man unjustly accused; this it can do with ever-increasing efficiency[3]. It will be seen that, in practice, unless the problem is one of choosing between two or three candidates for parenthood, the man has little to lose and perhaps everything to gain from blood testing; the mother of the child has, by contrast, comparatively little expectation of advantage.

Scots law has taken little cognizance of blood tests for parentage and the statutory basis of such tests, the Family Law Reform Act 1969, applies only to England and Wales. Under s. 20(1), the Courts may give a direction for the use of blood tests to see whether or not a person is excluded from paternity on application from any party to the proceedings; in practice, blood tests are generally agreed between the parties and court orders are very seldom required. Consent is necessary, the age of consent being 16 (s. 21) but, under s. 23(1), the Court may draw inferences from the fact that a person has failed to take steps as directed.

There is nothing to stop such evidence being brought by agreement in Scotland but the admissibility of such evidence could be strongly challenged especially in relation to the taking of blood from a child. The law would not compel that this be done[4] and, in 1958, Lord President Clyde was of the opinion that there should be hesitation before allowing a course to be taken that might have a serious effect on the child[5]. One would feel, however, that the truth ought to prevail—'. . . there is nothing more shocking than that injustice should be done on the basis of a legal presumption when justice can be done on the basis of fact'[6]; modern serology is clearly an expression of fact.

Certain essentials must be met before the results of the tests can be admitted as evidence even in England and Wales. First, specimens must be obtained as a minimum from the mother, the child and any putative father. Secondly, the specimen must be suitably identified by the parties concerned and by their legal

---

[2] The complications introduced by modern reproductive techniques involving ovum donation, womb-leasing and the like are referred to on page 175.

[3] Inclusion of the HLA (Human Leucocyte Antigens) system will, of itself, exclude 98 per cent of all wrongly accused men. The HLA system is complex and, while it is of paramount importance in the field of transplantation, it cannot be said to be readily available for paternity testing outside specialized units. The status of the HLA system today is comparable with that of the MN system at the time of Imrie v. Mitchell (*see* footnote 7, page 185). It will not be further discussed save to note that the principles of inheritance are similar to those relating to the red cell antigens and serum factors.

[4] Whitehall v. Whitehall 1958 S.C. 252.

[5] In Imrie v. Mitchell 1958 S.C. 439 (*see* footnote 7, page 185). Attitudes are, however, changing; *see* Docherty v. McGlynn 1985 SLT (Reports) 237.

[6] Ormrod J. in Holmes v. Holmes [1966] 1 W.L.R. 187, at p. 188.

advisers. Thirdly, declarations of consent and agreement as to the validity of the specimens must be signed together with a declaration that neither party has received a blood transfusion within the last 3 months. Blood tests on infants less than 2 months old are somewhat less satisfactory than in the adult and, ideally, a child should be at least 6 months old at the time of testing. Verified photographs of the principals are essential if a doctor not attached to a testing centre is asked to take the samples.

Principles of paternity testing

The simple principles that govern the exclusion of paternity by blood testing can be summarized:

1. Save in conditions of extreme rarity, generally involving deletion of genes, blood-group genes and antigens are passed on 'true' by a parent to its off-spring.
2. One gene of an allelic pair is derived from each parent. Each parent has one of two genes to donate at random.
3. A blood-group antigen cannot be present in a child unless it is also present in at least one parent.
4. If one parent possesses a homozygous allelic gene pair, then that gene *must* be conferred on all his or her offspring.

The blood-group antigens are contained in a number of 'systems', each system containing a number of allelic pairs. Systems are distinguished in that they are segregated independently from each other—the more systems tested, the more likely is a wrongly accused father to be positively excluded from paternity. The 'value' of a system in this respect depends on several factors—the number of allelic pairs it contains, the relative distribution of the genes in the population and, not least important, the ease with which its component antigens can be demonstrated. This last point needs explanation. There is no true dominance or recessiveness in blood-group genes; the terms relate, in effect, to the ease with which they can be demonstrated. Antigens are of different 'strengths'—i.e. they react either strongly or weakly both in the laboratory and *in vivo* as to their capacity to provoke the formation of antibodies. They are demonstrated by different methods, some of which are complex; in the nature of things, the systems that were documented earliest contain the strongest antigens and are most easily defined in the laboratory. The determination of an antigen usually requires an antibody and the necessary test antisera vary from being universally available to being extremely rare or non-existent. It may, therefore, be beyond the technical ability of a laboratory to demonstrate some of the lesser blood-group systems.

For present purposes, it is proposed to deal only with the ABO, MNS and Rhesus (CDE) systems in detail—the use of these three systems alone could eliminate 59 per cent of wrongfully accused putative fathers.

The MNS system is the most 'efficient' individual system (*see Table 18.1*) and illustrates some points that are not easily appreciated in the better-known ABO system; it will be used as the main example of testing for paternity.

Use of the MNS system in paternity cases

The allelic antigens originally discovered were designated M and N. Antisera are readily available to both so that the genotypes MM, MN and NN can be distinguished with ease. The simple rules described on page 184 can now be applied:

Parents	Impossible children
MM × MM	MN, NN
MM × MN	NN
MM × NN	MM, NN
MN × NN	MM
NN × NN	MM, MN
MN × MN	None

However, the system also contains the alleles S and s. These are 'linked' to the M and N alleles so that the genes are always transmitted in a group of two. We therefore have the following possible 'system' gene profiles: MS, Ms, NS, Ns, and these can be combined to form 10 genotypes. This greatly increases the usefulness of the system. For example, there are no impossible children from the mating MN × MN; but if it is, in fact, MsNs × MsNs then any child containing the antigen S can be eliminated as a product of the union.

The MNS system also illustrates some of the difficulties in blood testing. In the first place, anti-s is an example of a rare antibody although it is obtainable commercially. If it were not available it would be possible to speak in terms of genotypes only when no S was demonstrable—the genotype would then be ss (*see* page 182). Secondly, the antigen M may occur as a variant that does not react with anti-M; the significance of this is illustrated in *Figure 18.3*. While all concerned should be aware of such rare variations, their significance must be interpreted in relation to their occurrence[7].

The Rhesus system

The Rhesus system differs from the MNS system in that it is basically composed of three, rather than two, allelic pairs: Cc, Dd, Ee. The most powerful antigen is D while, in contrast, d is so weak as to be non-antigenic. In common parlance, Rhesus-positive implies the possession of the gene D and Rhesus-negative its absence. The value of the whole system is, however, much greater as the individual genes of the three pairs can be combined in eight different ways to form 'system' genes[8] which are so closely linked that they are always transmitted as a group; although alterations in the group during the formation of the sex cells are theoretically just possible, the likelihood of 'crossing over' occurring so as to cause medico-legal difficulty is so infinitesimal as to be beyond practical consideration.

The Rhesus system has become more complicated than was originally described. Almost all the antigens have variants, one of which, C^w, is sufficiently common to be regarded as a standard antigen. Simply using the single genes CC^wDEcde, the groups of 'system' genes can be paired to form 78 potential genotypes. Such,

[7] But, even so, care must be exercised, especially when applying principle (4) on page 184. The decision in Imrie v. Mitchell 1958 S.C. 439, in which a 1:100000 chance of error was effectively regarded as sufficient to discredit a blood test result, is generally regarded as unreasonable. Yet the presence of an Mg gene, unheard of at that time, in the putative father could have produced the result illustrated in *Figure 18.3*. Ironically, the positive demonstration of such a rare gene would be as positive proof of paternity as is ever possible using antigenic analysis.

[8] That is: CDE, CDe, CdE, Cde, cDE, cDe, cdE, cde.

MATING	MM$_g$		MN	
	Father		Mother	
POSSIBLE	MM	M$_g$M	MN	M$_g$N
CHILDREN	1	2	3	4

Figure 18.3 Effect of a non-reacting variant of a gene. Mg is a variant of M that does not react with anti-M. Child 4 could, therefore, appear as NN and the putative could be wrongly excluded. Variants such as these are excessively rare, and anti-Mg is now available.

however, is the regularity of group transmission that 98 per cent of the groups consist of either CDe, cDE or cde. 32 per cent of Britons are of the genotype CDe/cde, 16 per cent are CDe/CDe and 15 per cent cde/cde—i.e. 15 per cent are Rhesus-negative.

In practice, the Rhesus system suffers from the inability to identify the potential antigen d. Thus, it is impossible to distinguish with certainty between the common genotype CDe/cde and the rare CDe/cDe because each can be defined only as the phenotype CcDe; the genotype is only inferred on a system of probabilities. This applies otherwise than in relation to d; thus, CDE/cDe is indistinguishable, save on likelihood, from CDE/cDE. The effect on paternity testing is, however, only marginal. The important feature is that a child cannot possess D unless one or both parents do so and this applies equally to C, c, E and e, all of which can be easily identified.

The Rhesus antigens are developed *in utero* and additional importance lies in their capacity to cause haemolytic disease of the newborn. Theoretically, all Rhesus antigens could cause this potentially lethal condition—C and E are not without a significant morbidity—but, in practice, the antigen D is mainly responsible. Cells from a fetus that is D positive by reason of the gene derived from its father may pass into a mother who is D negative. The mother reacts to the foreign antigen by forming anti-D which then passes back to the fetus, whose cells are destroyed. One medico-legally important aspect of the condition is that, nowadays, it would certainly be medically negligent to fail to identify the possibility of the condition and to take the necessary steps to protect the fetus and the mother.

The ABO system

Although it is by far the best-known and easiest system to demonstrate, the ABO system is slightly less easy to understand because, instead of one gene of a pair being available to fill the locus on the chromosome, there are three possibilities: A, B or O. There is no positive method of identifying the 'silent' gene O and it follows that the so-called blood groups A and B are phenotypes, the possible genotypes being AA, AO, BB and BO; the genotype AB is directly definable and the genotype OO is indicated by the absence of A and B. Certain absolute exclusions can be accepted in paternity testing—first, a person of group O cannot parent a child of group AB and, conversely, if one parent is group AB, no child can be of group O; secondly, if the genes A or B are present in a child, they *must* appear in one or both parents; on the other hand, the group mating A × B can produce children of any group provided it is actually a genotypic mating AO × BO.

Proteins of identical structure to the antigen A and B are widely distributed in nature. As a result, within a few weeks of birth, individuals 'recognize' a foreign antigen; a person of group A then produces, as a natural process, the antibody anti-B, a group B person forms anti-A, a group O person forms both anti-A and anti-B but an AB person recognizes no foreign substances and forms no antibodies. Not only does this provide a ready source of testing agents but, also, a blood group can be checked by testing the serum as opposed to the cells.

There is some practical importance in this in that the gene A can appear in a number of variant forms known as A_1—which is the common presentation—A_2, A_3 etc. The further removed they are from A_1, the weaker are the antigens and this difference can be demonstrated in the laboratory; moreover, persons of group A_2 etc. may contain anti-A_1 in their sera. These features breed true and greatly increase the value of the system in excluding or, perhaps, in providing presumptive evidence of parenthood.

Secretor groups

The ability of those of similar blood group to secrete water-soluble forms of A and B antigens into the body fluids is determined genetically; so-called 'H substance' is also secreted in pure form by those of blood group O and to a variable extent by those secreting A or B substances. 'H substance' can be demonstrated by using anti-H which occurs in certain plants. Secretion is dominant to non-secretion; 76 per cent of persons secrete the antigens and 24 per cent fail to do so[9].

While secretion has a minor part to play in testing for parentage, far greater medico-legal importance lies in the resultant ability to identify the blood-group antigens in body fluids that either contain very few cells—e.g. saliva—or in which the cells have been fragmented—e.g. old blood or seminal stains. Thus it may be possible to exclude—or strongly to corroborate—identity in any criminal case involving the spillage of body fluids; sexual assault provides the most obvious example[10]. The matter is discussed further at the end of this chapter.

Other cellular blood groups

Many other antigenic systems are present in the blood cells. The genetic distribution of some of these shows such disparity as to render them comparatively valueless as test systems; the necessary antisera are often rare; and, occasionally, special techniques are needed for their demonstration.

The *Kell system*, which may cause haemolytic disease of the newborn as does the Rhesus system, the *Duffy system* and the *Kidd system* are widely used in paternity testing although their individual capacities to exclude wrongly accused fathers are limited. The *Lutheran system* can also be used if antibodies are available.

Systems that have been well studied but are not used in paternity testing because of their complexity or instability include the *P system* which, again, may be responsible for fetal death, and the *Lewis system*, the main interest of which is that all persons of the phenotype Le(a+) are 'non-secretors'.

---

[9] This is a practical division. In fact, a minor degree of secretion can be demonstrated in some 'non-secretors' using very sensitive techniques.

[10] Note that 'non-secretion' refers only to non-secretion of water-soluble antigens; the cellular antigens A and B are determinable irrespective of the secretor status. Total deletion of the ABO antigens is excessively rare and results in the so-called 'Bombay' blood group.

Serum 'blood groups'

In addition to the antigens bound to the surface of the red cells, the blood plasma—or serum as it is when prepared for testing—contains protein substances that also appear as genetically controlled individual variants within systems. The principles of inheritance are similar to those described for the red cells. The serum groups are usually demonstrated by electrophoresis—a variant of chromatography (*see* Chapter 26) which measures the movement on paper of different proteins under the influence of an electric potential; the Gm system is an exception.

These systems include the *haptoglobins* which are concerned with the body's reaction to challenge and, as a result, differ in quantity, but *not* in quality, in disease states.

The *Gm system* is extremely complicated and is difficult to demonstrate. At least three alleles and other variants have been discovered but, no matter how the system actually functions, the principle remains that a child cannot produce a Gm factor that does not appear in the phenotype of either of its parents.

The *Gc system* is of similar type to the haptoglobins but is inherited independently.

The enzyme systems of the red blood cells

The functions of the red cells—those of absorbing, transporting and giving up oxygen—are performed through enzyme systems which, being of protein nature, can, again, be demonstrated as genetically controlled variants. The lawyer may, therefore, be confronted with such terms as 'phosphoglucomutase' but needs to know no more than that their use in paternity testing is based on principles identical with those already described.

The assistance available from a major laboratory

The value of the various systems is additive in excluding parentage; the effect of their combined use is shown in *Table 18.1*.

Thus, in the hands of a specialized laboratory, nine out of 10 wrongly accused men will expect to be excluded from paternity but these probabilities are based on the common alleles that make up the systems. The finding of an antigen of considerable rarity within the system will greatly increase the value of that particular system and, if it is discovered in both a man and a child, it opens up the possibility of identifying, as opposed to excluding, a male parent.

This aspect of paternity testing is allowed for in Section 20(2)(c) of the Family Law Reform Act which directs the laboratory performing the tests to indicate, in the event of non-exclusion, the value of the tests in determining whether a man *is* the child's father. In practice, the proportion of the population that would qualify for paternity is calculated and expressed as a percentage of the total population. Proof of paternity then becomes a matter of probability and the smaller the percentage of the population satisfying the criteria, the more likely is the man to be the father; the size of the percentage depends not only on the commonness or rarity of the antigens discovered but also on the number of systems examined. Lord Reid[11] put it that if 50 per cent of men could supply the necessary antigen, the test

---

[11] In S. v. S.; W. v. Official Solicitor [1970] 3 All E.R. 107(H.L.) at p. 110.

would be valueless in proof of paternity; if only one in 1000 could do so, the result would go a long way to proving the man was the father; but if the figure was 1 per cent or 10 per cent the test might go some way to making paternity probable. Even so, the Courts seem reluctant to employ the principle of probability particularly when a well-established presumption is involved; in one Scottish case[12], a statistical chance of 500000:1 against parenthood was considered insufficient to upset a circumstantial inference to that effect[12a].

TABLE 18.1. The maximum possibility of exclusion on a false paternity charge*

	System	Individual exclusion rate	Combined exclusion rate	
Red-cell antigens	ABO	0.176	0.176	
	Rhesus	0.280	0.406	
	MNSs	0.321	0.597	
	Kell	0.033	0.610	
	Duffy	0.048	0.629	
	Kidd	0.045	0.645	
Serum proteins	Gm	0.065	0.065	
	Gc	0.145	0.201	
	Hp	0.175	0.341	0.765
Red-cell enzymes	PGM	0.145	0.145	
	6PGD	0.025	0.166	
	AK	0.045	0.204	
	ADA	0.045	0.240	
	Acid phosphatase	0.210	0.400	
	GPT	0.190	0.514	0.890
TOTAL CHANCE OF EXCLUSION				89%

* The exclusion rate for each system is based on the gene frequencies in Great Britain. (Details kindly supplied by Professor B. E. Dodd.)

In fairness to all parties, paternity testing must be done by a specialized laboratory and Section 22 of the Family Law Reform Act provides that it is to be undertaken only by appointed practitioners. There are no such centres in Scotland and the limitations thereby imposed on any tests done must be appreciated.

Ethnic variations in blood groups

The genetically controlled blood-group antigens would be expected to vary in incidence in different ethnic groups and this is found to be so in practice. The more stable the population the more likely are single genes to predominate, major migrations should show as gene transferences and a gene may be actually advantageous in a given environment and therefore prosper locally. Thus, the incidence of the gene O is extremely high in South America and in most island communities, while the gene B is present most commonly in central Asia, getting less frequent as one moves westward and being relatively uncommon in the Americas. Similar variations are seen in the distribution of genes of other

[12] Sproat v. McGibney 1968 S.L.T. 33. The principle was firmly upheld although there was an additional doubt as to identification.
[12a] Our concepts of parentage testing are likely to be completely altered as a result of the demonstration of specific DNA profiles; *see* Jeffreys, A. J. *et al.* (1985), Individual-specific 'fingerprints' of human DNA, *Nature, London,* **316**, 76.

blood-cell antigens, serum groups, enzyme variants and abnormal haemoglobins[13]. There are significant differences even within the United Kingdom—43 per cent of those in Southern England are of group A as compared with only 34 per cent of Scots.

This apparently academic subject has to be mentioned because of its practical importance when considering the probability of paternity as discussed above. Racial variations must be taken into account in making any calculations and a valid assessment can be made only if large numbers of the particular relevant population have been studied. For practical purposes, Western Europe can be regarded as homogeneous in this context although the Basques form a markedly distinct enclave. It should be noted, however, that ethnic differences are never absolute. It is impossible to derive the race of an individual simply by analysing his blood-group spectrum.

The examination of stains

The examination of stains is a matter for the science laboratory. None the less, the subject is so entwined with blood-group genetics that it does not seem out of place to include a short description so as to complete the picture for the lawyer.

The 'depth' of identification of a blood stain depends very largely on its age—a fresh blood stain can be dealt with much as a specimen taken *in vivo*, whereas an old stain, in which the cellular structure has disintegrated, is greatly limited as to use and putrefactive changes may lead to erroneous results. Thus, A antigen appears to behave in certain circumstances as a B-reacting substance. In one case of the author's, 10 putrefied bodies recovered from the sea were blood grouped; eight appeared to be of group B—an incredible result[14].

The basic steps in the examination of a blood stain are, first, to prove that it is blood—a matter of either direct vision under the microscope or of a sensitive chemical test—and, secondly, to prove its human origin—a comparatively simple exercise.

The ABO group can nearly always be ascertained, even when the test has to be performed on blood-stained threads only, but the problem of degenerative change discussed above is a real one. The Rhesus antigens are probably the next most stable, while modern immunoelectrophoretic techniques are so sensitive that the serum blood groups may be as useful indicators of identity as are those attached to the cells. Given a square centimetre of blood-stained material, experienced workers can often identify some eight or nine genetic systems; the chances of association with a given individual with reasonable probability or for excluding a suspect are very high.

The identification of other biological stains—of which semen is the most important—follows much the same lines. Recognizable spermatozoa will remain on fabric for several months and direct positive observation under the microscope is certainly the most acceptable proof of a seminal origin. The enzyme acid phosphatase is highly developed in human semen and can be differentiated from the same enzyme which may be found in vaginal fluid; the activity of the enzyme is,

---

[13] The sickle-cell gene, which probably protects against malaria, is very common in Africa.
[14] *See* Jenkins, G. C. *et al.* (1972), The problem of the acquired B antigen in forensic serology, *Journal of the Forensic Science Society*, **12**, 597.

however, often difficult to demonstrate other than in fresh stains. The human origin of a seminal stain is seldom in doubt but can be shown with the same ease as in the case of a blood stain.

The individual identification of a seminal stain depends on the secretor state of the donor. As described above, water-soluble blood-group antigens will be found in the body fluids of only approximately three-quarters of the population; even so, the correlation of a 'negative' stain with a non-secreting suspect is not without value and increasingly sensitive testing diminishes the proportion of 'non-secretors'. Secretion of blood groups is limited to A, B and H substances; it follows that the chances of failure to distinguish between two individuals on the basis of seminal 'grouping' are of the order of 45 per cent of secretors—the medico-legal usefulness of such testing is, therefore, virtually confined to exclusion.

It is self-evident that stains may be mixed—the tights of a rape victim, for example, may be contaminated both with vaginal and with seminal fluids and may, therefore, give the reactions of both. Only in very exceptional circumstances would it be possible to distinguish between them.

There are strong indications that the science of stain identification may soon be revolutionized by the application of modern DNA genetic techniques. DNA profiles, which can be derived from blood or from semen, may be as specific to the individual as are his fingerprints (n. 12a, above).

19

Unnatural death of the fetus and the newborn: abortion, child destruction and infanticide or child murder

The law on abortion, child destruction and infanticide

In England and Wales

Changes in public attitudes to induced abortion have been dramatic. It was certainly regarded as one of the more serious crimes in the early medico-legal codes and it is specifically referred to in the Hippocratic Oath. Yet, today, the extent of abortion services provided is regarded as something of a measure of the community's state of civilization and the inevitable conflict of views arouses much emotion. The historical background to the present position in relation to both abortion and neonatal killing is most easily described through the statutory English law.

The basic law on abortion in England and Wales is contained in the Offences Against the Person Act 1861 which states:

> *Section 58.* Every woman, being with child, who with intent to procure her own miscarriage, shall unlawfully administer to herself any poison, or other noxious thing, or shall unlawfully use any instrument whatsoever with like intent, and whosoever, with intent to procure the miscarriage of any woman, whether she be or be not with child, shall unlawfully administer to her, or cause to be taken by her, any poison or other noxious thing, or shall unlawfully use any instrument or other means whatsoever with like intent, shall be guilty of an offence[1].
>
> *Section 59.* Whosoever shall unlawfully supply or procure any poison or other noxious thing, or any instrument or thing whatsoever, knowing that the same is intended to be unlawfully used, or employed, with intent to procure the miscarriage of any woman, whether she be or be not with child, shall be guilty of an offence.

This Act has not been repealed—recent legislation has done little more than to define the word 'unlawfully'. There is no mention in the 1861 Act of therapeutic abortion which was not recognized until the passing of the Infant Life (Preservation) Act 1929. This enacted (s. 1) that child destruction is committed when any person, with intent to destroy the life of a child capable of being born alive, by

---

[1] Amended by the Criminal Law Act 1967, s. 12(5).

any wilful act causes a child to die before it has an existence independent of its mother; provided that the prosecution must prove that the act was not done in good faith for the purpose only of preserving the mother's life. For the purposes of the Act, evidence that a woman had at any material time been pregnant for a period of 28 weeks or more shall be *prima facie* proof that she was at that time pregnant of a child capable of being born alive.

The Infant Life (Preservation) Act introduced some important legal concepts. It recognized the legal right of a child to a separate existence after the 28th week of intrautcrine development and, at the same time, established the unusual crime of child destruction. A child being born naturally cannot be the subject of criminal abortion; on the other hand, a fetus that has had no separate existence cannot be murdered. The 1929 Act, in establishing an offence that included killing a child during the process of birth, closed the door on what was, admittedly, more of a permissible defence than a practical likelihood.

The Act also introduced for the first time the statutory possibility of a legally performed abortion. Two phrases stand out. 'In good faith' are words of great importance in both permissive and prohibitory senses; they still form an essential element in the law regulating therapeutic abortion. The qualification 'for the purposes only of saving the life of the mother' is restrictive and for many years it was left to case law[2] to establish the limits within which a doctor could legally terminate a pregnancy; the Abortion Act 1967 was enacted mainly to clarify the position.

Some terms of the Infant Life (Preservation) Act may cause confusion as between medical and legal interpretation. The first involves 'viability' or a 'viable fetus'. A viable fetus to a medical practitioner is one that can be kept alive in both an intra- and extrauterine existence; to the lawyer, it is one that is presumed to be capable of independent survival—i.e. one that has reached 28 weeks' gestation. Similar confusion may arise in relation to a 'live birth' and a 'separate existence'. To the doctor, a live birth is represented by a child who showed signs of life at some point in the delivery; the legal definition of a separate existence insists, in addition, that it 'should have completely proceeded in a living state from the body of the mother'. Thus, it is theoretically possible to have a medical live birth of a child who has not reached the development of legal viability while the reverse situation may well arise in practice as a result of complications in delivery. It is, indeed, important to appreciate that the Infant Life (Preservation) Act does *not* define *non-viability*. An infant who has proved his or her will to live by breathing after birth has been born alive irrespective of the gestational age.

These considerations also apply to the law protecting the infant shortly after birth. The Infanticide Act 1938 provides that the offence of infanticide is committed when a woman by any wilful act or omission causes the death of her child, being under the age of 12 months, but, at the time of the act or omission, the balance of her mind was disturbed by reason of her not having fully recovered from the effect of giving birth to the child or of lactation consequent upon the birth. The legal concept of viability has no relevance to a charge of infanticide; all that is required is that the child should have been capable of being murdered—that is, had achieved a separate existence.

When such a charge is made, it is presumed that the child was born dead unless

---

[2] The most important being R. v. Bourne [1939] 1 K.B. 687; also R. v. Newton & Stungo [1958] Crim. L.R. 469.

the prosecution can show proof to the contrary; any doubts that may exist must be resolved in favour of the mother. The pathological evidence thus assumes paramount importance and will be discussed later in this Chapter. For the present, it is simply emphasized that it may be impossible, even in the presence of only early decomposition, to give positive evidence in respect of a live birth. In such cases, Section 60 of the Offences Against the Person Act allows for an alternative charge of concealment of birth. This section makes it an offence for any person to endeavour to conceal the birth of a child by secret disposition of its dead body—that is, disposition in a place where there is no normal access for the public—whether the child died before, at or after its birth; the questions of viability and separate existence are, therefore, immaterial.

The comparative law in Scotland

With one exception, there are no comparable statutes in Scots law, the relevant offences being subject to common law.

In general, it seems that abortion has been regarded as less of a problem in Scotland than is the case in England and this applies particularly to operations performed by medical practitioners. Despite the fact that there was no case law to support the concept of therapeutic abortion before 1967, it is doubtful if Mr Bourne would have achieved his object of clarifying the issue had he performed a 'test' abortion in Scotland because the authorities would not have prosecuted him[3].

In both England and Scotland, a woman must be shown to have been pregnant before she can be charged with self-inflicted criminal abortion. The intention on the part of an outsider to procure an abortion is criminal in both countries—the fact that the attempt is unsuccessful is immaterial; the main difference is that it is necessary in Scotland that the woman be pregnant and it is the responsibility of the prosecution to prove that pregnancy. It would be a defence in both England and Scotland to show that the fetus was dead prior to abortion.

There is no Scottish equivalent to the English Infant Life (Preservation) Act. Some very old case law[4] covers the possibility of destruction of the fetus during birth; it was regarded not as homicide but as a serious, albeit unnamed, crime but this view was later disputed[5]. Smith[6] thought that, provided the child had breathed, a defence that its death took place before it was fully extruded would not be valid in Scotland. Fortunately, the need for such a charge must be excessively rare.

The Infanticide Act of 1938 is also inapplicable to Scotland; the comparable crime under Scots law is child murder. None the less, it has long been appreciated that the special conditions surrounding the killing of the neonate merit leniency and, in practice, diminished responsibility is always assumed; the crime of child murder is thus reduced to one of culpable homicide. It goes almost without saying that, under both jurisdictions, the extenuating conditions can be applied only to the mother.

The Concealment of Birth (Scotland) Act 1809 is the only statute relevant to

[3] Gordon, G. H. (1967). *The Criminal Law of Scotland*, 1st edn., p. 383. Edinburgh; W. Green & Son. Mr Bourne aborted a woman made pregnant as a result of rape, having informed the authorities that he was to do so; he was prosecuted and acquitted although the mother's life was not in immediate danger.

[4] H.M. Adv. v. M'Allum (1858) 3 Irv. 187.

[5] H.M. Adv. v. Scott (1892) 3 White 240.

[6] Smith, S. and Fiddes, F. S. (1955) *Forensic Medicine*, 10th edn., p. 339., London; Churchill.

Scotland in the present context and provides that a woman may be convicted if she 'conceals her being with child during the whole period of pregnancy and does not call for and make use of help or assistance at the birth and the child be found dead or be amissing', the presumption being that the child would have been born alive and would have lived unless it had been concealed. This enactment is, in practice, more difficult to apply than is s. 60 of the English Offences Against the Person Act, principally because the concealment must be total and must be maintained for the whole pregnancy—it must, moreover, be shown that the child was viable not only in the legal but also in the medical sense. A prosecution can succeed in the absence of a body.

Criminal abortion

Infanticide or child murder, child destruction and criminal abortion are closely related, as all are ultimately referable to an unwanted pregnancy. The pattern and incidence of the basic offence of abortion—and, indirectly, of the other two—has been completely altered by the Abortion Act 1967, which applies throughout the United Kingdom with the exception of Northern Ireland. None the less, the number of abortions currently sought and the legal inadmissibility of some, even under the very wide terms of the 1967 Act, result in a sufficient surplus of cases to maintain the presence of criminal abortionists. The motivation of the Act can scarcely be appreciated without an understanding of the conditions it was designed to eliminate. A short consideration of criminal abortion is, even now, appropriate.

Approximately 20 per cent of pregnancies end prematurely. The proportion of these terminated illegally before 1967 cannot, for obvious reasons, be accurately assessed and has been estimated as being anything from 10 per cent to 70 per cent; the most widely quoted figure in the United Kingdom is 40 per cent given, with reservation, by the Inter-Departmental Committee on Abortion in 1939[7], although more recent observers have concluded that this figure is too high.

Given the almost invariable sequence of suspicion of pregnancy, confirmation of suspicion and failure of near natural attempts at abortion—e.g. hot baths, gin or feverish equestrianism—it is to be expected that the great majority of criminal abortions are attempted at between 2 and 4 months of pregnancy. The risks escalate beyond this point and only ignorant abortionists are likely to put themselves in jeopardy. Apart from the pregnant woman herself, an abortionist is, or was, generally of the 'Mrs Gamp' type, a member of the paramedical professions, a nurse or student or, occasionally, a registered medical practitioner—though doctors whose names have been erased from the Register should also be included. The general methods of choice used by each category will be evident from the following description (*see Figure 19.1*).

Abortifacient drugs

There are essentially three categories of drug used in attempts to procure abortion[8].

[7] Ministry of Health and Home Office, para. 26. London; HMSO.
[8] The perpetuation of this type of list might well be considered anachronistic. However, preparations, particularly of the emmenagogue variety, are still widely sold; the curious Gallic association of many of their trade names testifies to their time-worn origins (*see* David, T. J. (1974). The composition and current use of abortifacients *Medicine, Science and the Law*, **14**, 120).

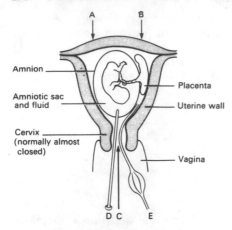

Figure 19.1 Methods available to the abortionist. Drugs that cause the uterus to contract may be used (A) or direct violence may be applied to the womb (B). The cervix may be dilated by instruments or hygroscopic tampons (C) inducing the uterus to contract. The amniotic sac may be penetrated by sharp instruments (D) causing direct or indirect death of the fetus. The fetus may be separated from the uterine wall by the injection of fluids or pastes (E)

Purgatives and Emetics—These are used in the mistaken belief that all smooth muscle will contract if one part—the bowel—is stimulated.

Emmenagogues—These are substances that increase the menstrual flow. Presumably, the rationale for their use is that substances that will provoke excessive normal menstrual flow will stimulate some flow when it is inhibited by pregnancy. It is probable that many of these drugs, including the more sophisticated female hormones (oestrogenic substances) which are often used with similar intent, owe their reputation to the fact that they produce a dramatic result when inhibition of the menstrual period is due to causes other than pregnancy. The advertisement of any drug in terms that might lead to their use to procure abortion was prohibited under the Pharmacy and Medicines Act 1941 (replaced by the Medicines Act 1968).

Ecbolics—These are drugs that actively promote contraction of the uterine muscle. Since most of them have a genuine pharmacological action and are therapeutically valuable, they can constitute a temptation to the medical practitioner. Two substances in this group that are well-known to the general public are lead, which is restricted under Schedule 1 of the Poisons Rules and by the Medicines (Prescription Only) Order, and quinine which is readily available in low-dosage units; both may cause severe symptoms of poisoning. The most efficient agent is ergot—which is used quite properly to ensure contraction of the uterus after delivery. Hormone preparations include pituitary extract which may, again, be rightly used to induce labour and, recently, prostaglandins have been introduced as therapeutic abortifacients.

The use of drugs draws attention to the interpretation of the term 'noxious thing' used in the Offences Against the Person Act. Theoretically, any substance having any unusual pharmacological effect might be regarded as noxious. For the purposes of the Act, however, it has been established that, to be relevant, the drug must be known to have abortifacient properties; otherwise it would be hard to prove intent. Moreover, the dosage must be taken into consideration in case the doctor is open to accusation every time a potential abortifacient is properly prescribed for the treatment of unrelated conditions.

Abortion by direct violence

Little need be said on this other than to remark on the resistance of the fetus to direct violence. The main medico-legal implications of this 'method' of abortion are that a husband who is prepared to subject his pregnant wife to such abuse is likely to do so in the absence of pregnancy and, secondly, that severe attacks on the gravid uterus are as likely to result in rupture with death of the mother as in simple expulsion of the fetus.

Criminal instrumentation

By far the most common form of criminal abortion involves the use of instruments of some sort. The function of these can best be understood by reference to normal pregnancy and delivery.

The fetus obtains its nourishment from an interwoven network of blood capillaries on the uterine wall which, at 3 months, is condensed into the placenta. If this connection is broken the fetus becomes a non-viable foreign body and may be expelled. This mechanism forms the basis of the injection of pastes or of the use of the infamous enema syringe to procure abortion.

The fetus is maintained in a fluid medium within the amniotic sac. Drainage of this fluid results in compression of the fetus by the uterine muscle and ultimate expulsion. Any instrument that perforates the amnion may precipitate abortion and there can be few pointed objects—from quill-feather pens to surgical catheters—that have not been employed for the purpose. Bundles of wax tapers have also been used.

Dilatation of the cervical canal initiates the normal discharge of a fetus. Artificial dilatation may, in effect, deceive the uterine muscle into believing the time for contraction to have arrived. Certain vegetable substances will absorb water and swell when placed in the cervical canal which is thereby opened. This is the mode of operation of slippery elm bark which was such a favourite of the abortionist because it was likely to leave no trace of interference.

The truly professional abortionist may, of course, combine these methods in the surgical operation of cervical dilatation and curettage or suction of the uterine cavity.

Death following instrumentation

An attempted abortion may fail or succeed; in either case, the woman may be unaffected, may require medical treatment or may die. A case resulting in less than fatal injury to the woman will come to light only in exceptional circumstances. But death will always be investigated and the lawyer needs an understanding of the various causative mechanisms.

Death may ensue immediately, it may occur fairly soon after the event or it may be delayed further. The practical significance of this classification is that, in the first instance, the body may well be found at the locus; in the second, death may occur at some distance from the scene of the abortion; while, in the third, it may even be difficult to associate the fatality with an abortion. Deaths associated with poisoning by drugs are not considered further at this point.

Immediate death

Vagal inhibition of the heart—This is the characteristic 'death on the couch', the abnormal sensory stimulus precipitating cardiac arrest being contact with the inner surface of the cervical canal. As previously discussed, the pathologist's major difficulty is that the post-mortem diagnosis of the condition is based almost entirely on the circumstantial evidence and on exclusion of other pathological states.

Air embolism—Separation of the fetal from the maternal circulation, which is the purpose of the enema syringe, results in the opening of blood vessels. It is possible for the receptor nozzle of the syringe to be withdrawn from the fluid during the process of forcible douching and air is then delivered instead of, or along with, fluid. The circulation finds it hard to deal with large gas bubbles and death from air embolism may result—generally in about 10 minutes which is the time taken for a lethal concentration of bubbles to accumulate in the arteries of the heart and brain. The amount of air needed to kill depends on the degree to which the vital organs are embolized—10 ml have been lethal while, in other cases, the injection of 100 ml has been survived. Although death from air embolism is usually rapid, cases have been reported of survival for 2 hours; the subject does not, therefore, always die where the abortion was performed.

Moderately delayed death

Fluid embolism—Even if air is not pumped into the circulation, the fluid used, often containing strong soap or toxic antiseptics, can be introduced. Death may then be fairly rapid but is as likely to be delayed until the effects of tissue necrosis or blood haemolysis have become evident.

Haemorrhage—The cervical opening is small and the vaginal and cervical canals do not run in a straight line. Moreover, the majority of lay persons are remarkably ignorant of the size and position of the pregnant uterus. It is not surprising that many attempts at instrumentation result in laceration not of the fetal sac alone but, additionally or alternatively, of the vagina, of the cervix or of the uterus itself. Laceration implies haemorrhage which may be sufficient to cause death. This does seem, however, to be surprisingly uncommon—the woman generally seeks medical assistance before the situation has got out of hand.

Delayed death

Sepsis—Sepsis was the commonest cause of death after criminal abortion before the advent of antibiotics and the occurrence of sepsis following an abortion could be taken as a strong indication that the condition was unnatural. Three features contributed in the main to this. First, the instrumentation was either unhygienic from the outset or became so during the process of procuring an abortion. Secondly, the uterus was often not cleared properly and this left a dead nidus of infection. Thirdly, the closeness of the lower bowel to an area frequently injured resulted in local sepsis or in septicaemia caused by organisms normally present in the faeces. The most dangerous of these were those causing gas gangrene and tetanus—they remain so even in the antibiotic age because of the very severe toxic effects they may exhibit and the often fulminating nature of the infection.

Acute renal failure—As described in Chapter 1, any condition that results in surgical shock may well have a profound effect on the kidneys. Many of the complications of criminal abortion are essentially 'shocking' and renal failure may ensue even if a woman has survived the original crisis.

The legal position of the doctor in criminal abortion

The relationship between the doctor and his patient is under considerable strain whenever a patient is involved in criminal activity, particularly when that criminality derives from acute mental distress as must most often be the case when illegal abortion is attempted.

The position is statutory when death results. In both England and Scotland the Registrar will, by regulation, report the matter to the Coroner or to the Procurator Fiscal. At any subsequent hearing, the doctor may properly protest his right to professional secrecy but, under both jurisdictions, he must ultimately provide evidence and answer questions that are put to him.

The concept that professional confidentiality takes precedence over the disclosure of criminality in life has also been disapproved. Lord Justice Inglis[9] was quite clear; 'I care not for professional etiquette or rule; there is a rule of life and a consideration far higher than these, and that is the duty of every citizen . . . to prevent the destruction of human life.' An English *obiter dictum* which is commonly quoted is that of Avory, J (1914)[10], who stated, 'there are cases where the desire to preserve [the confidential relation which exists between the medical man and his patient] must be subordinated to the duty which is cast on every good citizen to assist in the investigation of a serious crime'. This view was challenged by the Royal College of Physicians, who issued a statement in 1916 which still represents authoritative medical opinion on this question. Briefly, this statement concluded that every medical practitioner has a moral duty to respect the confidence of his patient; that, when convinced that criminal abortion has been practised on his patient, the doctor should urge her to make a statement as evidence against the person who performed the operation; that he is under no legal obligation either to so urge his patient or to press the point should she refuse; that, in any event, he should obtain good legal and medical advice before taking any action that might lead to legal proceedings; and that he should inform the Coroner should the patient die.

Times change as do attitudes. No practitioner would now be likely to report a criminal abortion in which no second party was involved. Yet there is surely sufficient violence in the world today without, by remaining silent, effectively conniving at the survival of criminals whose activities may well result in culpable homicide. The basic wrong lies not so much in the niceties of medical jurisprudence as in the fact that such cases should ever occur. It was against this background that the Abortion Act 1967 was passed.

The Abortion Act 1967

The bones of the Act are contained in Section 1 which states:

(1) . . . a person shall not be guilty of an offence under the law relating to abortion when a pregnancy is terminated by a registered medical practitioner if two medical practitioners are of the opinion, formed in good faith:

[9] In Roughead, W. (ed.) (1906). *Trial of Dr Pritchard*. p. 283. Glasgow; W. Hodge & Co. The trial took place in 1865.
[10] Reported in: The duties of medical practitioners in cases of criminal abortion, *British Medical Journal* (1916), **i**, 206.

(*a*) that the continuance of the pregnancy would involve risk to the life of the pregnant woman, or of injury to the physical or mental health of the pregnant woman or any existing children of her family, greater than if the pregnancy were terminated; or

(*b*) that there is substantial risk that if the child were born it would suffer from such physical or mental abnormalities as to be seriously handicapped.

(2) [In making a decision under Para 1 (*a*)] account may be taken of the pregnant woman's actual or reasonably foreseeable environment.

As has already been stressed, this is not the definitive law on abortion; indeed, the Act states that 'anything done within intent to procure the miscarriage of a woman is unlawfully done unless authorized by Section 1 of the Act'. Furthermore, s. 5 specifically retains the provision of the Infant Life (Preservation) Act 1929; the effect of this is to retain the illegality of abortion performed after the 28th week of pregnancy unless done for the sole purpose of preserving the mother's life[11]. The intention of the 1967 Act was to clarify the law in relation to therapeutic abortion.

That it was never intended to be a licence for 'abortion on demand' seems clear from the number of regulations that must be satisfied to make the operation legal. Not only must a legal abortion be carried out in a hospital of the National Health Service or in a place specifically approved for the purpose, but standardized forms must be used for recommending the abortion and for reporting that an emergency abortion has been performed—in which case, the need for two opinions is waived; a statutory form must be completed for notification of the termination of pregnancy within 7 days of the event. Part II of the latter form contains a number of questions designed to improve the statistical basis of any future legislation (Abortion Regulations 1968; Abortion (Scotland) Regulations 1968).

Nevertheless, the phrasing of the Act is very open and the scope for legalized abortion is considerable—it has been argued that the risks of normal pregnancy are greater than those of early abortion and that, consequently, any termination carried out in an approved place must be legal. Such a proposition is not easy to assess particularly as there has been a marked improvement in abortion mortality since the 'high' of some 27 deaths from legal operations in England and Wales in 1969. Other factors that might affect the mortality rate are the gestational age—the rate rises markedly after the 12th week of pregnancy—and the maternal age—childbirth is certainly more hazardous than abortion in older women but the reverse applies in young 'first-time' mothers unless the procedure is completed in the first 8 weeks of pregnancy[12]. Although such arguments must run contrary to the intentions of the original legislators, they serve to illustrate how those intentions have been subjected to erosion over the years.

The number of legal abortions performed is now higher than ever before. Over 140 000 operations were carried out on residents of England and Wales in 1985, giving a rate per 1000 women of child-bearing age of 12.97. The comparable figures for Scotland are interesting—there were 9838 terminations in the same year giving a rate of 8.8 per 1000 women. However, whereas 2 per cent of Scottish terminations were performed in approved places other than hospitals within the National Health

[11] But, since the 1929 Act does not run to Scotland, it must be assumed that this restriction does not apply there.
[12] The locality might also make a difference. This is an Edinburgh opinion (Myerscough, P.R. (1975). *Journal of Medical Ethics*, **1**, 130).

Service, the comparable figure for England and Wales was 59 per cent or 50 per cent if only residents were taken into account. When NHS hospital cases are considered alone, the abortion rate in Scotland is rather higher than that in England. The reason why half the women who have abortions in England do so at their own expense is a subject of debate beyond the scope of this chapter[13].

While a return to the situation that existed before 1967 is unthinkable, it has been argued that the Act as it stands is too lax. Nevertheless, repeated attempts to introduce amending legislation have failed and the Lane Committee[14], which sat at the time of greatest use of the Act, recommended very few changes, the most important positive recommendation being that the upper time limit for operations under the Act should be 24 weeks' gestation; on the negative side, the Committee declined to recommend altering the status of women non-resident in Great Britain.

The problem of non-residents highlights the doubts that have been expressed as to the 'good faith' of doctors. Over one third of the abortions performed in England in 1973 involved foreign women. The numbers fell as other countries adopted more liberal laws but the proportion was still 20 per cent in 1979; 99 per cent of these operations were carried out privately. The facts that the patronage of foreign girls has been actively solicited and that their total stay in Britain is currently of the order of 3 days must raise doubts in the minds of the medical profession. In the event, there has been only one prosecution relating to the Act and only one name has been erased from the medical register—that was on the grounds of advertisement rather than on operation practice. It must be assumed that the situation satisfies the authorities.

Although, in practice, very few legal abortions are performed after the 20th week of pregnancy, the problem of the gestational age is of more immediate concern. Many fetuses of 24 weeks' gestation will survive given modern neonatal intensive care and it is difficult to see how a deliberate failure to support such viable entities can, in theory, escape being an offence, including the possibility of manslaughter. On the other hand, the gynaecologist performing an abortion has effectively contracted to eliminate a fetus and may, therefore, be in an ambiguous position.

Difficulties also arise at the beginning of gestation. The Act makes no reference to the duration of pregnancy and it is, therefore, possible that the use of intrauterine devices, which are believed to displace the fertilized ovum, might be illegal. The practice of menstrual extraction, in which the possibility of pregnancy is anticipated by the gynaecologist, is, on the face of things, even more open to question but has, in fact, been declared on rather tenuous grounds to be protected by the Abortion Act[15]. All such situations deal, in the main, with the theoretical criminality of actions taken by doctors acting from the best clinical motives. Medical technology and expertise are overtaking the law; the process should be reversed for the benefit of both the profession and the patients.

An example of this dissonance is shown by the current technique of aborting by means of an infusion of prostaglandin rather than by surgery. It has been argued that, in such a situation, it is the nurse who administers the infusion over a period of

---

[13] Some 3500 women resident in Scotland and Ireland combined have legal abortions in England each year. The Abortion Act 1967 does not apply to Northern Ireland.

[14] *Report of the Committee on the Working of the Abortion Act* (1974). Cmnd. 5579. London; HMSO.

[15] These two aspects of the Act are well argued by Tunkel, V. (1979), Abortion: How early, how late, and how legal? *British Medical Journal*, ii, 253. There is an interesting innovative reference to an offence of attempted child destruction.

hours who is performing the abortion thus contravening the requirements for termination by a registered medical practitioner. It has now been resolved that termination of pregnancy is a team effort, the instructions of the doctor being the effective instrument; but it is interesting that, in sum, a majority of five to four judicial opinions were of the opposite view[16].

The subject of abortion engenders much emotion which is activated, first, by the doctor's 'Hippocratic conscience'. Not only is abortion specifically condemned in the traditional 'Oath' but the Declaration of Sydney, adopted by the World Medical Association in 1968 as a modern restatement of the Hippocratic Oath, includes: 'I will maintain the utmost respect for life from the time of conception'[17]. Surprisingly, however, by far the greatest publicity is given to religious principles—in particular, to those regulated by Roman Catholicism. I have obtained an opinion from a leading Roman Catholic philosopher particularly as to the apparent priority given by the Church to the well-being of the fetus when this affected the life of the mother. He wrote:

'On a subjective level, I can fully appreciate the position of the doctor or surgeon faced with the woman with serious complications which make it unlikely or impossible that her baby will come to term before she dies. He is bound to feel that [in failing to terminate the pregnancy] he has not done all he can for her and that therefore he is guilty of her death.

'On an objective level, two things seem to me rather clear. The first is that this attitude, entirely admirable as it is, does somewhat presuppose that the mother's life is more important than the child's and that, therefore, if the mother is to be saved, the child has to be sacrificed. But would it work the other way round? Would it be right and proper for the doctor to end the mother's life in order to give a viable child a decent chance of survival? Clearly not. You may answer that the eventuality is not in fact practical because it wouldn't arise. But if it did, no doctor would countenance it and no moralist allow it. Why? Because it would be plain murder. And that is the crucial second point. If it is plain murder in the case of the mother, why is it not in the case of the child?

'Which brings us back to the dilemma. Objectively, the doctor is not entitled to kill either in order to save the other. His job is to save both. He is bound to do all in his power to save the mother, short of doing what is wrong—and killing the baby is wrong.

'I would have to add that, if he still felt in conscience bound to terminate the pregnancy, I would not and could not blame him—because that is in the subjective order, and he is entitled to follow the dictates of his own conscience.'

The practical importance of the last paragraph is self-evident. Inevitably, this moral conflict dictated a 'conscience clause', excusing persons of a duty to participate in abortions, and this is provided in s. 4 of the Act. Paradoxically, this element in the Act has led to justifiable criticism of its operation to the effect that local medical prejudice has led to the formation of regional pockets where the rules are applied more stringently than elsewhere; equally, the employment potential of those invoking their moral right is severely jeopardized.

It is, however, important to understand than no conscientious objection to terminating pregnancy is allowable under the Act when the operation is necessary

---

[16] Royal College of Nursing v. Department of Health and Social Security [1981] 2 W.L.R. 279.
[17] The full text is available in *The Handbook of Medical Ethics* (1984); London: British Medical Association.

to save the life of, or to prevent serious permanent injury to, the woman; a doctor, or a medical ancillary, could also be held negligent in failing to provide or arrange such treatment for lesser reasons. Whereas, in Scotland, a simple statement on oath establishes the doctor's legal position, the burden of proof of conscientious objection in England rests on the person claiming it. Irrespective of conscience, any doctor is at risk of civil action should a decision not to terminate be shown in the end to have been wrong, the risk being greatly extended by the Congenital Disabilities (Civil Liability) Act 1976, s. 1(5). Even allowing for sincere conscientious objection on the doctor's part, it would obviously be improper for him to attempt to influence his patient on any grounds other than those he believes to be in accord with current medical practice and, if necessary, he must himself act according to these principles; while the Act excuses the medical profession from participating in the treatment authorized, there is no exemption from advising a patient as to the correct medical course. On the other hand, the doctor has to appreciate that his patient too may have a strong conscience and it goes without saying that, except in relation to emergency procedures, it could amount to serious professional misconduct to procure an abortion other than with the full consent of the patient; it would, perhaps, be ideal to obtain also the consent of the husband but the husband has no paternal rights to prevent a legal termination[18].

Finally, s. 4 does not absolve the doctor from treating conditions that have arisen by virtue of an abortion; his duty of care to his patient remains irrespective of his disapproval of the cause of ill health.

Potential evidence from the expert witness

Abortion

For reasons previously discussed, prosecutions for criminal abortions are unusual unless the woman dies. Should she do so, important pathological evidence may be obtained under four main headings.

First, the fact of pregnancy or of delivery must be established both under English and under Scots law—particularly the latter. Evidence of these may include the signs of response in the breast, although they are poorly developed at the elective time of criminal abortion. Discharge or haemorrhage from the vulva may be evident. Internally, the persistence in an ovary of a corpus luteum—the hormonal response to ovulation and subsequent pregnancy—may be noted; this atrophies in some 10 days in the absence of pregnancy but persists for approximately the first 20 weeks of gestation. The major evidence, however, comes from the uterus which will still contain a fetus in the case of unsuccessful attempted abortion. Otherwise, there will almost certainly be enlargement of the organ; the normal uterus measures some 7×4 cm ($2\frac{3}{4} \times 1\frac{1}{2}$ in) while at 3 months the size is of the order of an 8-cm (3-in) globe. Internally, the lining will be haemorrhagic and furry for a few days and a recognizable placental area may persist for 2 months. An attempt should be made to prove the presence of placental tissue microscopically. These signs are so general in nature that the pathologist can give no more than an estimate as to when delivery took place. The longer the interval, the more imprecise must be that estimate and, at 2 months, even the fact of delivery may be in doubt.

Secondly, evidence of interference will be sought. If there is any suggestion of

---

[18] Paton v. British Pregnancy Service Trustees [1978] 3 W.L.R. 687; (1980) 3 EHHR 408. *See also* C v. S (1987) Times, 24 February QBD, 25 February CA.

the use of 'noxious substances', specimens of blood, bowel content and tissues will be sent for analysis. Direct violence may be evidenced by abdominal bruising. The greatest significance will, however, be attached to the finding of lacerations which are commonly in the posterior vagina, the cervix or the uterus itself. The peritoneum lining the abdominal cavity may be penetrated and injuries of any sort may be complicated by haemorrhage or by sepsis. The presence of the latter is strong, but not conclusive, evidence of unnatural abortion; the type of the infecting organisms should be established in every case not only to indicate their origin but also for possible comparison with cultures made from suspect instruments. In addition to evidence of the use of penetrating instruments, the post-mortem may also show local signs of abortion by injection. Thus, frothy soapy fluid or paste may persist within the uterus and may even be found in the abdominal cavity in the event of very unskilled use.

It is equally the responsibility of the pathologist to exclude the possibility of natural abortion. A full autopsy is necessary to exclude such conditions as nephritis, diabetes, heart disease or placental abnormalities—accidental placental haemorrhage, although generally occurring late in pregnancy, is a natural phenomenon that may closely simulate illegal interference.

Thirdly, the cause of death may have a great bearing on the case, and although the pathologist can generally make a confident assessment it may, on occasion, be surprisingly difficult to do so. Thus, it has already been noted that vagal inhibition is essentially a post-mortem diagnosis of exclusion; haemorrhage may appear inconspicuous although copious quantities of blood have been lost elsewhere; purulent exudate involving the genitalia may, even when of apparently severe degree, be no more than of incidental significance.

Embolic modes of death may involve extra interpretative and technical skills. The production of apparent bubbles in the cerebral circulation is a common artefact induced by removal of the skull at post-mortem dissection; the competent pathologist is, however, aware of this and well able to distinguish such a localized abnormality from the full-blown picture of fatal air embolism with characteristic churning of the blood in the chambers of the heart. Most pastes used in abortion contain a fatty base; should such pastes be embolized to the lungs or brain, their presence should be demonstrable by special microscopic techniques. An expert chemical and spectrographic examination of the blood might well be of value in death supposed to be due to the introduction of toxic solutions by syringe.

Finally, evidence as to whether an abortion was self-induced or was the result of interference by an outside party can seldom be given unequivocally on the basis of the post-mortem examination alone. The pathologist will be led by the general assumption that the greater the injury produced, the more likely was it to have resulted from the woman's own efforts. It is of course possible that an abortionist may be very unskilled—only practice makes perfect—but it is far less likely that a woman, even given some special knowledge, will perform a clean surgical operation upon herself.

The 'patient' of the competent abortionist is likely to die only from those conditions that are unpredictable—vagal shock and embolism. It is in these cases that the circumstantial evidence—the place of death, the presence or absence of equipment, etc.—becomes so important and dictates the need for a visit by the pathologist to the scene. Even then, the wide variations in pathological processes must be taken into consideration and exceptions to general rules must sometimes be admitted as possibilities.

Concealment of birth or of pregnancy

Only the mother may be available for expert medical examination in cases involving these unusual charges and proof of recent delivery will depend largely on the clinical findings. The child is likely to have been close to or at full term and manifest enlargement of the uterus may well be found together with evidence of recent stretching of the abdomen—the typical recent red *striae gravidarum*. The uterus remains easily palpable for about 10 days after giving birth and the cervix may be flabby and/or torn. A typical bloody discharge, the lochia, persists for some 3 days to be replaced by a more normal appearing post-partum discharge which lasts for a further week; microscopy of this may prove its nature. Evidence of tearing of the perineum can be of great value—it need not necessarily occur and tears could conceivably be due to causes other than the passage of the fetus; but this is the most likely cause and the extent of laceration may suggest the maturity of the child.

Some time can elapse in cases of concealment—or of infanticide or child murder—before the need for examination becomes apparent. There will, then, be wide variation in the findings as some women return to normal much faster or slower than the average; it is generally accepted that positive proof of delivery, sufficient to satisfy the Court, will be difficult to obtain in the living person after a lapse of 8–10 days.

If the body of the infant is discovered its examination will follow the lines indicated below, in the sections Child Destruction and Child Murder, but it should be noted that there is a presumption of a live birth in the Scottish offence of concealment of pregnancy.

Child destruction

The main medical evidence peculiar to this charge concerns the legal viability of the child—has it or has it not achieved the 28th week of intrauterine life? The evidence is based on two main sets of observations—the general appearance of the fetus and the presence of centres of ossification in various bones.

By the 28th week, the fetus will have developed easily recognizable external sex organs but the testes are not descended into the scrotum; it will have head and body hair together with eyebrows and eyelashes; the skin will be developed and creased; and the nails will almost have reached the ends of the digits. The length from crown to heel is classically 35 cm (14 in). This is based on the formula that, after the fourth month, the length of the fetus in centimetres is five times the month of gestation (or, in inches, twice the month). There will be significant variations about this mean—at 7 months the possible scatter is likely to lie between 33 and 38 cm (13 and 15 in). The weight at this point is generally between 1.1 and 1.6 kg (2½ and 3½ lb).

Centres of ossification have been explained in Chapter 1. Many centres appear early in fetal life and are of little legal significance. Those that appear at or around the critical period include:

20th week:	calcaneus bone of heel;
24th week:	manubrium (upper end) of breast bone;
28th week:	talus bone of heel, first segment of the sternum (breast bone) proper;
32nd week:	last segment of breast bone;

At term: lower end of femur (thigh bone); cuboid bone of the foot, upper end of tibia (shin bone).

In general it is the presence of ossification centres that has the greatest significance; the negative evidence of their absence is less valuable.

Infanticide or child murder

The great majority of instances of child murder or infanticide occur during the first 24 hours of the infant's life. The basic pathological problem is, therefore, to distinguish between wilful killing and stillbirth, which has been defined on page 60. Since it is for the prosecution to prove a live birth, the medical evidence divides logically into two main categories—first, as to whether the child was, in fact, born alive and achieved a separate existence and, secondly, as to indications of an unnatural death.

Evidence of a live birth simply in the sense of full extrusion from the mother is almost impossible to give from a pathological examination but it may well be possible to assert that a live birth was, at least, improbable. Thus, it is unusual for an immature infant of less than 7 months' gestation to be born live; monstrous abnormalities of various sorts—in particular anencephaly (lack of a brain)—may be incompatible with life and the pathologist can generally give a firm opinion; maceration is certain evidence of this type as it constitutes *aseptic* degeneration of the fetal tissues following death *in utero*.

Positive evidence of a separate existence may also be derived from the post-mortem examination.

Major interest centres on the condition of the lungs which, as described in Chapter 1, are not only without function *in utero* but are relatively isolated from the general blood circulation. Fetal lungs are, therefore, virtually solid organs, homogeneous in consistency and colour. The effect of reflex inspiration of air at birth is to expand the lungs, a process which, in turn, initiates the true pulmonary respiratory blood circulation; both these processes take time—a matter of minutes—and, until they are fully established, the lungs may vary from place to place as to the degree of aeration and of vascularization. Thus, as the lungs fill the chest cavity they change in colour from purple to mottled pink and they increase in weight. These general changes can be further demonstrated by the so-called hydrostatic test or by microscopy.

The basis of the hydrostatic test is that an organ that contains air will float in water whereas one that does not will sink. Since aeration may be irregular, the lungs must be tested one by one, then lobe by lobe, and finally, and if necessary, piece by piece.

It is customary to decry the hydrostatic test. It appears to me to be a good practical test which has suffered from being given too great a 'scientific' significance as a single observation; this has resulted in the elaboration of theoretical objections that would be invalid if the post-mortem findings were taken as a composite whole. It is true, for example, that a child could have a separate existence and then develop disease of the lungs of such a type as to make them sink in water; but it has been pointed out that such disease would constitute a natural cause of death and despite a 'false' result no harm would be done because the charge of infanticide would rightly fail. The occurrence of a spurious flotation of the lungs is a far more important, and a more practical, objection to the test. It might arise in two ways. First, there is the possibility of artificial mouth-to-mouth respiration having been given. It is said that satisfactory aeration of the fetal lung by this means is difficult to achieve and that, even if it is effective, the pulmonary circulation would not be started—the appearances of the lungs would, therefore, be different from those of normal breathing. It could, however, be a difficult pathological decision to make. Secondly, there is a very real problem of putrefaction and aeration of the lungs by gas-forming bacteria. Compression of the lung tissue, which fails to remove inspired air but does discharge putrefactive gases, has been recommended to distinguish the two but the manoeuvre is clearly open to misinterpretation. It is a matter in the main of common sense and looking at the overall picture—if there is putrefaction of the lungs there will be putrefaction elsewhere, but the near impossibility of diagnosing a separate existence from the pulmonary findings in the presence of even early decomposition is stressed by all authorities. The most objective differentiation is to be made through microscopy; there is little histological similarity between freshly aerated and markedly putrefied lungs but the appearances of aeration *and* putrefaction may be very confusing. Some of the microscopic changes that indicate the occurrence of normal breathing are subtle while others depend upon survival for some time; there is no space for their detailed discussion here and the interested reader is referred to the classic article by Osborn[19].

Although the condition of the lungs has been discussed in detail, 'some other signs of a separate existence' must also be sought. Thus, the presence of gulped air in the stomach and intestine has been suggested as being valid evidence; anoxic convulsions are not, however, evidence of life and this sign could only be acceptable when combined with evidence of aeration of the lungs. Presence of food in the stomach or bowel would, of course, be evidence of a separate existence but this would imply long-term survival. The main evidence of this degree of survival is to be found in the umbilical cord which characteristically shows an inflammatory disposal reaction at the abdominal wall approximately 2 days after birth. The cord is shed on the 5th or 6th day but the time may be longer or shorter; the umbilical scar is healed in 10–12 days.

There remains the evidence to be drawn as to whether the infant's death was, in fact, due to 'some wilful act or omission'. There are very few limits to the way in which an infant may be murdered—widespread generalized violence, suffocation in its many forms, strangling, including the use of the readily available umbilical cord, drowning and wounding by one method or another are the commonest methods of infanticide. The pathology of all is described elsewhere and needs no repetition here.

It should, however, be stressed that the differentiation of homicide from accident or from natural disease is exceptionally difficult in the newborn period. Thus, the distinction between death due to natural asphyxia of central origin and that due to the application of a pillow to the face may be impossible, while frightened mothers can and do suffocate their infants accidentally; intracranial haemorrhage due to natural birth trauma may be indistinguishable from that due to deliberate violence, precipitate labour does occur and newborn infants *can* slip through the hands to the floor; an infant *may* drown in its own amniotic fluid; the umbilical cord *does* sometimes entangle with the child's neck and, in a distraught state, mothers may

[19] Osborn, G. R. (1953). Pathology of the lung in stillbirth and neonatal death. In *Modern Trends in Forensic Medicine*. Ed. by K. Simpson, Ch. 2. London; Butterworths.

attempt to kill a baby that has never lived. So much depends in each case on the circumstantial evidence and, again, it is the total picture that counts; it would be a brave pathologist who was convinced that he could correctly diagnose every newborn death on his unsupported post-mortem findings alone.

Nothing has been said about infanticide by omission, and it is the experience of most authorities that deliberate killing of babies by abandonment alone is surprisingly rare. A large proportion of embarrassing dead newborn infants are, however, hidden and this is irrespective of stillbirth or of whether death was due to natural or unnatural causes. Discovery is often delayed and in many instances changes due to putrefaction or animal scavengers may be so severe that the pathologist can do no more than state that there is no way of proving a separate existence. The possible procedures then include a charge of concealment of birth or, far more often, the issue of a certificate of stillbirth.

20

Injury and death in infancy and childhood

Although only a small proportion of deaths in infants and children are of criminal origin, many of them are obscure and may give rise to suspicion. Lawyers and doctors may find the pathological, sociological and criminological aspects more complex than appears at first sight.

Natural death in childhood

Natural death in the first 2 or 3 days of life is especially important as it is in this phase that child murder is most probable. The proportion of 'neonatal deaths'[1] that arise in the first 24 hours of life is high, varying between 30 per cent and 40 per cent largely according to the medical skills available; a further 15 per cent occur between 24 and 48 hours after delivery. Thus, approximately half of all such deaths take place within the first 2 days of life. There is a very close association with prematurity—a premature infant being defined as one with a birth weight of less than 2.5 kg (5½ lb). Over 50 per cent of all stillbirths and neonatal deaths occur in premature babies and the smaller the infant, the less are its chances of survival. Only some one in 20 or 30 babies weighing less than 1.25 kg (2¾ lb) will survive for 28 days despite the fact that approximately half are born alive—generally to die within a few hours. It requires only a small increase in birth weight to improve the prospects of survival very markedly and, within the weight bracket 1.5–2.0 kg (3⅓–4½ lb), nearly three-quarters should survive given modern medical attention.

Lack of oxygen resulting from damage to the placenta or cord is a common cause of stillbirth but the signs of hypoxia (see Chapter 13) are found in only some 10 per cent of neonatal deaths due to natural causes. Indeed, an autopsy indication of oxygen starvation in a mature infant should give pause for thought. However, deaths due to birth trauma make up what is probably the most important group from the medico-legal aspect because they may be difficult to distinguish from homicidal injury. These are rare in well-conducted obstetric practice and probably account for less than 5 per cent of deaths that follow live birth. Prematurity plays its part here too—the brain of a small baby is particularly susceptible—but, obviously, the unusually large infant is also at risk. Although

[1] The 'neonatal' period is defined as the first 28 days of extrauterine life.

subdural haemorrhage is rare in fetal fatalities taken as a whole (it has a general incidence of about 4 per cent), it is an almost invariable finding in death due to birth injury; since this lesion also results from homicidal injury to the infant's skull, its forensic significance needs no emphasis. In the end result, the true interpretation of a fatal injury discovered in this period may depend upon the combined evidence of the obstetrician, the pathologist and the police authority[2].

After the immediate postnatal period, the majority of infant deaths are the result either of infection or of congenital abnormalities. The former are being rapidly eliminated as a result of improved antenatal and postnatal care; syphilis, for example, used to be a prominent cause of neonatal death but is by now virtually non-existent. Congenital defects that may result in sudden death of the neonate are confined in practice to the cardiovascular and central nervous systems and to biochemical abnormalities that are not apparent on ordinary post-mortem dissection.

Congenital abnormalities of the cardiovascular system are mainly associated with failure of the heart to establish its four chambers with normal relationships—if, for example, the interventricular septum (see page 6) is inadequately developed, one is left with the classic 'hole in the heart' baby. Alternatively, the distinction between systemic and pulmonary circulations may not be achieved or the intrauterine cardiac anatomy (see page 7) may persist into extrauterine life.

The main abnormalities of the central nervous system include anencephaly—that is, absence or partial absence of the brain—which often results in stillbirth. Otherwise, there may be obstruction to the normal flow of cerebrospinal fluid that results in hydrocephalus ('water on the brain'), or the protective skeletal covering of the spinal cord may develop inadequately which leads to herniation of the spinal cord or of its surrounding membranes—so-called 'spina bifida'.

Anatomic abnormalities of all sorts account for at least 15 per cent of neonatal deaths.

Biochemical defects may be concerned with the metabolism of carbohydrates, of proteins or of fats; when they occur in the neonate they are known as 'inborn errors of metabolism'. Some of these—for example, phenylketonuria—may cause severe and irreparable damage, including injury to the brain.

Congenital disease may be due to chromosomal disorders, to genetic abnormalities or to environmental factors. Although it is convenient to speak of the last two as distinct categories, there is, in practice, something of a continuum between the conditions—from monogenetic, through multifactorial to purely environmental disease.

Environmental factors may interfere with the development of the fetus by reason of a specific insult, the end result depending greatly upon the actual time of the adverse stimulus. Basically, the more primitive the tissue at the time of attack, the more profound will be the effect; hence, infection in the mother—particularly by the rubella (or German measles) virus—or by drugs that interfere with the proper development of the fetus—of which thalidomide is the prime example—will have maximal effect in the first 3 months of pregnancy. By contrast, the effect of environmental factors that act upon the developed fetus as opposed to the

---

[2] The figures quoted for natural death are based on those kindly provided to the author by Dr J. C. H. Dunlop who analysed the records of the Simpson Memorial Maternity Pavilion, Edinburgh. They therefore represent the experience of a major obstetric unit that has ideal facilities but, at the same time, accepts many cases that are referred because of their difficulty.

developing embryo, will increase *pari passu* with growth; in such conditions, of which Rhesus incompatibility is a good example, premature birth may be a positive advantage.

The inheritance of genes has been described in Chapter 18. Only very occasionally is a harmful gene transmitted as a dominant characteristic—that responsible for Huntingdon's chorea is one example. Otherwise, recessive genes only express themselves because they are sex-linked or because they meet as an allelic pair. In either case, the chances of a repetition of the occurrence can be predicted statistically. More often, however, congenital disease is determined by a combination of factors. A familial abnormality of low penetrance will appear clinically only if the total hereditary environment is propitious. When this occurs, an abnormality is likely to recur in later pregnancies. For example, some 10 per cent of families with one child suffering from spina bifida will have a recurrence. But such assessments are no more than well-founded approximations and the parents' dilemma is epitomized if one turns the statement round—90 per cent of such families will *not* have a second affected child.

The same applies when considering chromosomal disease, the chances of which can be predicted only in vague terms. Changes in the number or characteristics of chromosomes may be induced but the influence of ionizing irradiation on gene mutation is, at present, of uncertain significance. Currently, the most important factor determining chromosomal abnormality is maternal age; Down's syndrome, or mongolism, is some 15 times more common in the children of mothers aged over 40 years than it is in the general child-bearing population.

A major modern medico-legal interest therefore centres on the application of the Abortion Act 1967, s. 1(1)(b) (*see* Chapter 19). What, in effect, are the chances of accurately predicting—and preventing—the birth of a seriously handicapped child?

Prenatal diagnosis of congenital defects

Much current research is being undertaken in this field. The available methods are divisible into so-called non-invasive techniques and those that involve penetration of the fetal environment—the amniotic sac.

On the non-invasive methods, the use of X-rays to examine the fetus is certainly contraindicated and studies by ultrasonic scanning have not been proved to be innocuous. Estimation of the levels of α-fetoprotein in the serum of the mother may demonstrate severe defects of the fetal central nervous system before 20 weeks' pregnancy but, at present, the technique is of uncertain value and a proportion of cases will be missed.

Invasive techniques that involve the withdrawal of amniotic fluid from the fetal sac (*see Figure 19.1*) are more promising. The fluid obtained can be used for:

1. Direct diagnosis, by biochemical analyses, of open lesions of the fetal central nervous system—in particular, anencephaly and spina bifida.
2. Culture of cells from the amniotic fluid to detect chromosomal abnormalities—which can be identified after 10–20 days in tissue culture—or to demonstrate inborn errors of metabolism which may entail culture for 6 weeks before adequate enzyme assays can be made.

All of these techniques have their difficulties. First, there is a 10 per cent failure rate in obtaining fluid in the early—and, therefore, useful—stage of pregnancy and this may necessitate repeated amniocentesis (puncture of the sac). Secondly, every amniocentesis carries with it the risk of miscarriage which follows the procedure in about 0.5 per cent of cases, and elective abortion, if proven to be advisable, must be performed rather later in pregnancy than is desirable. Thirdly, and perhaps of greatest medico-legal importance, neither positive nor negative accuracy can be guaranteed; although about 95 per cent of the diagnoses of central nervous system lesions and of chromosome abnormalities are correct in skilled hands, enzymatic testing still has some way to go before achieving such accuracy[2a].

The medico-legal problems posed in the event of an error in diagnosis include the possibility of an action for damages on the part of a deformed fetus for an enforced inadequate life; the normal definitions of medical negligence will then apply (*see* Chapter 30), although actions for 'wrongful life' on the part of the infant are unlikely to succeed[2b]. Amniocentesis is a procedure that demands from the diagnostic subject a full understanding of all its hazards, whether these are actual or implied. Consent of a special nature is needed; a suitable form of consent is reproduced in Appendix L.

Good sense must also protect the genetic counsellor, who, with or without the benefit of amniocentesis, can only advise as to the wisdom of child-bearing on the basis of probabilities. The terms of the Congenital Disabilities (Civil Liability) Act 1976 ensure that well-considered advice will be protected provided that it is given in accordance with current medical practice and knowledge.

Sudden death in infancy

At one time it appeared that the number of 'cot deaths' was declining. The trend may have been more apparent than real as much depends on definitions and on the availability of diagnostic resources; my experience is that, currently, one in 400 live-born infants will die suddenly and unexpectedly. This particular form of sudden natural death still poses a baffling problem to forensic pathologists, so much so that it is now customary to give no more specific cause of death than 'sudden infant death syndrome' (SIDS). Briefly, the condition presents as an apparently healthy child being put to bed by unsuspecting parents and being found dead either at the next feed or at normal waking time. The process may be extremely rapid and silent; in one case that I have examined, an apparently healthy infant was placed in its carry-cot on the back seat of a car—it was found to be dead at the end of a 40-minute journey.

Cases may occur between the ages of 2 weeks and 2 years—the main incidence is at 3–4 months. They are reported all over the world but always have a seasonal association, the majority of deaths being in the colder months. There is a rather indefinite association with the lower socioeconomic groups but no type of family is immune—the children of doctors are often stricken. With some 25 000 deaths due to SIDS occurring annually in the USA and over 3000 in the UK, the condition presents as a major health problem. It also has great social importance. The tragedy in losing an infant child needs no emphasis; added to this, the death, being unexplained and of uncertain cause, attracts a medico-legal inquiry by definition.

The search for a 'cause' of SIDS has been world-wide and intensive, yet no satisfactory answer has been reached. Many explanations—ranging from trace-metal deficiency to allergy to cows' milk—have been proposed but no theory stands up to critical analysis. Much attention is currently being paid to 'sleep

---

[2a] A combination of the modern techniques of chorionic villus sampling and of recombinant DNA methods is now significantly altering the picture.

[2b] The case of McKay and another v. Essex Area Health Authority and another [1982] 2 All E.R. 771 has been decided against the infant plaintiff on the grounds, *inter alia*, that non-existence could not be shown to be preferable to an impaired life. The child was born before the application of the Congenital Disabilities (Civil Liability) Act 1976.

apnoea'—a periodic failure to breathe during sleep that occurs in adults and may be exaggerated in infancy—but such a physiological death cannot be proved by normal autopsy techniques. Acute viral infections have been suspected and viruses may, indeed, be isolated from the lungs; the problem of whether the organisms are causative of death or are present in a purely incidental role remains. One difficulty of interpretation of this and other laboratory findings lies in the merciful shortage of control cases—that is, infants of a similar age killed accidentally—which can be examined in parallel. There may be no common cause but rather a common presentation of a number of abnormal states that provide no anatomical evidence of their origin.

There are three definable groups of SIDS. In one group the death is wholly inexplicable. In the second group, which is the largest, some minor abnormality—often in the form of a mild upper respiratory tract problem—can be recalled in retrospect. In the third and smallest group, a manifest illness, unsuspected in life, is detected at post-mortem dissection. In the heat of emotion, it is not uncommon for parents to blame their medical practitioner for the death but seldom, if ever, is this justified in the face of the triviality of symptoms. As a corollary, parents may have intense feelings of guilt on their own part; sympathetic counselling is, therefore, called for[3] and the medico-legal investigation must be designed so as to cause the minimum additional distress. At the same time, it has to be said that post-mortem dissection is essential in every case to exclude the possibility of unlawful killing. The 'cot death story' is now widely known; four out of 200 deaths examined in Edinburgh were found to be unnatural in origin and the description given by the parents in all four was typical of SIDS[4].

Interestingly, the condition of 'overlaying', which occupied so prominent a position in the forensic pathology of 50 years ago, is now virtually unknown. It is arguable that many such cases were, in fact, examples of SIDS.

Accidental death in childhood

Many forms of accidental death that are likely to occur in childhood are discussed in specific terms under the various headings in this book. These deaths do, however, form a special group—first, because there is a volume of legislation aimed at protection of the very young and, as a consequence, an offence may have been committed despite the undisputed fact that death was accidental while, secondly, the most common defence against a charge of infanticide, child murder or homicide of a young person is to suggest that the fatal injury resulted from an accident—the pathological distinction is of major importance and may be very difficult to make.

Many accidental deaths in this age group are asphyxial in nature and, of these, death from burning is comparatively common. Infants and children may be left unattended and be killed as a fire engulfs a whole house or hotel. More commonly, children accidentally pour boiling liquids from the stove on to themselves as a result of curiosity or they are exposed to an unguarded fire from which their clothes are accidentally lit. It is an offence for any person of the age of 16 or over having charge of a person under the age of 12 (or 7 in Scotland), without taking reasonable precautions, to allow the child to be burned or scalded by reason of being in a room containing an open-fire grate or any heating appliance insufficiently protected to guard against the risk of the child being injured[5].

[3] The advice of the Foundation for the Study of Infant Deaths is invaluable and is readily available.

[4] Without wishing to complicate the situation unduly, the possibility must be included of true cot deaths occurring in infants who have been accidentally injured during life—the Edinburgh series of cases contains one such instance.

[5] Children and Young Persons Act 1933, s. 11 as amended; Children and Young Persons (Scotland) Act 1937, s. 22. Should death or serious injury result, the penalty on summary conviction is a fine not exceeding £50!

The same Acts[6] also refer to the relationship of acute alcoholism and suffocation by overlaying in bed, a charge of neglect being possible if a child under 3 years old has been overlaid by a person aged 16 years or more who was under the influence of drink; even in the absence of drunkenness, true accidental overlaying may occur, particularly in the appalling housing conditions that still persist in many major cities. Asphyxial deaths in sleeping accommodation—be it crib, pram, cot or parents' bed—pose special problems. They may, as discussed before, be natural and they may be accidental. It has, however, to be reiterated that accidental asphyxia in infancy must be accepted as a cause of death with caution; it may be difficult, if not impossible, to distinguish pathologically between a baby that has been accidentally trapped face down on its pillow and one that has been held in that position so as to leave no mark on the back of the head or body; cot deaths themselves pose the same basic problem. Similar difficulties surround the occasional case in which an infant is strangled by its restraining harness; only rarely can the pathologist do other than describe the cause of death leaving the circumstantial evidence to indicate the way in which it arose.

Accidental drowning in children may, of course, occur amongst the older age group while at play. Drowning in infancy happens not uncommonly in the bath and, when accidental, death is often due to vagal inhibition of the heart—the baby slips backwards and water contacts the nasopharynx and larynx; as in adults, the finding of the conventional signs of drowning after death in the bath should arouse suspicion.

Asphyxia of central nervous system origin is usually a result of drug overdosage and is a tragically common cause of accidental death in younger children. The subject is discussed in greater detail in Chapter 22.

Death due to accidental injury may cause very great forensic difficulties when occurring in infancy and early childhood. Infant deaths due to road-traffic accidents are relatively rare due mainly, one suspects, to the improbability of drivers being drunk when transporting the baby. In older infancy and early childhood, automobile tragedies occur through inadvertent opening of car doors; child safety locks provide problems of their own, particularly in relation to escape from a post-crash fire, and the importance of adequate harness restraint for children in cars has received some of the attention it merits in the Transport Act 1981, s. 28. Death due to cervical spinal fracture is common in children subjected to quite minor deceleration trauma while standing unrestrained in vehicles. The frequency of pedestrian deaths in childhood needs no emphasis; they are doubly distressing in their emotional effects not only on the bereaved parents but also on the driver who, especially where this age group is concerned, may well have been blameless. Children may fall down the stairs or out of windows; again, the distinction between accident and homicide must depend very largely on the circumstantial evidence.

Children at play present a special problem. The provision of playgrounds is now expected and the apparatus is often used by children older than those for whom it was intended. Moreover, swings and roundabouts tend to be operated by the older children to an extent beyond the capacity of toddlers. Head injury and limb fractures are not uncommon results.

Perhaps the most difficult diagnostic area in accidental infant death concerns the isolated head injury. Such injuries are often explained as 'the baby slipped off my shoulder while I tried to turn on the light', or 'I fell down the stairs with the baby in my arms'. There is no doubt that such accidents do occur and it may be impossible to distinguish the resultant injuries from those caused by deliberate dropping of the

---

[6] Section 1(2)(b) of the 1933 English and s. 12(2)(b) of the Scottish Acts.

baby from comparable positions purely through the pathological findings. False explanations of this type are, however, used to cloak deliberate injury of a different type—homicidal head injuries in infancy are often caused by direct manual violence or by swinging the child by the feet against a wall or other solid object. Certain features may help to distinguish these injuries in the post-mortem dissection. First, there is the degree of injury that may be greatly in excess of that likely from the given explanation. Secondly, the position and external appearances of the injury may give rise to suspicion. Thus, a blow from the hand may leave no external mark and the resulting deep bruising and fracture may be markedly localized to one side of the head whereas injuries due to a fall, which are uncomplicated by bruising of the shoulder or arm, are more likely to be vertical in presentation. The most important cause for suspicion is the unexpected finding of a head injury in a death purported to be natural—the great majority of genuine accidental injuries will be reported immediately to the doctor.

Deliberate injury in infancy and childhood

There remains for discussion one important condition which is far more common than is generally suspected[7]—that is, the 'battered baby syndrome' which should, less emotionally, be referred to as 'repetitive non-accidental injury in childhood'. The term 'battered child' was chosen deliberately for its impact by Kempe to whom must be given the major credit for bringing the subject to public notice[8].

Non-accidental injury in childhood

From approximately 1945, a syndrome describing head injury and multiple limb fractures in children[9] was regarded as a clinical entity; only in the mid-1950s was it realized that these children were suffering from repeated injury inflicted by those responsible for their care—generally including one or both parents. Children often come to autopsy as a result of such treatment but the main bulk of sufferers present as clinical and sociological problems; one of the most disturbing features is that violence breeds violence—a high proportion of those who deliberately injure their children were themselves the objects of similar assault. Estimates vary as to the number of children who will die each year as a result of being 'battered' in Great Britain. It has been put as high as between 450 and 750 but a more realistic figure, supported by the NSPCC, is in the region of 100 per annum[10]. These derive from a

[7] Some 2 per cent of infant deaths between the ages of 4 weeks and 1 year are due to premeditated violence (*Memorandum of the Standing Medical Advisory Committee for the Central Health Service Council* (1970). London; DHSS).

[8] *See* the original paper: Kempe, C. H. *et al.* (1962), The battered child syndrome, *Journal of the American Medical Association*, **181**, 17. A recent collection of papers on the subject is contained in Franklin, A. W. (ed.) (1977), *The Challenge of Child Abuse*; London; Academic Press.

[9] Caffey, J. (1946). Multiple fractures in the long bones of infants suffering from chronic subdural hematoma. *American Journal of Roentgenology*, **56**, 163.

[10] The higher figure was given in 'A guide to management of non-accidental injury in children' prepared by a Working Party in the Department of Child Health, University of Newcastle-upon-Tyne. (*British Medical Journal* (1973), iv, 657.) The Report of the Committee on Child Health Services (Court, S. D. M. (Chairman) (1976). Cmnd. 6684, London; HMSO), quoted, without comment, figures from the British Paediatric Association indicating an annual mortality of 350–400. A far lower estimate is given in Jackson, A. D. M. (1982), Wednesday's children, *Journal of the Royal Society of Medicine*, **75**, 83, although he is not so optimistic about the future.

total of some 5000 affected: 20 per cent of these will be seriously injured.

The clinicosocial expression of the condition is difficult to summarize but, in general, the following may be found:

1. The family is often inadequate, maladjusted, immature and under social stress.
2. The child is usually aged less than 4 years and over half the cases, both fatal and non-fatal, are reported in the first 2 years of life.
3. There is often a delay in, or failure of, reporting the injuries to the medical practitioner and a false explanation of their cause is then given.
4. The commonest injuries are bruises and fractures, the latter being predominantly of the chest cage (especially the back), long bones and skull. Burns and bite marks are sometimes seen and severe injury to the abdominal viscera may occasionally be present. Injuries to the inside of the lips or the gums and dislocation of the teeth are almost diagnostic. Bizarre variations include deliberate poisoning or immersion. The child nearly always shows evidence of emotional and, sometimes, physical deprivation.
5. The most important diagnostic feature is that the injuries have been caused at different times.

Examination of the living should include, whenever possible, photography and radiography—these provide invaluable evidence of a permanent nature. A re-examination of a child suspected of being 'battered' some 24–48 hours after suspicions have been aroused is often helpful—bruises, in particular, may become more obvious and new ones may have appeared.

These classic clinical signs will be mirrored in fatal cases at post-mortem dissection, which must include a full X-ray study as a routine—the plates are invaluable not only as evidence of injury and its dating but also in assessing the possibility of bone disease as a causative or contributory factor. The examination should also include a microscopic study of the wounds in an attempt to establish their various ages. Death is often due to some terminal excessive injury resulting in cerebral or abdominal haemorrhage; a more difficult situation arises when it is effectively due to a combination of malnutrition and neglect which may be wilful or due merely to intellectual inadequacy—mothers tend to be young and intelligence quotients in one or both parents are, as a group, lower than in those who do not maltreat their children.

Considerable advances have been made in the care of children at risk, responsibility for the safety of whom rests with the local Director of Social Services. The social services, the NSPCC or the police may apply to the court to have a child placed in care. The police have emergency powers to keep a child in a safe place for up to 8 days without other authority and a Justice of the Peace may, on application by any person, make a 'place of safety order' lasting for 28 days[11]. Following, or alternative to this, there is the somewhat lengthy procedure for bringing care proceedings through the Juvenile Court which may make an order requiring the parents to take proper care of the child, make a supervision or hospital or guardianship order, or may make a care order bringing the child into the care of the local authority. The whole system is designed for the benefit of the child and, in the event of a conflict between the interests of the parents and of the child, the Court must arrange for the latter's separate representation[12]. Appeal against

[11] Children and Young Persons Act 1969, s. 1 and s. 28.
[12] Children Act 1975, s. 64.

the order of the Juvenile Court to the Crown Court is available to the child but not to the parent, although the parents may still act on behalf of an infant[13]. The evidence given by the person seeking a care order is confidential and the informant's name need not be divulged to the parents[14]. The care situation in Scotland is regulated by the Social Work (Scotland) Act 1968, part III (as amended by the Children Act 1975) under which much the same rules apply, the main administrative difference being the interposition of the children's 'Reporter'; cases are heard at a Children's Hearing and appeal, by child or parent, is to the Sheriff. Under both jurisdictions, the reporting in the newspapers or elsewhere of proceedings involving children is forbidden. In certain circumstances, local authorities may assume parental rights over children in their care and this includes the fact that they have been so placed for more than 3 years[15].

Non-accidental childhood injury raises questions of medical confidentiality. Doctors, possibly alerted by the health visitor, are likely to see the injured baby first and the medical profession cannot abnegate its obligations for eliminating a condition that, in mortality and morbidity alone, is a serious problem for society. Since the doctor's responsibility is to the patient, who is, in this case, the child, there can be no ethical contraindication to reporting the case but such reports should be made in the first instance to the Department of Social Services (or the children's department of the Area Health Services)—who have a clear 'right to know'—rather than to the police. The practical alternative is to arrange for admission to a paediatric hospital with the express purpose of protecting the patient[16]; the wide consultation that is regarded as of such importance in the management of the children[17] is best arranged from such a unit[18].

There are other practical problems in relation to repetitive non-accidental childhood injury which lie in the sphere of criminology. The predisposing conditions must be dealt with correctly and, in fatal cases, the pathological examination has its role to play in fully defining the nature and the sequence of the injuries discovered. This may affect the outcome of any criminal trial. A murderous attack on a child can seldom be excused on medical grounds; by contrast, the establishment of a true 'battered baby syndrome', which is widely accepted as the outcome of a psychosocial disorder, may rightly result in conviction for culpable homicide or manslaughter rather than murder and be followed by equally enlightened sentencing. However, while there was a move towards rehabilitation of the family rather than punishment a few years ago, some disillusionment is now evident among paediatricians. Certainly, there would seem to be two essentially different groups involved. On the one hand, there are those unstable parents who, in a perpetual state of exasperated inability to cope with family life, resort to violence as the only apparent escape from such pressures; these persons may well be treated as social invalids. On the other hand, parents who subject their children to deliberate torture by seating them on electric fires, burning them with cigarettes,

[13] B. v. Gloucestershire County Council [1980] 2 All E.R. 746.
[14] D. v. NSPCC [1978] A.C. 171.
[15] Children Act 1975, s. 57, s. 74; Social Work (Scotland) Act s. 16.
[16] Tunbridge Wells Study Group on non-accidental injury to children (1973). *British Medical Journal*, **iv**, 96.
[17] *Report of the Committee of Inquiry into the Care and Supervision provided in relation to Maria Colwell* (1974). London; HMSO.
[18] See also Arthur, L. J. H., *et al.* (1976). Non-accidental injury in children: What we do in Derby, *British Medical Journal*, **i**, 1363, for an account of the team approach.

biting and the like cannot be deserving of public sympathy. The pathologist makes a further contribution to criminology in distinguishing between these two types of injury.

The concept of what constitutes child abuse has been greatly extended in recent years—particularly so as to include sexual and emotional abuse. Whether as a result of this or because of a real increase in incidence, the number of reported cases of child abuse grows every year. Neither sexual nor emotional abuse is easy to demonstrate objectively and the diagnosis may, on occasion, be hotly disputed—especially if it is reached on a unilateral basis[19].

Deliberate injury to children is a social evil which cannot be solved by unilateral action—be it on the part of the medical profession, the health visitors, the social workers or the police. It is a problem that emphasizes particularly well the interdependence of forensic and community services in the protection of the individual. Emotion is, however, an uneasy motivator and it is well to remember the alternative view which is that the existence of 'at-risk registers' and the like may serve to frighten parents who have no cause for guilt; children who are genuinely accidentally injured may, as a result, be deprived of necessary treatment. Finding the correct balance of views may be less easy than appears[20].

[19] Dyer, C. (1987) First High Court judgment on sex abuse in Cleveland, *British Medical Journal*, **295**, 382.
[20] Child abuse: the swing of the pendulum. *British Medical Journal* (1981), **283**, 170.

21

Sexual offences

Expert medical evidence will be called in relation to a number of offences associated with sexual activity, among which the following will be discussed in some detail:

1. Rape.
2. Inflicting clandestine injury on a woman.
3. Indecent assault.
4. Lewd, indecent or libidinous practices.
5. Indecency with children.
6. Homosexual offences.
7. Incest.

The extent and value of such evidence will vary according to the charges laid.

The law

The majority of sexual offences are defined in England and Wales by the Sexual Offences Acts 1956 to 1976. There is a principally psychiatric medico-legal interest in the Indecency with Children Act 1960 (and with indecent exposure—dealt with by the Vagrancy Act 1824). Homosexual practices conducted between consenting adults in privacy are no longer regarded as criminal by virtue of the Sexual Offences Act 1967.

In Scotland, the more serious sexual offences are dealt with at common law. Otherwise, the earlier enactments of the Criminal Law Amendment Acts 1885 to 1928 are consolidated in the Sexual Offences (Scotland) Act 1976.

Consent and age in sexual offences

Rape has recently been redefined in England and Wales. A man commits rape if he has unlawful sexual intercourse with a woman who at the time of the intercourse does not consent to it and, at the time, he knows that she does not consent to the intercourse or he is reckless as to whether she consents (Sexual Offences (Amendment) Act 1976, s. 1). This definition derives from the Heilbron

Committee[1] which was established largely as a result of the decision that, when a man accused of rape honestly believed the woman to have consented, the reasonableness of the accused's mistake was irrelevant as a matter of law[2]; despite the resulting public indignation, the principle was approved by the National Council for Civil Liberties. In Scotland, rape is a crime at common law defined as 'the carnal knowledge of a female by a male person obtained by overcoming her will'. It follows that, so long as there is no consent, the age of the victim is immaterial to a charge of rape; age, however, becomes important in the event of apparent consent by a young person.

Irrespective of consent, intercourse with a girl under the age of 16 is unlawful. To have intercourse with a girl below the age of 13 years is a very serious, and distinct, offence and there is no defence on the basis of mistaking her age[3]. In Scotland, the common law age for constructive rape is 12 years; it might be possible to raise the defence of error as to age in the event of such a charge being laid.

The age of the victim between 13 and 16 years is significant under both jurisdictions. In England, having or attempting to have intercourse with a girl above the age of 13 and under 16 years constitutes the offence of having or attempting to have unlawful sexual intercourse, rather than rape. Section 4 of the 1976 Act defines a similar offence in Scotland. Under both codes it is a defence for a man under the age of 24, who has not been previously charged with a like offence, to prove he had reasonable cause to believe that the girl was aged 16 or over[4].

In England, a boy aged less than 14 years is presumed incapable of committing rape and this presumption is irrebuttable; such a boy could, however, be convicted of indecent assault. No such presumption exists in Scots law.

Irrespective of age, consent to sexual intercourse is considered impossible in the case of a mental defective as defined by the Sexual Offences Act 1956, s. 7 or the Mental Health (Scotland) Act 1984, s. 106 (6). The situation is similar to that of a normal girl below the age of 16. It is a defence for the accused to prove that he did not know and had no reason to suspect that a girl was a defective and any consent given, although invalid in law, would certainly mitigate the offence. The meaning of 'mental defective' in s. 7 of the 1956 Act as amended by the Mental Health Act 1959, s. 127 was further modified by the Mental Health (Amendment) Act 1982, s. 1 and Sch. 3.

Age and consent are relevant also in the offence of indecent assault—an offence that falls short of rape generally because of absence of penetration of the vulva, although this may not necessarily be the reason (see H.M.Adv. v. Logan, below). Under the 1956 Act it is an offence in England and Wales to commit an indecent assault on a man or woman[5]. Children under 16 cannot give legal consent and, therefore, indecent assault on them must always be an offence; s. 14 provides specific statutory support for this generalization. The potential defence of error as

---

[1] Report of the Advisory Group on the Law of Rape (1975). Cmnd. 6352. London; HMSO.
[2] Morgan and others v. DPP (1975). 61 Cr. App. R. 136; an extraordinary case involving connivance by the woman's husband. An equally surprising case was reported shortly afterwards (R. v. Cogan, R. v. Leak [1976] 1 Q.B. 217).
[3] Sexual Offences Act 1956, s. 5; Sexual Offences (Scotland) Act, s. 3.
[4] In the event of a man 'marrying' a girl below the age of 16 it is a defence throughout Great Britain, irrespective of the man's age or of the number of convictions, that he believed her to be his wife and had reasonable cause for that belief (Marriage Act 1949; Marriage (Scotland) Act 1977; Sexual Offences Act 1956; Sexual Offences (Scotland) Act 1976). A similar exception is made in connection with a charge of indecent assault.
[5] As compared with rape which, in the United Kingdom, can only be perpetrated by a man on a woman.

to age by a young man is not available against a charge of indecent assault, unless it should arise in association with 'marriage'.

An actual assault is necessary to establish a charge of indecent assault and, to cover those cases in which no assault was alleged, the Indecency with Children Act 1960 was applied to England and Wales; under the Act, it is an offence for a person to commit an act of gross indecency with or towards a child under the age of 14. In Scotland, these cases are loosely referred to as 'lewd and libidinous practices' which are an offence at common law when associated with children below the age of puberty (12 years in relation to girls). Between the ages of 12 and 16, the offence is defined in the Sexual Offences (Scotland) Act 1976, s. 5; consent is no defence nor is error as to age.

Age is important in relation to homosexual offences under the Sexual Offences Act 1967 and under the Criminal Justice (Scotland) Act 1980, s. 80 in which an adult is defined as any person more than 21 years of age. A boy aged less than 14 cannot be charged with buggery in England though he can be charged with indecent assault. The more serious homosexual offences are dealt with at common law in Scotland; in theory, though probably not in practice, there is no limitation as to age. Gross indecency between males is covered by the Criminal Justice (Scotland) Act, s. 80; a consenting child cannot be held guilty of such an offence.

Medical evidence in alleged rape

The medical evidence to be obtained in a case of alleged rape can be directed to answering the questions implied in the wording of the definitions—was there sexual intercourse, was there lack of consent and, if so, what was done by the man to overcome the woman's will? The evidence may be derived from a medical examination both of the victim and of the accused.

Unlawful sexual intercourse

Unlawfulness in relation to age and mental state has been discussed above. After the age of legal consent, unlawful sexual intercourse may be defined as intercourse out of wedlock and, from this, it has been extrapolated that a man cannot be charged with the rape of his wife unless, for example, there is a legal separation order in force[6]. The archaic nature of such a presumption and its consequent dubiety is beautifully argued by Gordon with particular respect to Scotland[7]. If there is such a thing as 'irrevocable privilege' for a husband, it is anomalous to suggest that he could be charged with assault in circumstances that, outside marriage, would constitute rape, yet there is no doubt that such a charge would be valid in England[8]. Medical evidence of sexual offence might, therefore, be called even within the confines of marriage.

Sexual intercourse is defined as intercourse intended to be within the vagina; by an extraordinary process of reasoning, a man cannot rape a woman in a deviate fashion nor is there such an offence as an attempt to do so[9]. The medical examiner

[6] R. v. Clarke (1949) 33 Cr. App. R. 216. See R. v. Steele (1976) 65 Cr. App. R. 22 for an extension of the exception.
[7] The Criminal Law of Scotland (1978), p. 888, quoting, in particular, Willis J. in R. v. Clarence [1888] 22 Q.B.D. 23, 33.
[8] R. v. Miller [1954] 2 Q.B. 282.
[9] R. v. O'Sullivan [1981] Crim. L.R. 406. But see, for example, recent Australian legislation (e.g. Crimes (Sexual Offences) Act 1980 (Victoria)) in which the concept of rape is greatly extended.

may well have little difficulty in saying positively that sexual intercourse has taken place when a previously virginal hymen has been recently penetrated, particularly if this has been accompanied by some force. The external genitalia are often bruised or swollen and obvious lacerations of the hymen, together with bleeding, may well be present, the main problem being to differentiate the latter from menstrual efflux. Difficulties arise when such typical signs are lacking as may well be the case in the non-virginal state. The absence of lacerations does not necessarily exclude penetration even when previous intercourse can be discounted; the hymen may be naturally lax and sufficiently patent to admit a penis or it may have been rendered so by the use of tampons or by masturbation. The certain sign of penetration is the finding of spermatozoa in the deeper portion of the vagina. It has been stated that recognizable spermatozoa can be found 3 days or more after intercourse and that morphologically perfect specimens with tails are present up to 16 hours after deposition[10]. In my experience, such survival is the exception rather than the rule; while being abundant at 2 hours, perfect forms are rare at 12 hours, the usual finding at that time being of 'scanty bodies indistinguishable from degenerating spermatozoal heads'. In any event, the taking of adequate swabs from within the vagina is an essential step in the examination of the suspected victim, certainly within 24 hours of the alleged offence. It is the positive finding that is of evidential value; a failure to identify spermatozoa is of little consequence as, in law, emission is not essential to sexual intercourse.

The difficulties facing the medical examiner have not yet been exhausted. Full penetration is not required to constitute rape, sexual intercourse being held to mean 'a degree of penetration of the vulva by the penis'; quite clearly, the doctor cannot, and should not be expected to, provide positive evidence on this point on the basis of a simple physical examination. Again, however, a search for spermatozoa may be of very great value; superficial swabs should be taken from the area between the labia in addition to those taken deeply as a positive finding in them would, save in exceptional circumstances, be very good evidence of intercourse within the legal definition[10a].

The examination of the suspect for evidence of sexual intercourse is generally unrewarding. The glans is very seldom found to be injured beyond what might be anticipated after legal sexual intercourse. Attempts to identify the woman's secretor substance on the male penis—somewhat after the fashion in the examination of bite marks (*see* Chapter 29)—would theoretically be useful, particularly in cases involving multiple potential assailants, but have proved disappointing in my experience. Others have suggested a search for cells from the vaginal epithelium, which have fairly individual staining properties, but the time during which they will be recognizable must be limited. During the process of the examination evidence of venereal disease may come to light and, in the event that the victim subsequently develops a similar disease, this might be useful supporting evidence. The alternative proposition, though less probable, might also hold good, the former state of chastity of the victim being no bar to a charge of rape.

The use of force or fear

Lack of consent is the basic ingredient of rape in England and Wales. The concept of lack of consent has been broadening so that it can now include what might be described as

---

[10] David, A. and Wilson, E. (1974). The persistence of seminal constituents in the human vagina. *Forensic Science*, **3**, 45. It is, perhaps, worth noting that these figures were obtained from studies following normal intramarital intercourse; see the very different results, in keeping with my own, reported by Sharpe, N. (1963), The significance of spermatozoa in victims of sexual offences, *Canadian Medical Association Journal*, **89**, 513.

[10a] Although rape is 'complete' on penetration, it continues until withdrawal (Kaitamaki v. The Queen [1984] 3 W.L.R. 137).

resigned acquiescence[11]. It follows that evidence of the use of force is not essential to a successful prosecution but it still represents very strong corroboration of lack of consent; it is, perhaps, now of particular relevance in relation to the definition of rape in Scotland.

The ultimate evidence of force is the death of the victim[12]. A careful pathological assessment of the mode of dying is then essential both to the prosecution and to the defence. However, the remainder of this section will be confined to uncomplicated rape.

It used to be said that the victim's resistance must be 'to the utmost' but this absolute term must be interpreted in a relative fashion; the important feature is unwillingness to take part throughout the act. The medical examiner is often in great difficulty here, it being a frequent finding that there is little tangible evidence of force or resistance either in the victim or in the assailant—particularly if several men have been involved. I have seen a case in which the vulval damage to the woman was such that an urgent hospital appointment was arranged, yet the most that could be discovered in the accused was a small abrasion over one eye. In another instance, two young men were convicted of rape; no injuries were found in either and those in the victim could only be described as 'no more than could be anticipated as a result of aggressive lovemaking'.

Many potential injuries in the victim are prevented by the interposition of clothing, and examination of the clothes is an essential part of the complete medical inspection. All doctors will be aware of the possibility of artefacts induced by the accuser herself but real difficulty occurs surprisingly seldom. An association with blood or seminal stains is evidence of genuineness but it is particularly important to examine with care the precise relationship between stains and tears as these may demonstrate anomalies as to timing; the scientific investigation of clothing is a matter for the laboratory but the doctor must be allowed to make his own assessment at the time of examination.

Injury to the accused may be minimal for the same reason. There may also be a gross disparity in size between victim and rapist and, as indicated above, less injury will be anticipated if there is more than one assailant. An element of subjectivity is almost inescapable and the medical evidence as to a struggle seldom carries more weight than does that derived from the circumstances.

Resistance to rape may be modified by fear, say, of reprisals against a third party, and there can be little or no medical evidence to be drawn on this score—other than a dubious inference from the lack of injury. There seems to be some difference in the English and Scots law on this point. In the former jurisdiction, a charge of rape would still stand under this type of duress. Scots law would, however, require threats of immediate harm rather than of future action; the Sexual Offences (Scotand) Act 1976, s. 2(1) prescribes a specific offence of procuring or attempting to procure by threats a woman to have unlawful sexual intercourse. Medical evidence might, however, be sought in the event that the will of the female is said to have been overcome by drugs—of which alcohol must be by

[11] R. v. Olugboja [1981] 3 W.L.R. 585. Suggestions that there may be such a thing as 'contributory negligence' to rape have been widely criticized. (*See* Lord Hailsham, L.C. reported in *The Times* (1982), Jan 12th, p. 1.)

[12] In England, the Homicide Act 1957, s. 1, abolished the concept of 'constructive malice' whereby the victim's death as part of the process of rape would have amounted to murder. In Scotland, death during rape would be murder only if the cause of death was unrelated to the act of rape (*see The Criminal Law of Scotland*, p. 745).

far the commonest. In practice, the medical examiner would be unlikely to be able to do more than take the necessary samples for laboratory analyses. The law is, again, of interest and importance. It is an offence under the Sexual Offences Act 1956, s. 4, 'to administer any drug, matter or thing to a woman with intent to stupify or overpower so as thereby to enable any person to have unlawful sexual intercourse with her'; there is a similar provision in the Sexual Offences (Scotland) Act 1976, s. 2(1)(c). It is accepted under common law in Scotland that rape itself can be committed by drugging a woman so that she becomes incapable of resisting the accused—drugging, in that it constitutes a means of overcoming the will of the victim is, in effect, a loose form of force. Only alcohol can have any real relevance and the prominent points would seem to be, first, that the woman must be plied with drink *in order* to overcome her resistance—the mere process of 'softening up' by excessive social drinking would be insufficient to substantiate a charge of rape[13]—and, secondly, that the woman must be deprived of the ability to consent or refuse consent to intercourse.

It is not rape in Scotland to have intercourse with a woman who is insensible through alcoholism of her own making or who is asleep[14]—if such a thing is possible. The reason given is that since the helplessly intoxicated woman is incapable of consenting or refusing consent, there can be no rape because rape involves intercourse against the woman's will[15]. Such cases provide examples of the Scottish offence of inflicting clandestine injury to a woman; they would constitute rape in England due to the absence of positive consent, the alternative of indecent assault being precluded by the act of intercourse. Medical evidence would certainly be called but since there was, by definition, no resistance and previous virginity would be unlikely, the evidence would probably be limited in practice to the demonstration of spermatozoa in the vagina.

Intercourse by fraud

Examples of rape by fraud include impersonation of the woman's husband, an offence defined as rape in both the Sexual Offences Act 1956, s. 1(2) and in the Sexual Offences (Scotland) Act 1976, s. 2(2). Obtaining intercourse by pretending to be giving medical treatment has been regarded as rape in England[16] but would probably be regarded as only fraud in Scotland. Again, the medical evidence would be likely to be limited to demonstration of emission in such cases.

Scientific evidence of a medical nature in rape

During the medical examination, the doctor will seek and retain certain specimens for laboratory study and analyses; these may be of non-human or of human biological nature.

The former need not be dealt with here as they will lie in the province of the forensic science laboratory—obvious examples would be the retention of any loose fibres, grass or seeds about the person or clothing which might provide rebutting or corroborative evidence of circumstantial detail.

[13] H.M.Adv. v. Logan 1936 J.C. 100.
[14] H.M.Adv. v. Sweenie (1858) 3 Irv. 109.
[15] H.M.Adv. v. Grainger and Rae 1932 J.C. 40.
[16] R. v. Flattery [1877] 2 Q.B.D. 410.

Although the biological specimens will probably be examined in a science laboratory, the interpretation of results may well fall to the medical witness. Those that may most often be of value include:

1. Blood stains and seminal stains from the clothing of both male and female. Seminal stains can be grouped on the ABO system in secretors while blood may well be fresh enough to demonstrate additional group antigens, 'serum groups' and specific enzyme systems. For these investigations to be of maximal value, blood and saliva samples must also be obtained from the female and from a suspect when this is possible. If the bloods are of different groups, the distribution of the stains between the couple may be of evidential value. The greatest caution must be maintained in interpreting results if victim and suspect are of the same group; this implies that both must be fully investigated as a routine. The use of the precise antigenic groups of both blood and semen to exclude or incriminate a suspect follows the pattern indicated in the section on paternity testing (*see* Chapter 18). Apparent seminal stains will also be examined for the presence of spermatozoa which may remain recognizable for long periods—up to 6 months—on fabric; admixture with other body fluids may, however, result in their early disappearance.
2. Pubic hair combings from both victim and accused. The presence of foreign hair will at least show proximity. Hair known to be from the two principals—i.e. obtained by plucking—must also be available for comparison.
3. Nail scrapings. To be examined for blood or tissue from the other party.
4. Any potential bite marks should be examined for the presence of saliva as described in Chapter 29. The use of similar preparations from the glans penis has been discussed above.

The nature of consent on the part of the person being examined is important (*see also* Chapter 30). An examination without consent is a potential assault and of, at least, doubtful evidential value. In cases of rape, there is little difficulty as to the woman because she will generally appreciate that an examination is an essential adjunct to her accusation; even so, it is well that the doctor should specifically warn her of the intimate nature of the examination as this may, albeit surprisingly, not be understood, particularly when the prime complainants are her parents. It is also important to emphasize that there is no confidentiality as regards the findings. The problem is more complex in the case of the accused, to whom the advantage of examination may be in doubt. Knight[17] says that 'consent must be obtained without fail after telling the accused person the object of the examination'. Glaister[18], who must be regarded as the Scottish authority, advises that 'it is not sufficient that the person to be examined offers no resistance or objection, for that may result solely from ignorance of his or her rights. The proper procedure is to inform the accused, in the presence of a third party, that the examiner has been asked by the authorities to make an examination, but that he can only do so after obtaining consent, which can be withheld, and that he will report the results of his examination whatever they may be'. No one would deny that the taking of blood or even the removal of pubic hair requires consent as the person examined sustains injury in the process—this principle will apply equally to the female. In addition, such investigations require the active participation of the suspect. The corollary is that,

[17] In *Legal Aspects of Medical Practice*, 3rd edn., p. 201.
[18] In *Medical Jurisprudence and Toxicology*, 13th edn., p. 56.

in the absence of consent, an examination must be confined to observation; such observation may, however, be tactile as well as visual[19]. Even so, increasing regard is being given to the interests both of the victim and of the public—particularly in relation to evidence that may be ephemeral. This is especially so in Scotland where it is extremely probable that an examination undertaken without consent but on the authority of a Sheriff's warrant would be regarded as a fair procedure[20]. The amount of force that might properly be used in making an examination under warrant is, however, still in dispute. The proper course would seem to be for the doctor to insure himself against a charge of unethical practice by requesting the Crown to seek a warrant on his behalf and to obtain the advice of the Procurator Fiscal on any subsequent points of difficulty; it would then be for the Court to decide on the admissibility of the evidence[20a].

Charges against practitioners

Charges of rape, of attempted rape or, more commonly, of indecent assault are not infrequently made against doctors and dentists in the course of their practice. The more serious charges almost invariably result from delusions, possibly wishful, arising under anaesthesia; dentists are, therefore, particularly at risk when they operate and anaesthetize single-handed, while the practice of 'horizontal dentistry' is psychologically predisposing to sexual fantasy on the part of the patient. The general medical examination would go far to exclude the possibility of rape but, in the event of deliberate premeditated fabrication, the 'patient' would be likely to inflict damage on her clothing and person. An interesting situation could arise in the event of the charges being substantially true. It would clearly be rape to give a woman an anaesthetic in order to have intercourse; on the other hand, Gordon[21] suggests that it is not rape to have sexual intercourse having drugged a woman for a lawful purpose such as to give an anaesthetic for an operation—*Grainger and Rae* would presumably apply.

The doctor is particularly open to charges of indecent assault—some of which arise from a genuine misunderstanding of the nature of an intended examination. It was once a truism that a doctor should not allow himself to be isolated with a female patient; such are the present economic conditions, however, that the counsel of chaperoning at all times cannot always be followed. It would, however, be foolhardy for a doctor to undertake an examination of the genitalia or even of the breasts in the absence of a female witness.

Medical evidence in attempted rape or indecent assault

The examination of a victim of assault with attempt to commit rape would follow the lines of investigation of any case of assault. Medical evidence would be called to assess the severity of the assault and this might derive from an examination of both parties.

Indecent assault, which is not a specific offence in Scotland, may be perpetrated homosexually or heterosexually by either sex. It must be overtly sexual, with an element of immodesty, and may be accompanied by violence ranging from severe

[19] Forrester v. H.M.Adv. 1952 JC 28 per Lord Carmont at p. 35.
[20] See H.M.Adv. v. Hay, discussed in Chapter 29, and H.M.Adv. v. Milford 1973 S.L.T. 12.
[20a] The taking of 'non-intimate' and 'intimate' samples is now governed in England and Wales by the Police and Criminal Evidence Act 1984.
[21] p. 886.

to mere touching—indeed the assault need only be psychic if physical contact is threatened; medical evidence becomes of decreasing value as the element of assault diminishes. The least traumatic offence is the commission of lewd or libidinous practice for which no physical contact is required. It may well be that the medical examination that is often required in such cases does more psychological harm to the very young girls who are involved than does the occurrence itself; the offence is limited to practices against girls under 16 and boys under 14 years, the only alternative in the case of offended adults being a charge of what is loosely known as 'indecent exposure'.

Incest

Incestuous relationships differ in England and Scotland. In England the Sexual Offences Act 1956 makes it an offence for a man to have intercourse with his mother, sister, daughter, granddaughter or half-sister; there may, of course, be further charges if the female is aged below 16 years[21a]. Similar relationships with the sexes reversed are also forbidden but a girl must be over 16 years old to be guilty of incest. The law in Scotland has taken a major step forward in the Incest and Related Offences (Scotland) Act 1986 which inserts new provisions in the Sexual Offences (Scotland) Act 1976. The prohibitions by way of consanguinity are still wider than those in England and include intercourse with a grandmother, aunt, niece, great grandmother and great granddaughter. Incest cannot now be committed by those related only by affinity and the absurdity of incest being impossible between bastard relatives is removed. The Scots incest and marriage laws are brought into conformity in that incest may be committed with an adoptive mother or daughter and a new separate offence of having intercourse with a stepchild under the age of 21, who has cohabited with the stepparent when aged below 18 years, is introduced. More significantly and farsightedly, a person aged over 16 years who is in a position of trust or authority over a child and who has sexual intercourse with that child when aged less than 16 years commits an offence which is punishable by imprisonment up to and including for life. The element of an abuse of trust, which is so essential to the concept of incest, is thus given due notice.

The conditions for proof of incest are the same as those for rape—there must be penetration but this need only be vulval. Medical and medico-scientific evidence in incest is largely confined to establishing the fact of intercourse in the female and either not excluding or excluding the suspect male. Cases seldom come to light immediately and it may well be that pregnancy provides the evidence of intercourse. In addition, the relationships might be tested as described in Chapter 18. Both parties are equally guilty of the crime but, in practice, the female is very rarely prosecuted. Deviate intercourse cannot be incest.

[21a] *See* Criminal Law Act 1977, s. 54 for incitement of a young girl to incest.

[22] Lev. 18:6–18. But the express prohibitions therein are regarded as examples of degrees of forbidden relationship—the Law of Scotland is, therefore, more strict as regards incest than is the Old Testament.

[23] H.M.Adv. v. R.M. 1969 J.C. 52.

[24] *The Law of Incest in Scotland* (1981). Scottish Law Commission Report No. 69, Cmnd. 8422. Edinburgh; HMSO.

Homosexual offences

Homosexual relationships between consenting women do not constitute an offence unless one of them is under 16 years of age and is, therefore, unable to consent to an indecent assault.

In England, sodomy is a form of buggery and consists of connection per anum with any other person; the term is slightly more restrictive in Scotland and refers to unnatural carnal connection between men.

Buggery is an offence in England under the Sexual Offences Act 1956, s. 12, but the Sexual Offences Act 1967, s. 1, provides that it is not so when performed in private by consenting parties who have both attained the age of 21. Merchant seamen and members of the armed forces have no such licence. Sodomy in Scotland is a separate common law crime. The Criminal Justice (Scotland) Act 1980, s. 80 now allows for private homosexual practices between consenting adults as in England.

Proof of penetration of the anus is needed to establish unnatural carnal connection but proof of emission is not required. As in rape, therefore, the examining doctor may be in great difficulty in the event of incomplete penetration but, in practice, serious resistance by the passive partner is unlikely to occur—full distension of the anus is probable. The signs likely to be discovered depend, therefore, on the habituation of the passive partner. In the case of a first offender, tenderness, oedema and, perhaps, laceration or bruising will be present around the anus. The orifice of the habitual passive sodomist by contrast becomes dilated and smooth, the sphincter is lax and, of greatest importance, loses its elasticity; the surrounding skin may become horny and may also show scars from earlier lacerations. The presence of traces of lubricant may provide suggestive evidence and the finding of spermatozoa on swabs prepared either from within the canal or from the anal mucosa will prove the act almost beyond dispute. But it must be admitted that, in many cases, there will be insufficient evidence for the doctor to reach a firm conclusion that unnatural intercourse has occurred. The pathologist examining a dead man may have difficulty in distinguishing true sodomy from the effects of post-mortem change; cases are often seen, particularly in young persons, where an apparently grossly patulous anus could only be ascribed to a post-mortem phenomenon.

The examination of the active partner is unlikely to provide much firm evidence. Certainly, the glans may be damaged—but this is not proof of anal connection; remnants of faeces or lubricant may be present beneath the foreskin in the unlikely event of a suspect not having washed himself before examination. In practice, convictions are more likely on a charge of gross indecency than on a charge of sodomy.

Transvestism and trans-sexualism

Although by no means an offence, transvestism—that is, changing into clothes of the other sex—or trans-sexualism—a psychiatric change which includes attempting to simulate the sexual appearances of the other sex—are of forensic significance on occasion. The close association of transvestism with the sexual asphyxias is discussed in Chapter 13; the problems of trans-sexualism and marriage are discussed in Chapter 17. Extremely sophisticated measures to alter the sexual characteristics of the body may be undertaken and have even caused considerable difficulty in the identification of mass casualties[22].

[22] *See* Stevens, P. J. (1970), *Fatal Civil Aircraft Accidents*, p. 149; Bristol; Wright.

Intercourse with animals

The English offence of buggery includes bestiality which can be committed by either a man or a woman with an animal[23]. Bestiality consists of intercourse per vaginam although Gordon (at page 895) believes that it can also be committed per anum. It is a common law crime in Scotland to have 'unnatural carnal connection' with an animal; it is doubtful if a woman could be so charged.

The offence is committed when there is penetration; emission is not essential. Veterinary evidence would be important if a small animal was used but the only medical evidence likely to be led in most cases would relate either to the presence of human sperm in an animal or to demonstrating an animal origin of sperm in the human vagina. Spermatozoa differ in size and shape according to species[24], some cells are, however, very similar to the human and the origin of stains and material on diagnostic swabs would probably be most easily demonstrable by serological methods (*see* page 40). Most acts of bestiality are conducted in privacy and there can, therefore, be little forensic medical experience of the offence; but the emphasis on bestiality in 'hard' pornography suggests that the subject may exert a surprising fascination.

[23] Sexual Offences Act 1956, s. 12.
[24] A readily available illustration is to be found in Smith, S. and Fiddes, F. S. (1955), *Forensic Medicine*, 10th edn., p. 305; London: Churchill.

22

Poisons and poisoning

Poisoning is of two main types—that which affects large sections of the community and that which involves individuals only. Environmental and industrial poisoning are the main components of the former category; the number of deaths and the extent of disability directly attributable to poisoning of the community reaches serious levels in most industrialized countries—their limitation is often a matter of legislation. Individual intoxication may be accidental, iatrogenic, suicidal or homicidal. While the last has certainly the greatest medico-legal significance, it is now rare compared with some decades ago; far more individuals die from accident or suicide.

Environmental poisoning

Basically, environmental poisoning results either from the effects of smoke pollutants in the air or from the presence of specific substances or elements in the surroundings as a whole. The major contributors to the former are coal fires and motor car exhausts.

The production of factory smoke is controlled through the activities of the Alkali and Clean Air Inspectorate and contributes surprisingly little to the total smoke pollution of the urban atmosphere. Most pollution comes from domestic coal fires the products of which, when reacting with a simple fog in windless conditions, produce the classic London 'pea-souper'. If the fog is not dispersed, there is a massive build-up of smoke particles and of the gas sulphur dioxide. Mortality and morbidity are related closely to the combined concentration of these substances, the majority of deaths occurring in those already suffering from disease of the lungs or heart. There were some 4000 excess deaths during 4 days of fog in London in 1952.

The most effective way of controlling this type of poisoning is through the limitation of smoke—it is doubtful if sulphur dioxide, which is the main industrial atmospheric contaminant, is harmful by itself. Local authorities are now empowered to regulate smoke production in their area[1] and it is a matter of general

---

[1] Clean Air Act 1956, s. 11. There is specific authority to try to control the level of sulphur dioxide by limiting the sulphur content of heating oil (Control of Pollution Act 1974, s. 76).

observation that the incidence of 'pea-soupers' has steadily declined; concurrently, there has been a reduction in the associated cardiopulmonary diseases which can, therefore, be regarded as controllable by legislation.

The effects of motor car exhausts stem from several factors. Depending on the efficiency of the engine, the exhaust gases contain between 2 per cent and 10 per cent carbon monoxide and this is reflected in the carboxyhaemoglobin levels in persons such as policemen on traffic duty. Although the levels reached—of the order of 5–6 per cent—will not cause deterioration in function, the condition is of minor medico-legal importance in that it has been claimed that carbon monoxide derived from smoking—and, therefore, also from other environmental sources—is to some extent responsible for the development of coronary heart disease[2]; it is thought, however, that this view would get little general support. Other important forms of carbon monoxide poisoning are discussed later in this section but, in the present context, the main significance of the gas when derived from motor car exhausts lies in its potential as a cause of vehicular accidents, especially in a synergistic role; this has been discussed in Chapter 10.

The hydrocarbons liberated in exhaust gases due to incomplete combustion of the fuel are more important from the environmental aspect. The interaction of sunlight and exhaust vapour produces an atmosphere that is irritating to the nose and eyes—the characteristic 'smog' of the Western USA. Unlike the British fog, 'smog' has little permanent effect on human beings but has been reported as being damaging to crops.

Motor car exhaust gases also contain lead, which forms a link with the second aspect of environmental pollution—that is, pollution by specific elements. Apart from radioactive pollution (discussed in Chapter 27), the outstandingly significant substance in this class is lead. Lead poisoning is, in the main, a matter of industrial medicine but outbreaks of subclinical poisoning occur at an environmental level particularly in areas close to lead works. Lead present in the soil, as well as that present in the air, then constitutes a significant part of the health hazard and children, who are more susceptible to the metal, are at greatest risk[3]. The contribution of motor cars to this risk is not clear. Certainly there is more lead in the atmosphere of urban streets than there is in country areas but absorption into the body is not proportionately increased; nevertheless, all industrial countries are legislating to reduce the amount of lead in motor car fuels[4].

Industrial poisoning

Industrial poisons may be absorbed through the skin, they may be ingested or they may be inhaled; inhalation is by far the most important source not only on physiological grounds but also because it is largely outwith the control of the individual. Much of the preventative legislation is, therefore, concentrated on the maintenance of a pure atmosphere.

Industrial poisons are given threshold limit values (TLV) which are expressed as

[2] *See*, for example, Wald, N., *et al.* (1973), Association between atherosclerotic disease and carboxyhaemoglobin levels in tobacco smokers, *British Medical Journal*, i, 761.
[3] A lead level of 40–50 μg/100 ml blood in a child is regarded as requiring investigation whereas the level at which an industrial worker is considered in danger of developing lead poisoning is 80 μg/100 ml.
[4] Control of Pollution Act 1974, s. 75. The lead content of petrol used in the United Kingdom must now be reduced to 0.15 g/l. (Motor Fuel (Lead Content of Petrol) Regulations 1981, S.I. No. 1523).

the airborne concentration of the given substance to which it is believed that nearly all workers may be repeatedly exposed without ill effects. Such values, which are expressed either in weight per cubic metre or in parts per million, are to some extent artificial and are well compared with the 30 mph speed limits on roads—not all accidents will be prevented by such a limit but it is an arbitrary standard below which it is impractical to go; in industry, the TLV is the level thought likely to be injurious if exceeded.

When dust or fumes of a potentially dangerous character are present to an extent that exceeds this limit, then all practicable measures must be taken to protect the persons employed against their inhalation[5]. The Act stipulates all practicable measures, not merely some, and practicality refers only to the technical possibilities within the limits of current knowledge[5a]—cost, for example, does not enter into the definition. The measures taken may include substitution either of the offending substances or of a particularly dangerous process; they may take the form of purely passive prevention as by the use of masks and hoods; active elimination by extraction is, however, incomparably the best means of preventing industrial poisoning and it must be used, ideally sited as close to the source as possible, when the conditions make it practicable. It scarcely needs emphasis that the extraction cannot be haphazard and care must be taken to ensure that contamination of the local community is kept to a minimum. The Factories Act also deals with the possibility of ingestion of industrial poisons; s. 64 prohibits the eating of meals where a toxic process is carried out.

The early identification of cases of poisoning forms one check on the lack of efficiency[6] of a factory's preventive methods. It is for this reason that a number of conditions (listed in Appendix K) are scheduled as Notifiable Diseases—notifiable, that is, to the Health and Safety Executive. These diseases must be distinguished from Prescribed Diseases (see page 152); although nearly all Notifiable Diseases are also Prescribed, the method and purpose of reporting are different. Many of the notifiable conditions are specific; others—for example, 'toxic anaemia'—are usefully non-specific in that they open possibilities for clinical notification of dangerous conditions before they are specifically defined by regulations.

Poisoning in industry is a vast subject which is constantly changing in emphasis and growing in extent—for example, attention has recently been focused on the carcinogenic potential of vinyl chloride, a substance that is essential to the manufacture of plastics[7] (see Appendix I). The subject will, therefore, be dealt with only in general terms, attention being drawn to the main categories of hazard.

First, there is poisoning by heavy metals of which, as has been seen, lead is the outstanding example; industrial processes involving lead are subject, in particular, to the Factories Act 1961—of which ss. 74 and 128 limit the employment of women and young persons in lead manufacturing processes—and the Control of Lead at Work Regulations 1980 (SI 1980/1248); several other statutes and regulations touch on the subject[8]. Industrial intoxication by lead is almost entirely a matter of inhalation although ingestion is also considered hazardous. The main danger of lead lies in its cumulative effect; industrial cases are all examples of chronic

[5] Factories Act 1961, s. 63.

[5a] Brooks v. J. & P. Coates (U.K.) Ltd [1984] I.C.R. 158.

[6] Efficiency is positively identified by monitoring or measuring the atmosphere at regular intervals.

[7] Some 35 pages are devoted to the problem in *Proceedings of the Royal Society of Medicine* (1976), **69** (No. 4).

[8] The Alkali, etc., Works Regulation Act 1906, s. 7, for example, includes the control of fumes from lead smelting works.

intoxication—colic, joint pain, anaemia, muscle paralyses and generalized brain dysfunction (encephalopathy) may result and are probably due to the fact that lead is basically a poison to enzymes.

Other metallic poisons that are dangerous mainly by way of inspiration include beryllium and cadmium, which are intensely harmful to the lungs, and manganese and mercury, chronic poisoning from both of which causes extensive abnormality of the central nervous system—the latter metal giving origin to the term 'mad as a hatter'. The effects of chronic metallic poisoning may be delayed for many years; much responsibility rests on the medical profession in establishing a cause-and-effect relationship.

The second major group of industrial poisons consists of the hydrocarbons, of both aromatic and of aliphatic type. Again, intoxication is generally by inhalation but absorption through the skin plays a significant part in many cases.

Poisonous aromatic hydrocarbons include benzene itself, which in its chronic form causes an anaemia of very specific type; nitrobenzene, which may be acutely fatal if splashed on the skin; nitroglycerine, again absorbed rapidly through the skin and capable of causing a fatal fall in blood pressure; and trinitrotoluene, which was responsible for a large number of industrial deaths in both World Wars, the outstanding features being cyanosis, anaemia and, occasionally, toxic jaundice—jaundice, or yellowness, being a visible indication of liver failure.

Aliphatic hydrocarbons may be dangerous industrial chemicals when halogenated—that is, combined with chlorine or bromine. The simplest of these compounds—methyl chloride and methyl bromide, which can be used as refrigerants or, in the case of the latter, as a fire extinguisher—are acutely poisonous to the brain. Otherwise, the common characteristic of this group of poisons is their action on the liver and, to a lesser extent, the kidney. Halogenated hydrocarbons are used principally as cleaning agents or industrual solvents. Most have a narcotic action and the least toxic can be used as anaesthetics. Carbon tetrachloride, tetrachlorethane and, especially, dichlorethane are severely damaging to the liver and are the main sources of industrial toxic jaundice. Tetrachlorethane was a serious cause of illness in early aircraft workers when it was used to tighten the fabric of aeroplanes. The variations in toxicity of the halogenated hydrocarbons offer wide opportunities for substitution and, as a result, the extent of the industrial hazard is diminishing.

Finally, attention is drawn to the potential association of cancer with some industrial processes. Many of these conditions are of historic interest—for example, the 'mule spinner's' cancer induced by chronic friction between the skin and clothing impregnated with mineral oil. Others, as discussed above in relation to vinyl chloride, are only beginning to appear. For an association with occupation to be clear, a cancer must, generally, be of a fairly rare type; it is possible that some common tumours are related to specific substances—the association of carcinoma of the lung with asbestosis and smoking is an example (*see* page 157)—but, for purposes of the Social Security Act, it may be difficult to show that they 'do not constitute a risk to the whole population'. Examples of unusual cancers that are prescribed include carcinoma of the nasal membrane in workers exposed to nickel fumes (disease No. C.22) or to wood dust (disease No. D.6); mesothelioma (disease No. D.3) is sufficiently rare to be firmly attributable to asbestosis. Disease No. C.23, cancer of the bladder, is interesting as the most common industrial association of this tumour is with workers in aniline factories; the condition is, in fact, due to the presence as an impurity of the prescribed substance naphthylamine. Vinyl chloride monomer is associated with angiosarcoma of the liver.

Agricultural poisons

Agricultural poisoning merits isolation from other industrial hazards because, apart from potential effects on the workers, there may well be secondary ecological effects; the community as a whole may also be at risk if a toxic substance is distributed widely in the environment or is incorporated in foodstuffs. Excluding manifest abuses such as using defoliation as a weapon of war, potential agricultural poisons may be either of the insecticide, the fungicide or the herbicide groups[9]. To be effective, those agents must be toxic; the art of their production and use lies in limiting that toxicity to the species it is intended to destroy.

Control of the problems of non-specificity now lies with the Advisory Committee on Pesticides[9a]. The Committee must be provided with full details of a proposed pesticide—including its justification for use, its toxic properties and its potential residual effects in foodstuffs; particular importance is placed on possible harm to the human users and consumers of treated crops, to livestock and to wildlife. Products so notified are given trials clearance—usually for a limited period—which may involve destruction of all treated material until the remaining safety measures have been taken. Following trials, there is usually a period of limited clearance during which regulated sales may be permitted; if this is passed satisfactorily, a provisional commercial clearance is granted which allows the product to be marketed commercially for a defined period. If the exhaustive inquiries demanded during these phases have indicated that the product is safe to use[10] and is free from serious ecological ill-effects, a full commercial clearance may be given subject to recommendations as to labelling, as to the method of treatment and the choice of crops and as to the protection of man, livestock and wildlife. The Committee keeps any chemical under review and may vary the regulations in the light of any fresh evidence that accrues during normal use.

In addition to this monitoring system, several statutory controls are imposed. Those chemicals that are most toxic to the user are specified under the Poisonous Substances in Agriculture Regulations 1984 (S.I. 1984/1114)[11]; a main danger of the specified chemicals is that, in addition to inhalation, entry to the body through the skin is a common method of poisoning. The Regulations are, therefore, very much concerned with the provision of protective clothing. Other chemicals, which constitute a hazard if improperly used, are listed in the Farm and Garden Chemicals Regulations 1971 (S.I. 1971/729); the main purpose of the Regulations is to ensure that toxic chemicals are adequately labelled and carry appropriate warnings. Less specifically, certain chemicals that may be used as pesticides are subject to the Poisons Rules made under the Poisons Act 1972; the Act is described in greater detail in Chapter 23[12].

---

[9] Rodenticides will not be discussed at this point. All such agents are known collectively as pesticides.
[9a] Food and Environment Protection Act 1985, s. 16.
[10] Note that a chemical may be poisonous but, when used in a specific way taking normal precautions, it may not necessarily be hazardous—paraquat is a prime example of such a substance (*see* below).
[11] These include the dinitrophenol compounds; endrin; the organophosphorus compounds; fluoroacetic acid compounds; organomercury sprays; arsenic; the organotin compounds; nicotine; and sulphuric acid.
[12] Numerous Acts have been passed with the intention of preserving the ecology in general or specific species of wildlife. These include the Protection of Animals Acts 1911 to 1962, the Rivers (Prevention of Pollution) Acts 1951 to 1961; the Protection of Birds Acts 1954 to 1967; and Control of Pollution Act 1974.

In assessing the poisonous properties of an agricultural chemical, due note must be taken of the advantages offered. Some of the organochlorines are theoretically if not actually poisonous[13]; but the massive benefits to mankind resulting from the widespread reduction of insect-borne diseases, including malaria, infinitely outweigh any such considerations. Similarly, paraquat (*see* below) has revolutionized the agricultural economy of many developing countries; an occasional suicide in such areas must be accepted as a price to pay for the community benefit. Certain insecticides or herbicides will, however, be specifically mentioned in view of their current medico-legal interest on other than industrial grounds.

The most important group among the insecticides is that of the organophosphorus compounds which can enter the body through the inspired air, the skin or even the eye. They owe they profound effect to altering the normal mode of action of the nerves on the muscle masses and to antagonizing the effects of the sympathetic nervous system. The most common preparation, parathion, has been used homicidally; because the action of the organophosphates is essentially physiological, the detection of such cases presents a formidable forensic challenge.

Nicotine is a common fungicide which when concentrated[14] is a powerful poison; it enters the body through either the lungs or the skin. I have been concerned with two deaths in children that could only be attributed to contamination with a nicotine spray.

The herbicide that has caused most recent public concern is paraquat. This remarkable substance is immediately destroyed on contact with the ground—used normally it is, therefore, remarkably safe and highly efficient. Unfortunately, and possibly directly associated with the publicity given to individual cases, it has become a frequent medium for suicide in farming communities; accidental poisoning is also common and there have been at least three convictions for murder by its use in the United Kingdom. Death from paraquat poisoning is singularly unpleasant and, currently, there is no proven antidote[15]. Its major action is on the lungs; the pathological appearances are so unusual that fatal poisoning can be diagnosed without recourse to the toxicologist.

One other slightly bizarre medico-legal aspect of chemical agriculture deserves mention—crop spraying is that type of aviation which has the highest mortality. This is related almost solely to the difficult flying conditions; actual poisoning of pilots by their chemical cargo is extremely rare, though minor effects, such as those of the organophosphates on the eyes, could be very dangerous in this situation.

Iatrogenic and suicidal poisoning

These forms of poisoning are interlinked and can be discussed under one heading.

Very large numbers of new medicinal compounds, which are of increasing complexity both as to their multiplicity of content and as to the effects of the

---

[13] In fact, the Research Committee on Toxic Chemicals reported in 1970 that no evidence had been produced of risks to man resulting from the use of DDT or dieldrin when these were applied properly nor when occurring as residues in a normal diet. Other members of the group—e.g. Aldrin—might be more hazardous.

[14] Nicotine is free from restrictions when sold in an insecticidal dust containing not more than 4 per cent nicotine (Poisons Rules 1978, Schedule 13).

[15] Paraquat is now restricted as to sale save in its weak, granulated form. (Poisons Rules 1978, Schedule 4.)

individual drugs contained, appear regularly on the market; doctors are under constant pressure to try new remedies; and, in the conditions of an overworked practice, there is a positive economy of surgery time to be gained by prescribing drugs in such quantity as will serve the patient for a considerable period. Accidental poisoning can occur, therefore, in the normal process of medical practice and, in essence, mishaps can be put down to one of four sources of error:

1. Overprescribing the quantity of a single drug.
2. The cumulative effects of drugs.
3. Adverse reactions on bodily systems other than that being treated.
4. Drug interactions with one another or with articles of diet.

The statutory defence against the majority of these mishaps is provided by the Medicines Act 1968 which is described in Chapter 23. The Act, *inter alia,* authorizes the establishment of a Medicines Commission[16]. The Commission, which now consists of a chairman and 13 members, advises the licensing authorities and, to this end, appoints Committee which are charged with overseeing the safety, quality or efficiency of medicines and with promoting the collection and investigation of information relating to adverse reactions to drugs on which such advice will be based[17]. The most relevant of the Committees so far established is the Committee on the Safety of Medicines[18]. This Committee meets monthly to review the position of drugs on trial and has a subcommittee to consider notifications of adverse drug reactions that have been made by practitioners. When satisfied that a hazard may exist, the Committee, on its own authority, dispatches warning notices drawing the attention of practitioners to areas of danger. All manufacturers of drugs are now required to circulate data sheets in association with advertisements sent direct to practitioners (Medicines Act 1968, s. 96); these data sheets must give all reasonable information as to dosage, effect, contraindications, adverse reactions and the like. The information is consolidated annually by the Association of the British Pharmaceutical Industry as a Data Sheet Compendium which is issued free to doctors. There is, therefore, now ample opportunity for doctors to appreciate the hazards of drug therapy and failure to heed the many warnings given is likely to be construed by the Courts as negligence.

It is unusual for a drug to act on only one system—for example, a high proportion of those usually prescribed for disorders of the central nervous system also have a profound effect on the heart and blood vessels; the danger here is that the prescribing doctor may fail to make himself aware of the patient's total condition. Occasionally, drugs may have serious side effects in humans that did not show up in preliminary animal testing. Unexpected cumulative effects may arise if the patient's capacity for metabolism or excretion of a drug is reduced by disease, say, of the liver or kidney that has passed unnoticed. Drug interactions are extremely common—they may be complementary or antagonistic, the effects may be dangerous or, on occasion, may be desirable; in many instances, a known effect can be counterbalanced by modifications of the dose. Occasionally, a catastrophe may occur because of unawareness on the part of the practitioner, but the most common cause of adverse interactions results from the use by patients of drugs remaining from a previous prescription—repeated self-medication may be

---

[16] The Medicines Commission and Committees Regulations 1970 (S.I. 1970/746).
[17] Medicines Act 1968, s. 4(2) and 4(3).
[18] The Medicines (Committee on Safety of Medicines) Order 1970 (S.I. 1970/1257).

dangerous if the patient is by then receiving another drug for another complaint.

This introduces the problem of overprescribing which may be unintentional as, for example, when a doctor prescribes two preparations each of which contain an element of the same drug. But the far greater problem lies in semi-elective overprescribing forced by pressures of work; a not uncommon pattern is of a large primary issue followed by repeated prescriptions without adequate confirmation of the patient's need. This can scarcely be regarded as professional negligence but, as a direct result, there are few households in which an excess of potentially dangerous medicines is not to be found; while some persons would take their own lives no matter how carefully their prescriptions were regulated, there is little doubt that a degree of responsibility for many deaths due to suicidal or accidental poisoning must be laid on the pressures of National Health Service practice.

The pattern of suicidal poisoning varies over the years but, at present, it is universal experience that the great majority of cases stem from the misuse of the barbiturate group of drugs. There can be no misuse without availability and, until recently, drugs were obtainable on prescription only—the majority of supplies must, therefore, have derived from legal prescriptions. It used to be said that some three persons died in Great Britain each day as a result of suicidal barbiturate poisoning; the virtually innocuous nitrazepam is therapeutically as effective as barbiturates, and strenuous efforts have been made to outlaw barbiturates from treatment schedules in much the same way as was successfully accomplished in some localities in respect of amphetamines. Barbiturates are now controlled under the Misuse of Drugs Act 1971[19] and the scene may change rapidly. It is problematical whether all or even the majority of fatal barbiturate poisonings are, in fact, suicidal; some may be accidental and the relationship with alcoholism is discussed in Chapter 25. Apart from barbiturates, the 'tranquillizers' as a heterogeneous group also account for a large number of suicides—again, these drugs must always be obtained on prescription and many diazapines are now classified as Class C controlled drugs; they are, however, relatively derestricted as to possession[19a].

One difficulty in establishing the cause of death in drug poisoning lies in the great variation in post-mortem tissue levels that have been reported in fatal cases; this problem is discussed more fully in Chapter 26. Certainly, there are obvious features that may make one person more susceptible to a drug than another—the route of absorption and the presentation of the drug (i.e. how it is dissolved or otherwise compounded) may be of significance; an unwell patient is likely to be less tolerant of a given poison than is one who is fully fit—a fact that emphasizes the importance of a full autopsy to assess the real significance of drugs in the mode of death; by and large, children and old persons are more susceptible to poisons than are those in other age groups. But very often these features will not, in themselves, explain apparently anomalous findings and both the pathologist and the toxicologist are dependent largely on the circumstantial evidence; certainly, attempts to estimate the dose taken that are based on a single post-mortem tissue analysis are liable to very wide error.

Other common suicidal poisonings relate to substances that are available on general sale, the most important group being the analgesics taken for headaches, etc. Despite the efficiency of modern treatment, there are still an appreciable number of deaths due to aspirin although paracetamol has largely displaced it as a

[19] Misuse of Drugs Act 1971 (Modification) Order 1984 (S.I. 1984/859)
[19a] Misuse of Drugs Regulations 1985 (S.I. 1985/2066, Sch. 4).

suicidal agent. The occurrence of sudden 'waves' of poisoning by specific drugs leads to the suspicion that it is publicity which determines vogues in suicide although, in fact, this subjective impression is hard to substantiate. I have been surprised at the number of deaths due to lysol or similar corrosive poisoning that still occur—these seem to be confined to the elderly. Other suicidal poisonings are rare and their individual nature often indicates severe mental derangement; many cases of suicidal paraquat poisoning exhibit this feature.

Ingestion of toxic substances is by far the commonest form of suicide and, in some areas, as many such victims are admitted to intensive care units as are derived from road-traffic accidents. Single men and, particularly, widowers seem to be at risk; the divorced and separated of both sexes are also especially prone to this form of suicide which seems to have aroused less public concern as a cause of death than it merits[19].

There remains carbon monoxide poisoning which, 10 years ago, was as common a method of suicide as was barbiturate poisoning. It has always been rare in the USA, where domestic gas supplies are almost universally of natural origin; the introduction of natural gas into British homes has, similarly, reduced the incidence of carbon monoxide suicides to negligible numbers. Such cases as occur are largely associated with motor-car exhaust fumes. Generally, some method of increasing the certainty of success—e.g. by passing a tube from the exhaust to the interior of the car—is used. In the absence of such apparatus, the distinction between suicide and accident may be very difficult to make; in fact, poisoning by exhaust fumes from motor cars is probably more often accidental than suicidal.

Accidental poisoning

Accidental poisoning is of considerable medico-legal significance; first, because of its commonness and, secondly, because of the not infrequent difficulty met in distinguishing it from suicide or homicide. It is best discussed in two phases—as related to children and as related to adults.

Children are most often poisoned by reason of genuine mistake. Perhaps the most dangerous factor lies in the similarity between some medicinal tablets and some widely advertised brands of sweets. Alternatively, poisonous berries growing naturally may be mistaken for fruits seen more commonly in the greengrocer's shop. Children may also be victims of their natural inquisitiveness—there is a strong urge to discover what is so pleasant about the 'sweets' kept beside the parents' beds. The prevention of accidental poisoning in children is a matter, first, of adequate security of containers[20], medicine cupboards, cleaning closets, garden sheds and the like, coupled with adequate surveillance when in an unusual environment—as, for example, on infrequent picnic outings. The determination and agility of children is well known; locks are essential wherever potentially poisonous substances are stored.

Accidental poisoning in adults is, again, of dual origin. First, there are incidents involving errors of perception—the dose of a drug is misread due to age or ill health, medicines are poured out in the dark or when half-asleep; such errors are potentiated by the effects of alcohol. It may be very difficult to distinguish genuine error from a deliberate act. Secondly, there is involuntary error—the taking of poison in the belief that that it is an innocuous substance. As in the case of children,

[20] See British Medical Journal (1976), i, 604, for a description of compulsory (with reference to paediatric presentation) or voluntary (adult presentation) use of child-resistant containers. For aspirin and paracetamol, see Medicines (Child Safety) Regulations 1975 (S.I. 1975/2000).

this may occur in nature or in the home. Examples in the former situation include the eating of the poisonous fungus *Amanita* in mistake for the edible mushroom *Agaricus* or the use of aconite root instead of horse-radish. Poisoning due to involuntary error in the home is almost always a matter of improper labelling—the frequency with which intensely poisonous substances are stored in open areas in beer or lemonade bottles while these still retain their original labels is astounding. Once again, the possibility of deliberate substitution has to be considered.

Carbon monoxide is a very common agent of accidental poisoning which may, on occasion, give rise to unusual findings at the scene of death. The subject has been discussed in detail in Chapter 13. The diagnosis often depends upon awareness of the possibility; curious mistakes, such as attributing death to food poisoning rather than to carbon monoxide, have resulted from inadequate post-mortem examination.

Homicidal poisoning

The pattern of homicidal poisoning also seems to have changed over the years. Not only have the types of poison used altered, but the condition as a whole appears to have become very uncommon. This must be due largely to steadily more effective legislation. The facilities of the National Health Service (see below) must have a considerable effect while, amongst other factors, the direction of social change is such as to reduce the overall need for the disposal of wives or husbands; when a poisoning occurs it is often found to have unusual background features such as a motivation on eugenic grounds.

Poisoning is a crime at common law in Scotland. The English Offences Against the Person Act 1861 is more precise and deals with endangering life or with causing grievous bodily harm by poisoning (s. 23) and even goes so far as to specify an intention to annoy (s. 24). No distinction is made under either jurisdiction between a drug and a poison; both may be noxious things but, as regards the former, the dose given is relevant to the definition as is its mode of presentation— that is, for example, whether or not the substance is in the form of a reputable pharmaceutical preparation. There is no attempt to specify a noxious substance; it is the intention of the individual user that is of paramount importance.

Very occasionally, homicidal poisoning may be associated with medical treatment, when the injurious substance may be introduced by injection. In the vast majority of cases, however, such poisons are administered by mouth and the victim must suffer to some extent from symptoms of gastroenteritis; the great majority of poisons used with intent to murder will cause vomiting with or without diarrhoea. This is particularly true of the well-known irritant metallic poisons, of which arsenic is the most infamous, and of phosphorus[21]. Nevertheless, natural food poisoning (*see* below) or diarrhoea and vomiting due to virus disease or to psychiatric causes are far more common than is homicidal poisoning. The

---

[21] Many of the poisons used in the famous cases of the past were incorporated in rodenticides—thallium is, perhaps, the most modern example and its supply is now strictly controlled. No rat poison may now contain strychnine, the use of which is authorized only for the killing of moles or foxes; the use of monofluoroacetic acid in rat control is mainly restricted to use in ships or sewers (Poisons Rules 1978, Schedule 12). Yellow phosphorous and red squill cannot be used for the destruction of any mammalian animal (Animals (Cruel Poisons) Act 1962). Rat poisons are now largely compounded of biological substances but acquired resistance may dictate a return to chemical control.

practitioner may well be excused for failing to diagnose such a case at first glance but when his suspicions are aroused he is faced with an ethical dilemma. He must have the interests of his patient as his main concern; yet, to take action that might be interpreted publicly as implying suspicion of foul play could result in serious charges in the event that it was ill founded.

The doctor in this position should continue to treat his patient but should take extra precautions against the time when his evidence may be needed in court. Thus, particularly careful notes ought to be made of statements, of relevant times and of specific points that are considered unusual. The normal specimens of vomit and faeces should be taken and labelled accurately; there would seem to be no reason why a toxicological analysis should not be arranged in parallel with bacteriological examinations provided confidentiality is assured. Ideally, specimens of food might be obtained and sent for similar analysis but this could be extremely difficult to achieve if a homicidal attempt were really being made. The ultimate test is to remove the patient to hospital and, in practice, this is what will usually happen in the conditions of a National Health Service. By the time a practitioner is sufficiently concerned to suspect poisoning, he will have been already anxious to obtain improved conditions for his patient on purely medical grounds; this will be particularly so if he finds, as may well happen, that he has been called in late to the case. The homicidal process is, thus, effectively aborted.

If deliberate poisoning is proved to the satisfaction of both the practitioner and the hospital consultant, then it would be right for a confidential report to be made to a senior police officer; few doctors would, however, like to do so without the support of their defence or protection society. In the event of a death that arouses suspicion, the doctor's duty is clear and unequivocal—the case must be reported to the Fiscal or to the Coroner; this applies also to deaths due to natural poisoning.

Natural poisoning

Food poisoning

Food poisoning as a cause of accidental death has been already mentioned as has its importance in the differential diagnosis of homicidal poisoning. This is probably its main forensic significance although actions for tort or delict might well be brought against suppliers, restaurants and the like when damage is suffered; conceivably, criminal charges could be brought in the event of death.

Acute poisoning may result from the ingestion of either living virulent bacteria or of toxins or toxic principles which, in turn, can derive from bacteria or may be normal components of the foodstuffs. An important distinction is that bacteria, unless present in the form of resistant spores, are killed by heat; toxins, however, may be thermostable, particularly when they are mixed with or are part of the food.

Strictly speaking, bacterial food poisoning will include any disease transmitted through food or water or by a food handler—for example, typhoid fever, cholera, or dysentery of either bacterial or of amoebic (protozoal) type. However, while a few other bacteria may cause very similar symptoms, the term is virtually confined to infection by organisms of the *Salmonella* group, virulent *Staphylococci* or *Clostridium welchii*—an organism that also causes gas gangrene. *Salmonellae* are essentially parasites of animals and may pre-exist in the foodstuff or be introduced by contamination; the food shows no evidence of putrefaction and symptoms may be due to the presence of preformed toxin or to proliferation of the bacteria in the human host. *Staphylococci*, on the other hand, are nearly always introduced from a human carrier during the processing of food such as ice-cream or bakery products. In either case, the symptoms of abdominal pain, vomiting and diarrhoea may closely simulate those of acute metallic poisoning. *Cl. welchii* typically contaminates raw meat, poultry or stews; outbreaks of food poisoning in institutions are often due to this organism.

Botulism is the classic food poisoning due to the presence of preformed bacterial toxin. The organism (*Cl. botulinum*) lives in soil and can, therefore, be transmitted in vegetables; it grows only in the absence of oxygen and will flourish in canned or bottled foodstuffs. Home bottling of vegetables is probably the least uncommon source of the condition but meat products are also implicated. The disease is generally of great severity and is often fatal; it causes paralysis of the central nervous system and the usual symptoms of food poisoning are absent. Cases are very rare in the United Kingdom.

Poisoning resulting from the nature of the food may come either from vegetables or from animals. The fungi, which are most likely to be eaten in error, are the best known of the very many vegetables that have poisonous properties. Fungi of the genus *Amanita*, eaten in mistake for the common mushroom *Agaricus*, contain toxins that may cause severe gastrointestinal upset with accompanying surgical shock or, through the action of the alkaloid muscarine, may interfere with the nervous stimulation of the muscles. The toxic principles of some fungi are hallucinogenic and are creating a modern social problem. The most dangerous fungus, *A. phalloides*, is toxic even having been cooked. On the other hand, many fungi apart from the common field mushroom are palatable and non-toxic.

Animal foods that are toxic in the absence of bacterial contamination mostly derive from fish[22]. The poisonous principle is neurotoxic and is concentrated maximally in the gonads and the liver at spawning time.

Poisonous fungi and poisonous fish are used both homicidally and suicidally in primitive societies.

Poisons naturally injected

Many animal species inject venom either as a defence mechanism or as a means of immobilizing their prey. Of these, snakes are by far the most important both medically and in the forensic context.

There are two main families of venomous snake—the *Viperidae*, all of which are poisonous, and the *Colubridae*, many of which are non-poisonous but which include the very dangerous cobras and kraits. Venom is injected reflexly through the fangs when the snake strikes or bites. All venoms contain a mixture of toxic principles but, in general, the colubride venom is neurotoxic and kills rapidly due to paralysis while that of the viperidae acts on the blood and kills slowly by destroying the red cells and altering the clotting mechanisms. Tragedies have occurred in mistaking the staggering gait and slurred speech of the victim of cobra bite for drunkenness.

---

[22] The dangers of most shellfish and molluscs stem not only from their primary toxicity at certain times of the year—perhaps due to the presence of commensals—but also from their lifestyle as scavengers and their frequent contamination with disease-producing organisms.

Snake venoms are not of equal potency nor is each injection equally efficient; but the concentration of the dose depends upon the body weight and it follows that snake bite, or any other venomous injection, is more dangerous in the case of children than in adults. The prognosis is also greatly influenced by the availability of efficient treatment.

The treatment of snake bite is both general and specific. It is the latter, in the form of antivenin therapy, which causes most medico-legal concern. Horses can be immunized against snake venom and thus provide antisera for the treatment of humans. The most specific antisera will be the most efficacious but their use depends upon accurate identification of the specific snake; in practice, therefore, the doctor is often forced to use a less efficient, 'wide-spectrum' antivenin. At the same time, there is always a risk of severe reaction by the patient to the 'horse' components of the injection (*see* page 68). There may well be a therapeutic dilemma. Little doubt would be raised in areas in which poisonous snakes abounded—provided that the patient was seen within 8 hours of being bitten, antivenin would be given without hesitation. At the other extreme, the only poisonous snake that exists in Great Britain, *V. berus*, injects a venom that is only slightly toxic—it has accordingly been concluded that its bite is less dangerous than is the use of the available antivenin[23]. The decision could be a hard one in the case of a small child; if antiserum was given, test dosing followed by very careful administration and desensitization (e.g. by the use of adrenalin) would be mandatory. It is believed that snake bite kills some 40 000 persons annually throughout the world, the most dangerous areas being Asia, Central America and Australia. Most Asian practitioners would probably agree, however, that a number of otherwise violent deaths are incorrectly attributed to snake bite.

The sting of the scorpion, which does not live outside the subtropics, is perhaps the second most common serious envenomation on a world-wide basis; at the very least, the sting is intensely painful while the venom of certain species is as dangerous as is that of some snakes. Dangerously poisonous spiders are far less common than is generally supposed. The most serious bite is that of the species *Latrodectus*—the 'black widow'—which tends to lurk on rustic latrine seats. Antivenins are available both for scorpion sting and for spider bite and, again, the seriousness of the prognosis is inversely proportional to the body weight of the person attacked.

Few insect stings are completely free from danger, particularly if they are multiple. The sheer pain may induce a vagal type of shock, whereas unduly sensitive persons may die from an antigen/antibody reaction. Between 1962 and 1971, there were 44 deaths due to bee and wasp stings in England and Wales; about 40 comparable deaths occur annually in the USA.

[23] Royal Society of Tropical Medicine and Hygiene (1962). Notes on the treatment of snake bite. *Transactions of the Royal Society of Tropical Medicine and Hygiene*, **56**, 93.

23

The law relating to drugs and poisons

The law relating to environmental and industrial poisoning is a wide subject very largely beyond the control of the individual. The purpose of this section is to outline only the statutory control of poisons and drugs that are dispensed through the pharmaceutical and medical professions.

Thus limited, there are three enactments of major importance. The Pharmacy and Poisons Act 1933 has been replaced by the Poisons Act 1972 and the Medicines Act 1968. The first of these is concerned entirely with non-medicinal poisons and, in the main, regulates the storage of poisons and their sale and supply to the public and to the health professions. The second large Act is, as its name indicates, related to medicinal drugs; it covers many administrative aspects of advertisement and sale and essentially regulates the standards of pharmaceutical practice. The Misuse of Drugs Act 1971 deals with only a limited list of drugs; nevertheless, it is that part of drug legislation that most closely concerns the individual doctor, the law enforcement officer and the drug taker.

Sale of non-medicinal poisons to the public

The Poisons Act 1972 takes over the main functions of the 1933 Act in dealing with non-medicinal poisons. It provides for:

1. The registration of sellers of poisons.
2. The categorization of poisons in relation to how they may be sold or supplied[1].
3. The drawing up of Poisons Rules and their review.

The last two provisions are amongst the functions of the Poisons Board which advises the Secretaries of State on both aspects[2].

The Poisons List is divided into two Parts. Part I poisons may be sold only by pharmacists from registered premises; Part II poisons may be sold only by

---

[1] Poisons List Order, 1978, S.I. No. 2; Poisons Rules 1978, S.I. No. 1.

[2] The Poisons Board consists of five members appointed by the interested Government Departments, the Government Chemist, five persons approved by the Pharmaceutical Society of Great Britain, four members appointed by echelons of the medical profession, one by the Royal Institute of Chemistry and any additional members thought necessary. It is probable that its function will be taken over by the Health and Safety Executive.

pharmacists or, from specified premises, by persons who are approved by the local authority as listed sellers of Part II poisons. The Poisons Board has authority to recommend the precise listing of poisons but, in general, Part II poisons are those to which it is reasonable for the public to have adequate access—they thus include those substances that, although poisonous if misused, are in everyday household use.

All listed poisons must be sold in impervious containers that show the name of the poison and the proportion contained in any mixture, the word 'Poison', sometimes with substituted specific warnings[3], and the name and address of the seller. Those poisons that are included in the first schedule of the Poisons Rules (see below) are restricted in that the retail purchaser must either be known to the seller or must provide a certificate signed either by a householder known to the pharmacist or by a police officer in charge of a Station; full details of the sale must be entered in a book kept for the purpose, and the purchaser must sign the entry. The permissive sections of the old 1933 Act whereby there was no interference with the sale of listed poisons to doctors, dentists, veterinary surgeons etc., no longer have any relevance, and exemptions from the provisions of the Act under s. 4 do not include exemption from signing the register or from keeping records.

The Act empowers the Secretaries of State, after consultation with the Poisons Board, to draw up Poisons Rules. Many of these rules are expressed in 14 Schedules, some of which are of limited application.

Schedule 1 lists those poisons subject to special restrictions as detailed above. Some Schedule 1 poisons also have a medicinal role and, when prescribed for that purpose, are subject to the provisions of the Medicines Act 1968 (*see* below). Schedule 4 is of interest on two counts. In the first place, it must be clearly distinguished from Schedule 4 of the 1972 Poisons Rules which concerned the restriction of barbiturate drugs and is now ineffective. Secondly, as it now stands, it restricts the sale of certain Part II poisons either to general sale by pharmacists of to sale by listed sellers only to persons engaged in the trades or businesses of horticulture, agriculture or forestry for the purposes of such trade or business; thus, the public distribution of many potent pesticides that are dangerous to humans is specifically controlled.

The Poisons Acts have undoubtedly been largely responsible for the decline in homicidal poisoning that has been so evident over the past 50 years.

The Medicines Act 1968[4]

This massive Act is concerned, in the main, with the regulation of the manufacture and supply of medicinal products, which are defined (s. 130) as any substances (not being instruments, apparatus or appliances) that are manufactured, sold, supplied, imported or exported for use by being administered to human beings or animals for a medicinal purpose or that are ingredients of a substance or article used for medicinal purposes. A 'medicinal purpose' implies treatment or prevention of disease, diagnosis, contraception, induction of anaesthesia or interference with a normal physiological function in either a negative or positive fashion.

---

[3] Poisons Rules 1978, Schedule 6.
[4] This Act repeals the Pharmacy and Medicines Act 1941, the Therapeutic Substances Act 1956 and the greater part of the Pharmacy and Poisons Act 1933.

Part II of the Act introduces licences and certificates relating to the sale, wholesale and manufacture of medicinal products with general exceptions from the restrictive regulations for doctors, dentists, veterinary practitioners and pharmacists; clinical trials on patients and medicinal tests on animals are also controlled (ss. 31 and 32). Part III deals with the sale of medicinal products. Part IV defines pharmacists and pharmacies and their registration. Part V deals with the labelling, packaging and identification of medicinal products and Part VI lays down criteria on the important subject of advertising—particular attention is paid to the problems of false or misleading advertisements and representations.

It is evident that, while the Act defines a number of offences, all of which may come within the ambit of the lawyer, very few of these involve directly the doctor or the dentist—indeed they are specifically excluded from the majority of the provisions; a detailed discussion is, therefore, beyond the scope of a text on forensic medicine which must, however, consider the special points concerning the supply of medicines to the general public.

The basic provision in this respect lies in s. 51 of the Act which introduces the category of General Sale List Medicines[5]. These drugs are of generally innocuous type and a few are listed as being saleable in automatic vending machines. Medicinal products used in eye drops or ointments or those intended for injection may not be on general sale (Schedule 3 of the 1984 Order). Unless a medicine is categorized as a general sale list medicine, it must only be sold or supplied from a registered pharmacy.

Section 58 of the Act defines the category of Prescription Only Medicines[6]. As the name implies, such drugs can be sold or supplied by retail only in accordance with a prescription given by a doctor or dentist as appropriate. The general classes of such drugs include all products containing one or more of the substances listed in Part I of Schedule 1 to the Order, medicinal products containing any drug specified in Schedule 2 to the Misuse of Drugs Act 1971[7] and medicinal products that are for parenteral administration, irrespective of whether or not they contain a prescription-only drug[8].

There remains a group of drugs that are covered by neither of the above sections. These are known as Pharmacy Medicines and can be offered for retail sale only through a retail pharmacy business.

There are very stringent rules governing the labelling of medicinal products and, in particular, pharmacy and prescription-only medicines must be clearly labelled 'P' and 'POM' as appropriate. All medicinal products must be labelled 'Keep Out of the Reach of Children'. A record must be kept of every sale or supply of a prescription-only medicine unless the medicine was prescribed through the National Health Service and this includes medicine dispensed in an emergency (q.v.); records and prescriptions must be preserved for 2 years.

Article 12 of the Order details the requirements for a valid prescription of a prescription-only medicine. These are that it:

[5] Specified in Medicines (Products other than Veterinary Drugs) (General Sale List) Order 1984, S.I. No. 769. The special provisions for veterinary practitioners are omitted from this text.
[6] Medicines (Products other than Veterinary Drugs) (Prescription Only) Order 1983, S.I. No. 1212.
[7] There are exceptions to this whereby certain drugs—e.g. codeine, morphine and medicinal opium—are excluded when present below a specified strength.
[8] The effect of the Act is that no one can administer a parenteral injection (other than to himself) unless he is an appropriate practitioner or is acting under the instructions of one. However, insulins are specifically excluded from the category of prescription-only drugs and certain others can be administered by anyone in an emergency (Articles 4 and 5 of the Order).

1. Shall be written in indelible ink.
2. Shall contain the following particulars:
   (a) the address and usual signature of the practitioner giving it;
   (b) the date on which it was signed by the practitioner giving it;
   (c) such particulars as indicate whether the practitioner giving it is a doctor, a dentist, a veterinary surgeon or a veterinary practitioner. `
   (d) where the practitioner is a doctor or a dentist, the name, address and the age (if under 12 years) of the person for whose treatment it is given; and
   (e) where the practitioner is a veterinary surgeon or a veterinary practitioner the name and address of the person to whom the prescription-only medicine is to be delivered.
3. Except where it is a repeat prescription, shall not be dispensed later than 6 months after the date referred to in 2 (b) above.
4. Where it is a repeat prescription, shall not be dispensed other than in accordance with the direction contained therein.
5. Where the prescription is not a repeat prescription but contains a direction that the prescription be repeated without specifying the number of times it may be dispensed, shall not be dispensed on more than two occasions.

If a doctor is unable to provide a prescription the pharmacist may supply the medicine subject to the doctor undertaking to rectify the position within 72 hours; no repeats are allowed and the medicine must contain no substances subject to full control under the Misuse of Drugs Act 1971. The pharmacist may also supply in extreme emergency at the request of the patient so long as he is satisfied that an emergency exists and that the patient had previously been prescribed the medicine requested. The total supply must not be sufficient for more than 3 days' treatment (excluding public holidays) and the medicine must not contain a controlled drug (Misuse of Drugs Act 1971, Schedule 2) other than a barbiturate for the treatment of epilepsy.

Otherwise, Part I of the 1968 Act—its administration—is apposite in that it establishes the Medicines Commission which, in turn, has the power to recommend to the Minister the setting up of committees with particular responsibility for the safety and efficacy of medicinal drugs. These functions have already been discussed.

Drug abuse

The Misuse of Drugs Act 1971 repeals the Drugs (Prevention of Misuse) Act 1964 and the Dangerous Drugs Acts 1965 and 1967. The major regulations in pursuance of the Act are the Misuse of Drugs Regulations 1985 (S.I. 1985/2066), the Misuse of Drugs (Safe Custody) Regulations 1973 (S.I. 1973 no. 798) and the Misuse of Drugs (Notification of and Supply to Addicts) Regulations 1973 (S.I. 1973 no. 799).

The 1971 Act does four things of major importance to the doctor:

1. It establishes an Advisory Council on the Misuse of Drugs.
2. It classifies certain drugs as Controlled Drugs.
3. It takes steps to regulate doctors who are deemed unsuitable to prescribe or administer controlled drugs (ss. 12 and 13).

4. It empowers the Advisory Council to advise on the establishment of centres for treatment, rehabilitation and after-care of persons affected by the misuse of drugs.

The Act is, therefore, far more than simply repressive in type and represents a great advance in social legislation over the statutes it repeals.

The Advisory Council, as presently constituted, consists of not less than 20 persons with wide and recent experience in the specialities of medicine, dentistry, veterinary medicine, pharmacy, pharmaceutical manufacturing, chemistry and social work involving the misuse of drugs. The remit of the Council has the very great advantage of flexibility. It must monitor the national situation in regard to drug abuse and can advise on measures to be taken in the light of changing circumstances. Drugs can, therefore, be controlled rapidly; alternatively, drugs that seem at any time to have ceased to be a problem can be released from restriction. Equally important functions of the Advisory Council include the promotion of co-operation between all the social services involved in the eradication of drug abuse and the education of the public—and especially the younger public—as to the dangers of the misuse of drugs.

Historically, dangerous drugs have been equated with narcotic drugs—as evidenced by the establishment of Narcotics Bureaux and Commissions in many countries. The pharmaceutical industry has, however, made such advances in recent years in the production of drugs that have powerful effects outwith their intended therapeutic roles that drug abuse has escaped from its previous confines. Stimulants, hallucinogens and the like may be just as dangerous or antisocial as are the narcotics, particularly when they are used as mixtures; it is this trend that Section 2 of the Act is designed to combat. Under this Section and its resultant regulations, certain drugs are listed as 'controlled'. Controlled drugs are classified into classes A, B and C, the classes being determined by the punishment specified for the offences of their production, supply and possession. The penalties are greatest in the case of Class A and least in the case of Class C drugs[9] and, in all cases, are more severe in relation to production and supply than as to possession. It is a logical consequence that, in practice, the most harmful drugs are placed in Class A. A distinction is made, however, in the case of drugs that are both harmful and have negligible therapeutic application; these drugs are listed in Schedule 1 of the 1985 Regulations. Whereas many professional persons—including doctors, dentists, etc.—may legally possess controlled drugs for the purpose of carrying on their profession, a special licence is needed for the possession of those in Schedule 1[10].

The lawful supply of controlled drugs is carefully regulated. A prescription given by a doctor must be in ink or otherwise indelible and be written in the prescriber's own hand and signed and dated by him; it must state the name and address of the person to be treated and of the prescriber unless it is written on a National Health Service prescription form; and the dose of the controlled drug must be written both in words and in figures. Repeat prescriptions are not permitted and, should it be the intention to dispense the prescription by instalments, the total amount of controlled drug to be given in each instalment and the intervals to be observed must be

[9] Rather surprisingly, the only difference between Class A and Class B drugs relates to the punishment for possession of a controlled drug (Schedule 4 of the Act).
[10] This is not stated positively but would appear to be so by a process of deductive reasoning—it is certainly the policy adopted by inspectors appointed under s. 23 of the Act.

stated. The pharmacist must either know the signature of the prescriber or must have no reason to doubt its genuineness. These restrictions are intended to detect or discourage forgery and to prevent the stockpiling of controlled drugs by individuals (*see Figure 23.1*).

The 1985 Regulations maintain the requirements for recording the supply and administration of controlled drugs. Unless the drugs are supplied to a patient on prescription, an entry must be made in a bound register of receipt and supply of all drugs in Classes A and B and of all those in Schedule 1 of the Regulations. A doctor must keep such a register and must produce this for inspection on request when so directed in writing by the Secretary of State. Controlled drugs must be kept in locked containers that can only be opened by the person legally in possession but there are relaxations in respect of many Class B and Class C drugs. A locked car would not be considered a locked receptacle for the purposes of the Regulations[11], but a locked glove compartment in a locked car would probably qualify.

The Misuse of Drugs Act includes statutory controls over the rights of doctors to prescribe and possess drugs. Under s. 12, the Secretary of State may direct that a doctor who has been convicted of an offence under the Act[12] shall be prohibited from possessing or prescribing controlled drugs; such a direction is operative once it has been served on the practitioner to whom it applies but can be cancelled or suspended at any time.

Sections 13 and 14 are of more practical concern to the lawyer. Under the former, the Secretary of State may prohibit a practitioner from possessing or prescribing controlled drugs either if the doctor prescribes controlled drugs to an addict without notifying the case as required or if he contravenes the Regulations which state that heroin and cocaine can only be prescribed under licence unless it be for treatment of organic disease or injury; a prohibition may also result if the Secretary of State believes that the practitioner has been prescribing controlled drugs in an irresponsible fashion. Section 14 describes the necessary procedure.

In the first instance, the case is referred to a Tribunal[13] who may find that there is no reason for a direction of prohibition to be made; in that case, the practitioner is so informed. Should the Tribunal find against the practitioner, a recommendation is made to the Secretary of State indicating those controlled drugs that he should be forbidden to possess or prescribe. The proceedings before the Tribunal are private, unless a public hearing is requested by the respondent, and the practitioner may be legally represented. An appeal against the findings of a Tribunal is referred to an Advisory Body which consists of a Queen's Counsel as Chairman, a medical (or dental or veterinary) practitioner in Government employ and a further member appointed by the respondent's profession; legal representation is again allowed. The Advisory Body may recommend a direction of prohibition either accepting or modifying the advice of the Tribunal, it may refer the case back to the Tribunal or another Tribunal, or it may advise that no further proceedings be taken.

A further disciplinary power exists when there appears to be considerable urgency over the need to suspend a practitioner's right to supply controlled drugs (Section 15). In these circumstances, the Secretary of State refers the case to a professional panel which consists of three members of the respondent's profession. In the event that the panel advises the need, the Secretary of State may issue a

---

[11] Rao v. Wyles [1949] 2 All E.R. 685.

[12] Or certain offences in connection with the Customs and Excise Act 1952.

[13] The Tribunal consists of a lawyer of at least 7 years standing as Chairman and four members from the medical (or dental or veterinary as appropriate) profession.

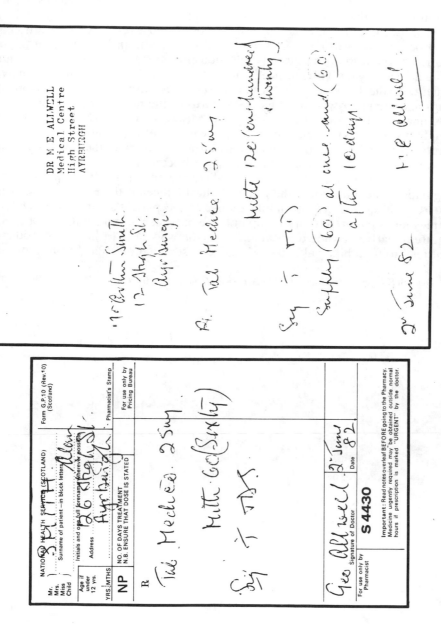

Figure 23.1 Typical prescription for controlled drugs in the National Health Service (left) and in private practice (right).

direction of temporary prohibition for a period of 6 weeks but must, at the same time, refer the case to a Tribunal. The temporary prohibition may be extended, subject to the agreement of the Tribunal, for periods of 28 days.

This control of a doctor's or dentist's practice by statute is a departure from the established regulation of professional conduct by the General Medical or Dental Councils (*see* Chapter 30); the seriousness of this step is reflected in the intricacy of the procedure. Nevertheless, it is noteworthy that, with the exception of the legal Chairmen, the respondent's case is still tried entirely by his peers. It is to be noted that a decision by the Tribunal need not necessarily be the same as that taken by the General Medical Council; the former is concerned with the misuse of controlled drugs and the latter with the ethical standards of the medical profession[14].

A final word is needed concerning the Misuse of Drugs (Notification of and Supply to Addicts) Regulations 1973, which are of additional medico-legal significance in that they constitute a new statutory erosion of the general principles relating to professional confidentiality. If a doctor has reasonable grounds for considering a patient he attends to be addicted to one of the drugs specified in the Regulations, he must notify the Chief Medical Officer at the Home Office (who is also responsible for Scottish notifications) of the patient's particulars. Only one notification is required from a group practice or from a hospital but renotification is required yearly. As noted above, the doctor who fails to notify an addict yet continues to treat him makes himself liable to severe professional restriction.

[14] Desrath Rai v. General Medical Council (1984). *Lancet*, **i**, 1420, PC.

24

Drug addiction

A. T. Proudfoot

For centuries most groups in society have used drugs for their pleasurable and relaxing effects, to facilitate communication with the 'spirits', for religious reasons or simply to make possible prolonged physical exertion in the face of hunger and adversities. Present-day society is no exception but, in addition to having access to a wider range of drugs (in the generally accepted sense of the word) than ever before, it has to contend with the interrelated problems of cigarette smoking, dependence on alcohol, overeating and gambling. The 'rules' governing the use of a drug are determined by the society concerned and its use outwith these rules is termed 'abuse' or 'misuse'. It is implicit in any definition of misuse that the drug is being taken apart from medical need but it is often difficult to decide where use ends and misuse begins, even when the drug is being prescribed by a doctor. For example, the nightly use of sleeping capsules for months or years by middle-aged women (a common occurrence) would be regarded as justified by some physicians and as misuse by others; likewise, the long-term prescription of tranquillizers to young women who have difficulty in coping with daily living is debatable practice.

Addiction and habituation

Repeated administration of some drugs leads to individuals becoming compelled to continue taking them and, as time passes, tolerance develops—the amount taken may have to be increased to obtain the effect produced by the initial dose. Psychological and physical dependence may soon develop and sudden discontinuation may lead to a complex sequence of withdrawal symptoms. Not every misused drug will produce all these features nor the same combination of them but they are, to many, the hallmarks of 'addiction' and were incorporated in early definitions of the term.

Addiction used to be distinguished from 'habituation', which was considered to be a less serious state. Though the habituated individual may have had the desire to continue taking the drugs, the element of compulsion to do so was absent; there was little or no tendency to increase the dose, no physical dependence and there were no ill effects on stopping the drug. However, the expression habituation has fallen into disuse and, although addiction is an unsatisfactory term because it has been used over the years with such various meanings, it is so much part of the vocabulary that it is unlikely to be dropped. Some definition is necessary if only from a legislative standpoint. The Misuse of Drugs (Notification of and Supply to Addicts) Regulations 1973 designate an individual an addict 'if, and only if, he has as a result of repeated administration become so dependent on the drug that he has an overpowering desire for the administration of it to be continued'. In the context of these Regulations the term 'drug' refers only to compounds such as cocaine and a dozen or so narcotic analgesics listed in a schedule to the Regulations. This definition is unsatisfactory in as far as it may be difficult to decide when an 'overpowering desire' for continuation of the drug exists.

Unfortunately, the nature of addiction is not understood. In some countries it is regarded simply as an undesirable habit and is managed accordingly, with attempts to re-educate addicts by a programme of strict military-type discipline and work after an initial withdrawal period. Other societies look upon addiction as a disease and have tried, with a conspicuous lack of success, to find a medical 'cure'. As a consequence, considerably more money and effort has been expanded 'treating' individuals than in education and prevention.

Routes of drug administration

Drugs may be taken in several ways. Volatile organic solvents arising from glues and dry-cleaning agents are inhaled deep into the lungs where they enter the circulation. Occasionally powdered or crystalline drugs are sniffed ('snorted') in the solid form or in solution into the nose and absorbed into the bloodstream through the vascular nasal lining. Absorption by this route is unreliable and the quantities of drug reaching the brain and the subsequent 'experience' are correspondingly unpredictable. Likewise, drugs taken by mouth may not produce an effect that is sufficiently intense to satisfy many addicts, although this route may provide background intoxication on which to superimpose other drug effects. Such methods tend to be used by those who are experimenting or are relatively inexperienced in the abuse of drugs. 'Skin popping', the injection of a solution of a drug under the skin, goes some way to magnify the effects of the drug because absorption is faster and more complete than after ingestion. It does not, however, have the impact ('rush') of direct injection into the bloodstream ('mainlining') and for this reason, and because of the development of tolerance, it is not widely used by hard-core addicts trying to recapture the intensity of earlier experiences with drugs.

The drugs involved

Many compounds have been misused over the ages but it is only in recent decades, with the advent of a rapidly expanding pharmaceutical industry, that the number of drugs having some property attractive to misusers has increased greatly. In general, drugs are taken to alter mood, thought or perception. It is important to appreciate that the effect of any drug varies from one individual to another and depends not only on its pharmacological properties but also on the personality of the consumer, his feelings and surroundings at the time of taking it and his preconceptions about its effects. The effects may also be enhanced or diminished by other drugs taken simultaneously.

Drugs that are misused fall into three main groups: those that stimulate, those that have a depressant effect and those that alter the senses, particularly perception (sometimes referred to as hallucinogens or psychedelics).

Stimulants

Cocaine, amphetamine and amphetamine-related compounds are the major constituents of this group. Cocaine is derived from the leaves of the coca plant, *Erythroxylon coca*, which is found in Peru and Bolivia. For centuries the natives of Peru have chewed coca leaves or drunk infusions of them partly for religious reasons but also so that they could work more readily in hostile environments. Coca exhilarates, increasing both physical and mental energy and, in addition, induces a sense of detachment from reality. The use of coca spread, and cocaine was isolated from the leaves towards the end of the nineteenth century.

Cocaine may be snorted as a snuff ('snow') or injected. The drug is rapidly broken down in the body and the 'flash' that addicts prize so highly and that can become the *raison d'etre* wears off quickly. For this reason repeated doses are often taken at short intervals (even as often as every 10 minutes) and very large amounts may be taken in the course of a day.

Amphetamine and its related compounds (commonly referred to as 'speed'), methylamphetamine, dextro-amphetamine, diethylpropion, phenmetrazine, phentermine and methylphenidate (Ritalin) stimulate the brain and suppress the appetite. They were widely used as pep-pills and more specifically for the treatment of depression and obesity. Like cocaine, these drugs make individuals more self-assured, lively and talkative and help them to keep awake but irritability, restlessness and impairment of judgment and reasoning supervene if they are taken in excess. Ideas of persecution, delusions and hallucinations may also occur and lead to irrational behaviour, features that characterize the severe psychotic state that may follow chronic consumption of large doses. Some addicts find the hyperexcitability induced by these drugs unpleasant and prefer to take them in conjuction with a depressant drug, e.g. cocaine with heroin, or amphetamine with a barbiturate. Death from misuse of amphetamine is uncommon and is usually due to cerebral haemorrhage or disturbance of heart rhythm.

Cocaine and amphetamines induce marked psychological dependence. Withdrawal is characterized by prolonged sleep, considerable increase in appetite, profound depression and apathy which may lead to attempts at suicide or to restarting the drugs.

The number of prescriptions for amphetamines is steadily falling and, with rare exceptions, there is probably no place for them in modern medicine.

Depressants

The main drugs in this group are the narcotic analgesics heroin, morphine, pethidine, methadone and dipipanone (as contained in Diconal) and the barbiturates of which there are numerous varieties.

Opium (the dried juice from the unripe poppy seed capsule) has been known for many centuries and in some societies was used socially as is alcohol today. It has been used medicinally for just as long; the beneficial effects of opium and its derivatives were well recognized at a time when most 'drugs' were, at best, ineffective. Even today, there are no more potent drugs than opiates for the relief of pain and the induction of euphoria. It is these very properties that make them so desirable to the addict and makes the British medical profession jealous to defend the right to prescribe them. In contrast, doctors in the USA are not permitted to prescribe heroin.

Opium may be smoked—though this is now not common in Britian—and there was a vogue for the ingestion of a liquid extract (laudanam) in the early nineteenth century. Morphine was isolated from opium in 1803 and, together with heroin (diamorphine), is one of the most extensively misused narcotic analgesics. Pethidine, methadone, dipipanone (Diconal) and dihydrocodeine (DF118) are synthetic compounds with similar properties. Most narcotic analgesics are usually mainlined, the 'fix' being prepared by dissolving the tablets in some water, gently heating, filtering, then drawing the solution into a syringe. Not everyone experimenting with these drugs finds them pleasurable. Nausea and vomiting are common with early use but these symptoms are usually followed by a feeling of calm detachment and invulnerability.

Dependence on narcotic analgesics is not a new phenomenon but it is only in recent years that the size of the problem has increased in Britain. Until about 1960, there were approximately 450 addicts known to the Home Office. The majority were middle aged or elderly people who had been given opiates during a serious disease and whom it was impossible to take off drugs once the illness ended ('therapeutic addicts'). Doctors, their wives and others working in related professions also comprised a substantial number of the addicts at that time (so-called 'professional addicts').

After 1960, however, the numbers began to rise steeply, reaching a plateau of about 3000 in 1972. The rise was in the number of non-therapeutic, non-professional addicts and was largely confined to persons between the ages of 20 and 35 years. The increase in the number of addicts below the age of 20 was less marked but was still a cause for grave concern. Later in that decade the number of addicts did not increase greatly and there was reason for cautious optimism that the problem was under control. Unfortunately, it is virtually certain that the official statistics are unreliable and recent reports from major cities indicate a much larger population of narcotic addicts than is appreciated by the Home Office. One encouraging aspect is that the average age of addicts appears to be increasing and some of those using heroin have been switched to methadone as part of treatment programmes.

Opiates rapidly induce profound psychological and physical dependence but, because of tolerance, the 'buzz' that the user obtains declines and he may find himself having to continue the drugs just to feel normal rather than to become elated. Sudden withdrawal of opiates without substituting other drugs leads to the well-known syndrome of 'cold turkey'. Running eyes and nose, sneezing, goose-flesh, feeling of cold, restlessness, muscle aches and pains are followed by nausea, vomiting and diarrhoea with abdominal cramps. These symptoms may last several days unless controlled by other drugs and, as the addict knows only too well, they may be rapidly relieved by a further fix.

Barbiturates are synthetic compounds which have been used extensively in recent decades for inducing sleep. The most popular include pentobarbitone (Nembutal), sodium amylobarbitone (Sodium Amytal) and a mixture of the latter with quinalbarbitone known as Tuinal. Misuse of barbiturates by young people came to light in the late 1960s. They were readily obtainable in public houses and from other black-market sources by youngsters experimenting with drugs. They were taken most commonly by mouth but a small proportion of addicts injected them intravenously. The hazards of barbiturate misuse will be discussed later: they produce marked psychological and physical dependence and tolerance. Sudden withdrawal may lead to serious illness lasting for several days and comprising convulsions, agitation, confusion, tremor and auditory and visual hallucinations.

Concern about misuse of barbiturates, the number of deaths from suicide using these drugs and the increasing availability of alternative sleeping preparations has led to a marked decline in the prescribing of barbiturates in the past 20 years. Some doctors continue to prescribe them but barbiturates are now controlled drugs and their availability to addicts is now due to thefts from chemists rather than to overprescribing by doctors. Some maintain that there is still a role for barbiturates in the management of severe insomnia but there is a considerable body of opinion that, with the exception of phenobarbitone which is used for the control of epilepsy, there is probably no place for barbiturate hypnotics in present-day medicine. Doctors are now resisting the pressure from many patients to continue to supply sleeping tablets and, when forced to do so, prescribe non-barbiturate varieties. With one exception (methaqualone, mainly as contained in Mandrax and Quaalude) more recent preparations have not held attractions for misusers. Moreover, marketing of Mandrax ceased in 1981.

Drugs altering the senses

The main substances in this group are cannabis, lysergic acid diethylamide (LSD) and 'magic' mushrooms such as the liberty cap (*Psilocybe semilanceata*) which contain psilocin and psilocybin. Others, such as mescaline and STP (serenity, tranquillity and peace), are much less commonly used. None of these substances has found a clearly defined place in medicine and any use is, thereby, misuse. They are sometimes referred to as 'hallucinogens' but this term is misleading since they more commonly distort what is actually present, albeit often in a vivid manner, than cause hallucinations. To call them 'psychedelics' is also unsatisfactory.

Like opium, cannabis, which is derived from the leaves and flowering top of the Indian hemp plant (*Cannabis sativa*), has been used by some societies for very many centuries. Nor is its use in the United Kingdom a new phenomenon although it is now probably the most commonly misused drug. The increasing number of convictions for possession of cannabis and cultivating the plant, together with reports of seizures of large consignments, reflects its widespread use in Britain. The more potent hashish (the resin exuded by the plant) is preferred to marihuana (the leaves) and is usually smoked mixed with tobacco though, in other civilizations, it was often eaten.

The effects of cannabis vary so considerably from one individual to another that it is difficult to detail them. Some are unaffected by it while others experience excitement, contentment, greater power of concentration and breadth of thought and sociability. Time passes more slowly, colours and sounds become more vivid than normal and the individual floats in and out of a joyful, dream-like state in which every thought or image may be grotesquely distorted. Laughing without reason is common in the early stages and, later, memory, reasoning and co-ordination may be impaired until restlessness gives way to drowsiness. The only physical effects may be a persistent cough or bloodshot eyes.

Cannabis users maintain that the drug is not addictive and that its long-term use is harmless. Moderate use undoubtedly impairs efficiency at work and school and heavy use may render the individual incapable of work. Whilst no serious physical symptoms follow abstinence, and many can stop smoking without difficulty, there are a small number of individuals who may become psychologically dependent. There is also some evidence that tolerance to cannabis occurs and overseas reports suggest the development of psychotic illnesses similar to schizophrenia with prolonged heavy use. Even single exposures have been said to produce panic attacks with paranoia; it is also claimed that psychotic illnesses after cannabis are much slower to clear once the drug is withdrawn than are those due to amphetamines. The existence of cannabis psychosis has been questioned but the evidence for the safety or otherwise of long-term cannabis use remains sufficiently scanty for the debate to continue for some years.

LSD ('acid') and its perception-distorting properties were discovered in 1943. Its effects are similar to those produced by mescaline but the amount required to evoke them is considerably smaller. The capacity of a minute quantity of LSD taken by mouth to induce a delirious state with vivid, distorted and fantastic visions is one of the most remarkable features of the drug. Hearing and appreciation of music may be enhanced. The company and surroundings in which it is taken determine to a large extent how pleasant or otherwise the 'trip' will be. One might have expected emotionally labile, insecure individuals to react to the point of panic in the face of such experiences but this is not common. On occasions, however, some 'trippers' prefer to have one of their number present, not to take the drug, but to act as 'guide' to comfort and reassure when necessary. Bad trips characterized by acute anxiety, panic, terror or ideas of persecution are infrequent.

There is no physical dependence on LSD but the rewards of the trip may be so gratifying that the desire to take it again is very strong. For this reason psychological dependence occurs in a small minority of users.

The centuries-old practice of eating mushrooms to alter consciousness and produce visual hallucinations has been enjoying a revival in Britain each autumn for the past few years, particularly among schoolchildren and young adults. *Psilocybe semilanceata* and *Paneaolus* species cause similar effects and are readily found in grassy parks, golf courses and fields. Booklets advising on identification and use are on public sale at little cost. Up to 30 or so mushrooms may be eaten raw. Cerebral excitation, distortion of perception and hallucinations may be accompanied by nausea and vomiting. To date no serious medical consequences have been reported after ingestion of 'magic' mushrooms but it is probably fortunate that highly toxic fungi are uncommon in this country and are unlikely to be picked in mistake for hallucinogenic types.

Phencyclidine (PCP, angel dust) is a relatively new drug of abuse but has rapidly become a major problem in the USA. As far as one can be certain, it has not yet reached Britain but it seems inevitable that it will do so at some stage. Phencyclidine was originally developed as an anaesthetic but was discarded because of a high incidence of psychotic reactions. It causes distortion of perception and hallucinations in low doses. For this reason, in street drugs, it often masquerades as LSD or the active principle of cannabis, both of which are considerably more expensive and more difficult to produce. Large doses of phencyclidine cause increasing agitation, stupor alternating unpredictably with violent behaviour, convulsions and finally loss of consciousness. It may be smoked, ingested or less commonly mainlined. Dependence on phencyclidine is psychological.

Solvent abuse

The term solvent abuse is less than completely accurate but is preferable to the older name 'glue sniffing'. The difficulties with terminology are, first, that the vapours from these substances are deeply inhaled rather than sniffed and, secondly, substances other than glues and organic solvents are abused in this way (e.g. the gas butane, from refill cylinders for cigarette lighters).

Solvent abuse was identified many years ago but has only recently increased to the extent that it has attracted public attention and concern. It is usually a group activity and predominantly involves males aged 8–30 years. Dry-cleaning agents are as popular as glues and are inhaled from a rag that has been soaked with them. Glues are usually emptied into a potato-crisp packet or polythene bag, the opening of which is gathered together and held round the nose. Inhalation may continue intermittently for many hours. The effects are similar to intoxication with alcohol but also include hallucinations.

Patterns of addiction

Discussion of drug addiction is, more than many topics, guaranteed to arouse heated argument and produce strong polarization of views. Unfortunately, the opinions held are not always based on facts since, often, the facts are either not available or are distorted by the preconceived views of those who collect them. Much of what has been written about drug-taking is based on surveys of schoolchildren, students and addicts who come to medical or legal notice. Almost certainly, none of these groups is representative of the whole drug-taking population and, while study of each has yielded much useful information, it would be foolish to extrapolate from them to drug-takers in general. It is difficult, however, to see how this deficiency in our knowledge can be remedied for, as long as drug-taking remains illegal, users, particularly those taking cannabis or other 'soft' drugs (the vast majority), will not openly discuss these subjects. Probably the nearest one will get to an overall view of the misuse of drugs is that reported by researchers working within the drug-taking community and having the confidence of addicts. Even then, the difficulties are formidable: a typical cross-section is probably impossible to obtain and study groups can only readily be formed by accumulating contacts over a prolonged period of time. The personalities of some of those under study may make them exaggerate or play down their activities.

Early experiences with drugs are probably very intermittent and are most likely to involve solvents, mushrooms, anti-sea-sickness pills, mild stimulant drugs that can be bought over chemists counters and minor tranquillizers, often taken in conjunction with alcohol at parties and discotheques. Some individuals may then repeat the experience on a more regular basis. Cannabis is one of the most widely used drugs but probably only a small proportion of users confine themselves to this drug alone. LSD and amphetamines are the most popular other drugs but it should be appreciated that the great majority of cannabis smokers also use tobacco and alcohol. Smoking cannabis has for some time been regarded as the first rung on the ladder to addiction to opiates and cocaine, though the evidence for escalation is slim. Cannabis smoking is generally a group activity and so much of the response to the drug is determined by the behaviour of one's fellow smokers that it has been suggested that it is a social rather than a chemical experience. Moreover, many students and so-called 'middle-class Bohemians' take care to time their use of cannabis so that its effects will not interfere with work, study and other responsibilities. These groups often dissociate themselves from the injection of drugs, but 'fixers' may be attracted to such gatherings and pressurize those present into experimenting with heroin and other dangerous drugs. Some evidence, however, suggests that those who experiment with injecting drugs probably only do so a few times and that it is a small minority that adopts this method regularly.

A survey of 60 male addicts[1] attending a treatment centre revealed that all had at some time used cannabis, amphetamines and non-barbiturate sedatives. Between two-thirds and three-quarters of them had taken hallucinogens, barbiturates, heroin and methadone, but only half cocaine. Poly-drug use is common but most addicts prefer to use selected drugs on a regular basis though anything may be tried if needs dictate or others are available. The concomitant use of alcohol and tobacco is usual.

The group of addicts who mainline drugs regularly, particularly narcotic analgesics, has been written about extensively and further discussion of the 'junkie' and his total preoccupation with the acquisition and use of drugs is unnecessary. Some mainliners manage to stop these drugs and cope with the withdrawal symptoms on their own initiative or with medical help but, of those who come to legal or medical attention, some 30 per cent or more are still using narcotics 4–7 years later. Studies of US servicemen in Vietnam revealed a high incidence of narcotic addiction but only a small proportion continued using drugs during the first year of repatriation.

Characteristics, background and lifestyles of addicts

The great majority of people who misuse drugs are between the ages of 20 and 35 years and men outnumber women by about three to one. Whereas addiction to narcotics and cocaine is largely confined to London and, to a lesser extent, other large cities, the use of cannabis is much more widespread. One community study suggested that students and 'Bohemians' were more likely to confine their drug use to cannabis whereas a wider and more dangerous range of drugs, often injected, was more likely to be utilized by low-status unemployed or manual workers. Most early experiences with drugs are the result of curiosity, bravado, pressure from peers, abnormal personality and sometimes a search for excitement, pleasure or relief from anxiety. It must be emphasized that social disintegration is not inevitable with regular use of drugs. Many habitual cannabis users function entirely satisfactorily in the community and even some narcotic addicts are maintained on a relatively small dose which fluctuates little and does not prevent a stable and useful life.

Most addicts are of average or above-average intelligence yet—whether because of immaturity, impulsiveness, liability to sudden swings of mood or some other factor—they do not reach the levels of achievement that might be expected. Their performance at school may be poor, truancy is frequent and they tend to leave at an early age, often only to drift from one job to another. Their personalities and their relative inability to cope with stress are important factors in producing dependence on drugs. Illness in the home is not uncommon and the family background tends to be disturbed; many of them are illegitimate, have had an institutional upbringing or come from broken homes. Even if the family is apparently intact, disharmony between parents can be such that the home environment is no less detrimental than if the family were dissolved. Perhaps not surprisingly, addicts are often involved in delinquency even before starting on drugs.

Schoolchildren seem to gather most of their information about drugs from

[1] Gordon, A.M. (1978). Do drug offences matter? *British Medical Journal*, **ii,** 185.

television and though they know many of the drug names they usually have little knowledge of their effects.

Addiction and crime

Many addicts attending drug treatment centres have received court convictions at some time in the past and it has often been questioned whether this high incidence can be attributed to drug dependence. The evidence is conflicting. Of 60 consecutive new male attenders at a London treatment centre almost half had been convicted before starting drugs and 90 per cent subsequent to drug use. Theft, motoring and violence offences are common before and after drug use, with drug offences comprising an important proportion once dependence is established. Convictions after drug use are no more frequent in those whose first conviction antedated drug use than among the others convicted for the first time after starting on drugs!

Similarly, 60 per cent of a group of female addicts in prison were first convicted prior to addiction[2]. A high proportion went on to commit further offences over the next few years and, in general, this paralleled continued drug use. It has been suggested, therefore, that addiction does not lead to crime but that both activities merely reflect the abnormal personality and disturbed social backgrounds of the individuals concerned. Not infrequently the father, or more commonly a sibling, of an addict may have been convicted for some crime. This, together with parental loss, tends to be commoner in those addicts whose criminal activities antedate their use of drugs.

While the majority of offences committed by addicts involve drugs or damage to property, several studies have shown an increase in the incidence of violent offences and offenders after drug use. In some cases the nature of the offences became more serious involving, among other crimes, assault, offences with weapons, inflicting bodily harm and robbery with violence.

The medical hazards of drug misuse

The misuse of any drug carries risks to health. Fortunately most adverse effects are relatively mild and may depend more on the personality of the user and his emotional reaction to the drug than on the toxic effect of the drug itself. Thus, some individuals may be unable to cope with the expected effects of a 'normal' dose and become sufficiently alarmed and disturbed in their behaviour to refer themselves to hospital or to be taken there by friends. More commonly, arrival at casualty departments is the result of an emergency ambulance call or because disturbed behaviour has attracted the attention of the police. Others end up in hospital because they have misjudged the amount of drug and they are suffering from accidental overdosage. As indicated earlier, death from overdosage from stimulant drugs is uncommon but large doses of depressant drugs may lead to deep coma, possible obstruction of the respiratory passages, gradual failure of respiration, shock and death. These problems can generally be dealt with effectively if the individual reaches hospital, and mortality is low. Unfortunately,

[2] d'Orban, P. J. (1973). Female narcotic addicts: A follow-up study of criminal and addiction careers. *British Medical Journal*, **iv**, 345.

many addicts suffering from accidental overdosage do not survive long enough to reach hospital.

Some deaths associated with narcotic misuse are due to accidental overdosage resulting from the variable potency of 'street' drugs which, depending on the ease of availability, may be adulterated to a greater or lesser extent with other materials such as milksugars, talc and quinine. The additives themselves may cause serious problems when injected intravenously. Fortunately there is an antidote for narcotic analgesics, and the life-endangering effects can be dramatically reversed within seconds. However, no such antidote is available for barbiturate overdosage. In severe cases it may be necessary to attempt to increase the elimination of the drug from the body but the majority will survive if a patent airway is maintained and respiration is supported (by mechanical means if necessary) until the body degrades and eliminates the barbiturates and the patient returns to consciousness. The duration of coma may be several days and complications such as respiratory infections add considerably to the risks. It is no coincidence that barbiturates have been implicated in the deaths of a substantial number of addicts.

Many of the other important medical complications of addiction are primarily attributable to the injection of drugs. At every state the preparation of the 'fix' is totally lacking in sterility; the drug is often in a form never meant for injection, the water in which it is dissolved may at best be obtained from a tap or at worst from a public lavatory and the equipment used to hold the solution and strain it may be no more than socially clean. The same comment could be applied to many of the syringes and needles used. It will be obvious, therefore, that bacterial and viral infections are common and may be transmitted from one person to another because of sharing of 'gear'. Most bacterial infections occur at injection sites with abscess formation, skin ulceration and inflammation along the course of veins resulting in the formation of clot on the damaged vein lining (thrombosis) and obliteration of the channel.

Infection of the heart valves and abscesses in the lungs may occur and, although the multiplication of bacteria in the bloodstream may potentially cause infection anywhere, there is a particular predilection for joints. A specific virus infection of the liver, causing liver inflammation (hepatitis) and jaundice, is not uncommon and may be trasmitted from one individual to another by contaminated needles.

As the veins on the arms and hands become obliterated from repeated use and infection, those in the legs are usually next to be attacked but eventually no vein, regardless of its situation, is sacrosanct. It is not unknown for those on the breast, tongue, penis and around the anus and vagina to be used by desperate addicts. Extremely dexterous as many are at injecting tiny veins, occasionally an artery is 'hit', leading to thrombosis and gangrene of the fingers or feet; amputation may be necessary.

Death from accidental overdosage and infection in addicts is common and suicide is several times more common than in the general population. A review of 66 Holloway addicts after 5 years (see footnote, page 259) revealed that 10 (15 per cent) were dead at an average age of just over 22 years. Another study of 108 narcotic addicts, 6–7 years after notification, showed a mortality of at least 18 per cent (some could not be traced). These and similar statistics justify the anxiety of many about the possibility of escalation from so-called 'soft' drugs such as cannabis.

Inhalation of solvents and use of drugs that alter perception are seldom fatal. The few deaths that occur are usually not due directly to the drug but to attempts to intensify the experience (e.g. asphyxiating while inhaling solvents with a plastic bag over the head) or to trying to swim or fly while intoxicated. Heavy solvent abuse occasionally damages the liver, kidneys, nerves and brain, sometimes irreversibly.

Treatment of drug addiction

The results of treatment of addiction are far from satisfactory, partly because the nature of drug misuse is not understood and partly because many addicts have sociopathic personalities that cannot be readily altered. Many have insight into what the future holds for them yet accept the risks so as to improve (in their estimation) the quality of the present. Others presumably know about the hazards but deny them. In recent years there has been a vogue for withdrawing heroin and morphine by replacing them with methadone, which has somewhat different pharmacological properties, usually under the supervision of a drug treatment clinic. Unfortunately, this has not always prevented addicts supplementing methadone with other drugs, and methadone itself is a drug of addiction. The value of this approach is, therefore, far from proven. Even under supervision in institutions, it is difficult to prevent addicts obtaining drugs and, in the community, it is clearly impossible. Ultimately, long-term abstinence is only possible with individuals who are strongly motivated and who have the support of their families and perhaps psychiatrists, social workers and therapeutic communities.

Control of drugs

For as long as drugs have been used, measures to control their use or availability have been advocated or introduced. In the fourteenth century an Arab ruler extracted the teeth of those guilty of chewing cannabis; coca was denounced by the Catholic Church in the sixteenth century and peyotl by the Inquisition a few decades later. James VI of Scotland on ascending the English throne increased the tax on tobacco by some 4000 per cent in the hope of reducing its use. There is little evidence, however, that these measures met with any more success than did the prohibition of alcohol in the USA earlier this century.

In the United Kingdom, morphine and heroin addiction were the subject of review by the Rolleston Committee (1926), whose recommendations were incorporated into the legislation on dangerous drugs. There was little activity from then until 1958 when the Brain Committee[3] was convened to consider whether any changes in legislation or facilities should be made in view of the increased number of potentially addictive drugs used to relieve pain and of developments in the treatment of drug addiction. It was concluded that the problem of addiction in Great Britain was very small, that special treatment centres and registration of addicts were unnecessary and that extension of statutory powers to control new drugs was not needed at that time. The recommendation that addiction be regarded as an expression of mental disorder rather than of criminal behaviour is still accepted and has been of paramount importance in determining attitudes and in fashioning legislation of drugs. Only now is this view being challenged.

[3] Brain, R. (Chairman) (1961). *Drug Addiction. Report of the Interdepartmental Committee.* London; HMSO.

Between 1959 and 1964, the drug misuse situation changed sufficiently for the Brain Committee to be reconvened in order to consider whether its earlier advice should be revised[4]. The total number of known addicts had risen, heroin addicts had increased fivefold, the use of cocaine had also increased and there was a trend towards a much younger age of addicts. The problem was found to be largely confined to London and to excessive prescribing by a small number of doctors. In its second report the Committee accepted the need for control measures and recommended that heroin and cocaine for addicts should only be prescribed by the medical staff of special treatment centres which were to be established. Notification of addicts was also advised. Overall, most of the earlier decisions were reversed, and the new recommendations formed the basis for various items of legislation up to and including the Misuse of Drugs Act 1971 and its subsequent regulations which came into effect in 1973.

The desirability and effectiveness of legal control of drugs have been often questioned but are difficult to assess. Official statistics, including the number of addicts notified to the Home Office and convictions for drug offences, are generally considered to underestimate seriously the extent of drug misuse. This is partly supported by the results of a study of 66 people from the south of England who were convicted for their first drug offence between 1967 and 1970 and were followed up after 3 years[5]. Only 18 had been reconvicted for a drug offence but it was learned from other sources that 49 (74 per cent) were still taking drugs and that the pattern of drug-taking had become more serious. Conviction for a drug offence therefore appears to have little deterrent effect.

'Magic' mushrooms contain proscribed drugs but clearly cannot be controlled any more than organic solvents can be.

[4] Brain, R. (Chairman) (1965). *Drug Addiction. The Second Report of the Interdepartmental Committee*. London; HMSO.
[5] de Alarcon, R. and Noguera, R. (1974). Clinical effects on drug abuse of a conviction for a drug offence. *Lancet*, **ii**, 174.

25

Medico-legal aspects of alcohol

The greatest social significance of alcohol rests on its being a drug of dependence. It has been estimated that there are some 90 000 alcoholics in Great Britain and the position is particularly serious in Scotland.

Alcohol is a cortical depressant. Since it is the higher and the most recently evolved brain functions that are first affected by depressants, the immediate effect of a dose of alcohol is to inhibit those cerebral functions that are associated with orderly community behaviour and with finer critical judgments; an illusion of cerebral stimulation is thus precipitated. Chronic alcoholism, however, almost inevitably leads to physical and social degeneration, inability to retain employment, disruption of the family and the like, followed by generalized cerebral deterioration. Dependence is often of extreme degree and the high cost of alcoholic drinks has two major effects—first, increasingly cheap and, concurrently, toxic forms of alcohol are consumed and, secondly, there is often a lapse into petty criminality designed to obtain and conserve supplies. The criminal alcoholic who develops has to be distinguished from the intoxicated criminal—that is, the person with criminal inclinations that are potentiated by consumption of alcohol.

While the distinction between the sporadic and the compulsive drinker is emphasized in this section, alcoholism as a disease state will be discussed in detail in Chapter 28; the present concern is, in the main, to discuss the association of acute alcoholism with injury and sudden death and the resulting legal consequences.

Physiology of alcohol

Alcohol is absorbed rapidly from the stomach and especially from the upper intestine—if the stomach empties unduly fast, as in persons who have had certain surgical operations, absorption is likely to be more rapid and the effects more obvious; conversely, the commonly observed 'sobering' effect of a full stomach is probably due to delayed emptying. Once absorbed, the alcohol is dissolved in the body water and distributed according to the water content of the tissues—thus the blood, in which there is much solid material, contains less alcohol, volume for volume, than does, say, the cerebrospinal fluid. The amount of alcohol in the body is expressed in the United Kingdom in terms of milligrams of alcohol per 100 millilitres of blood[1].

The greater part of the ingested alcohol is destroyed by the liver. Approximately 10 per cent is excreted in the urine, sweat and breath. The combined effect of destruction and elimination is to reduce the blood alcohol by an amount that is variously estimated but which can, for practical purposes, be regarded as 15 mg/ 100 ml blood/hour (see page 284).

Since alcohol diffuses uniformly in the body fluids, it will be present in the urine which is formed in the kidneys. But as urine contains very little solid material, there will be more alcohol per 100 ml of urine than per 100 ml of blood and, in order to compare the two fluids, a ratio of 1.3:1.0 is usually accepted. This, however, assumes that the urine and blood are in equilibrium, and this cannot be so in practice because urine is isolated and stored in the bladder. The nearest one can get to equivalence of blood and urine is to empty the bladder and test the smallest amount that can next be voided naturally—a matter of some 20 minutes' excretion by the kidneys. Direct comparison of urine and blood has been found to be so inaccurate that few forensic medical experts would nowadays be prepared to make the attempt—results are given either as urine alcohol or as blood alcohol. Breath, however, is another matter, as the alveolar air is in immediate contact with the blood in the capillaries; theoretically, a constant breath/blood ratio should be achieved and this is accepted as approximately 1:2000. While it is true that there is an inconstant amount of a breath sample that is tidal air and has not been in contact with the blood, this can be compensated for in testing. Modern 'breathalysers' are of such accuracy and constancy that it is feasible to use them as true measures of intoxication[2]. However, current legislation accepts that the result given by the breath should be checked by blood analysis when it is only marginally above any prescribed limit (see below).

The amount of alcohol present in the blood at any time is determined by many more factors than the simple measure of the quantity ingested. It depends on the method of dosing, on the rate of absorption, on the available water for distribution—which is reflected in the body weight and stature—and on the capacity of the liver to metabolize the dose. All these variables operate in the context of normal social drinking and, consequently, it is common practice to assess only the minimum alcoholic intake likely to correspond to an analytic finding; for this purpose, the tables prepared by the British Medical Association are generally acceptable to the Courts[3].

The expert witness will also be asked what was the likely practical effect of a given blood concentration of alcohol. Again, the answer to this can only be given in wide terms. Much depends on the conditions for drinking, the availability of food, etc; there is also no doubt that habituation to alcohol occurs—the reason for this not being entirely clear—and the same blood concentration will have a lesser effect on the regular drinker than on the novice. However, the following table repesents an acceptable average assessment:

---

[1] In all the EEC countries, the expression is in grams per litre ('Promille'); the result is that the bald number quoted in the United Kingdom is 100 times that quoted for a similar concentration on the Continent.

[2] Road Traffic Act 1972, s. 7 (as replaced by Transport Act 1981, Sch 8).

[3] Relation of Alcohol to Road Accidents (1960). London; British Medical Association. See R. v. Somers [1963] 3 All E.R. 808.

10–100 mg/100 ml: Loss of self-control, an increase in self-confidence, talkativeness and alterations in judgment.
100–200 mg/100 ml: Distinct loss of skill, slurring of speech and commencing loss of co-ordination.
200–300 mg/100 ml: Loss of equilibrium, decrease in pain sense, marked disturbances in vision.
300–400 mg/100 ml: Increasing dissociation, stupor and probably coma.
400+ mg/100 ml: Coma (with its attendant hazards such as hypothermia) and possible death.

These are, however, subjective criteria. Objective measurements show that even low concentrations—of the order of 50 mg/100 ml—cause a lengthening of the reaction time in response to a complex situation and a decrease in visual function. If one adds to this the impulsive psychological effects, there is good reason to suppose that the most dangerous person on the roads with respect to alcoholism is the man who is only moderately intoxicated; while he is not able to react in an emergency in the normal way, he is, at the same time, unable to appreciate his deterioration in performance.

Such subtle changes are not disclosed by normal clinical tests—probably only those with a blood level of more than 150 mg/100 ml are detected as being unfit to drive by this means. Most countries have accordingly settled on holding it an offence to drive or to attempt to drive a motor vehicle when the proportion of alcohol in the blood exceeds x mg/100 ml; the figure x is variously defined—in Ireland it is 125 mg/100 ml; it is 80 mg/100 ml in Great Britain. A double standard is often adopted, this being reflected in the statutory penalties.

Alcohol is of medico-legal significance in relation to accident, suicide, homicide and natural death. The first of these, which includes the topic of road-traffic legislation, is by far the most important.

Aircraft accidents and alcohol

A momentary digression to aircraft accidents is excusable since they illustrate an important point in relation to alcoholism.

TABLE 25.1 Intoxicating liquor and the general aviation pilot in 1971

Fatal accidents studied for ethanol	256
Number positive (more than 15 mg/100 ml)	52 (20%)
15–49 mg/100 ml = 25%	
50–99 mg/100 ml = 12%	
100–149 mg/100 ml = 21%	
150 mg/100 ml+ = 42%	

The proportion of 'Ethanol Positives' has remained stable since 1968 and the proportion of accidents with ethanol 50 mg/100 ml or more is fairly stable. However, the proportion of accidents with ethanol 150 mg/100 ml or more is higher since the introduction in 1970 of an 8-hour abstinence period before flying.

It is not generally appreciated that, just as in the case of cars, a proportion of light-aircraft accidents are alcohol associated. The figures shown in *Table 25.1* are extracted from a survey of such accidents ending fatally in the USA[4]. The fact that

[4] Ryan, L. C. and Mohler, S. R. (1972). Intoxicating liquor and the general aviation pilot in 1971. *Aerospace Medicine*, **43**, 1024.

13 per cent showed alcohol concentrations that would be significant in any circumstances is, in itself, interesting. However, the authors of the study noted that since the Federal Aviation Authority had introduced a regulation forbidding private flying within 8 hours of alcoholic intake, the proportion of fatal accidents associated with a *very high* blood alcohol had, in fact, risen. Only one conclusion is possible—that there is one cadre of drinkers who are amenable to reason and regulation—that is, the social drinkers; at the other end of the scale lie the hardened alcoholics who are indifferent to moral pressures or punitive measures. The same thing probably occurs in motorists[5] and it is difficult not to infer that, if there are two classes of offender, there should, on general criminological grounds, be two types of penalty[6].

It is an offence to fly anywhere any aircraft registered in the United Kingdom or any other aircraft within the United Kingdom while under the influence of drink or drugs so as to impair the capacity of the crew member to do so[7]. Surprisingly, there is no authority to test the biological fluids of living pilots for alcohol content comparable with that which exists for drivers of automobiles.

Motor-vehicle accidents and alcohol

There is abundant evidence that alcohol is a potent source of automobile accidents. The results of four well-controlled surveys are summarized in *Table 25.2;* although the figures differ in degree, the association of accidents with rising alcohol concentrations is clearly reproducible. Some minor interest attaches to the consistent finding that very small amounts of alcohol actually reduce the accident rate. It is submitted that this does not represent a beneficial effect of alcohol but rather that persons who know they may be at risk are at particular pains not to be discovered.

TABLE 25.2 Alcohol and traffic accidents

Approximate band of alcohol concentration (mg/100 ml)	Ratio of accident/non-accident drivers			
	I	*II*	*III*	*IV*
0–50	0.7	0.8	0.3	0.9
50–100	3.3	1.3	2.4	1.5
100–150	8.7	2.1	10.2	4.0
Over 150	33.1	8.1	41.8	18.0

The figures have been modified from the following reports: *I.* Holcomb, R. L. (1938), *Journal of the American Medical Association*, **111**, 1076. *II.* Lucas, G. W. H., *et al.* (1955), In Proceedings of the *2nd International Conference on Alcohol and Road Traffic, Toronto,* p. 139. *III.* Vamosi, M. (1961), *Traffic Safety and Research Review*, **4**.8. *IV.* Borkenstein, F., *et al.* (1964), *The Role of the Drinking Driver in Traffic Accidents*, Indiana University Department of Police Administration.

[5] Witness the study by McCarroll, J. R. and Haddon, W. (1962), A controlled study of fatal automobile accidents in New York City, *Journal of Chronic Diseases*, **15**, 811, in which 4 per cent of a controlled accident group had a blood alcohol in excess of 250 mg/100 ml, which must indicate a flagrant disregard of consequences.
[6] As the Blennerhassett Committee (*Report of the Departmental Committee on Drinking and Driving* (1976). London; HMSO) acknowledged.
[7] Air Navigation Order 1980, Article 47(2) (S.I. 1980/1965).

The current United Kingdom (excluding Northern Ireland) legislation is contained in the Road Traffic Act 1972 as greatly amended by the Transport Act 1981, Schedule 8. Section 5 of the 1972 Act, which prescribes the offence of driving or attempting to drive a motor vehicle on a road or other public place while unfit to drive through the action of drink or drugs, remains unaltered save as to powers of arrest[8]; Sections 6 to 12 must now be read as stated in Schedule 8 to the 1981 Act.

The basic effect of the 1981 Act is to introduce breath testing for alcohol as a definitive test rather than as a preliminary to blood or urine analysis as previously obtained. The various types of breathalyser have been studied extensively[9]; standard instruments which operate on the principle of infrared absorption are now in use in both England and Wales and in Scotland—the manufacturers are, however, different in the two regions. Section 6 now makes it an offence 'to drive or attempt to drive a motor vehicle . . . or be in charge of a motor vehicle . . . after consuming so much alcohol that the proportion of it in (the driver's) breath, blood or urine exceeds the prescribed limits'[10].

The procedure is laid down precisely but, in general, a constable can require any person driving or attempting to drive a motor vehicle who is suspected of having, or having had, alcohol in the body or has committed a traffic offence while the vehicle was in motion or any person who was driving and was involved in an accident to provide a specimen of breath for a breath test; the specimen can be taken at the site of the incident, nearby or in a police station and failure to provide a specimen constitutes an offence. If the breath test is positive or if the subject refuses a test, the constable can arrest him without warrant; the police in England and Wales can also enter a place by force in order to obtain a specimen when there is reasonable suspicion that injury has been sustained by another person[11]. During the investigation at the police station, the accused may be asked to provide two specimens of breath; if he cannot do so for medical reasons, or if he is suspected of being under the influence of a drug or if no breathalyser is available, he can be asked to provide a specimen of blood or urine. Again, refusal to provide a specimen is an offence tantamount to having alcohol in the specimen above the prescribed limit. Specimens required in hospital can only be obtained on the authority of the medical practitioner in charge of the case, who may object if the undertaking of the test or the warning given would be prejudicial to the care of the patient.

The choice of blood or urine as an alternative to breath is at the discretion of the constable. A blood specimen must be taken by a registered medical practitioner and only with the consent of the accused. A specimen of urine must be taken within 1 hour of the incident and after providing a previous specimen which is discarded; in this way, the possibility is avoided of the specimen being contaminated with urine secreted some time before the incident and therefore probably containing more alcohol than was exerting an influence at the relevant time. In either case, a part of the specimen must be given to the accused if he so requests and he can use this for a second analysis employing a qualified analyst of his choice. It is apparent that the use of definitive breath testing deprives the accused of this right; this is covered in two ways—first the lower of the two results from the two breath tests is used; and, secondly, the accused can demand that his blood or urine be used for analysis if the lower breath result is no higher than 50 μg alcohol/100 ml breath (s. 8(6)).

[8] s. 7(6) (not applicable to Scotland).
[9] An excellent review is given in Emerson, V. J. et al. (1980), The Measurement of breath alcohol, *Journal of the Forensic Society*, **20**, 3–70.
[10] The prescribed limits currently mean 35 micrograms (μg) of alcohol/100 millilitres (ml) breath; or 80 mg alcohol/100 ml blood; or 107 mg alcohol/100 ml urine (s. 12(2)).
[11] Fox v. Gwent Chief Constable [1985] 1 W.L.R. 33, D.C.; (1985) *The Times*, 18 October, H.L.

Although it is not specifically stated, it can be assumed that analyses for alcohol in blood or urine would carry no weight unless they were performed by gas chromatography (*see* Chapter 26). The doctrine of *de minimis*—that something is too small to be taken notice of—is specifically non-applicable to the Road Traffic Act; it follows that great responsibility rests on the analyst when dealing with blood or urine concentrations that are only slightly above the prescribed limits. Using the gas chromatograph, a skilled analyst should provide results that show a standard deviation of no more than 2 per cent from the actual concentration. To be absolutely safe, a possible scatter of three standard deviations is accepted. Thus, whenever a result is 100 mg/100 ml or less, an amount of 6 mg/100 ml is automatically deducted; above 100 mg/100 ml, the deduction is 6 per cent of the actual figure. The result is then expressed as 'not less than [the corrected figure]'[12]. The limitations of such a rule are discussed in Chapter 26.

The use of a motor car is almost essential for the discharge of many professions and the obligatory disqualification for driving consequent upon conviction for driving or attempting to drive with a blood alcohol concentration in excess of the prescribed limit can be draconian in its effects—it is not surprising, therefore, that a mass of case law has been built up on the basis of all conceivable methods of outwitting the statute—so much so that a substantial body of legal literature has been devoted to the subject[13]; a main purpose of the 1981 Act has been to simplify the procedures and thus avoid artificial defences.

One aspect—that of what constitutes reasonable excuse to provide a specimen— is of sufficient interest both to the medical and legal professions to merit comment. It is difficult to see any reasonable excuse for failing to provide a breath specimen other than one founded on obvious medical grounds such as injury. It seems unlikely that a person who was unable to provide a specimen by reason of natural disease should have had a licence to drive. Similarly, there can be few reasonable grounds for a fit person to refuse to provide a valid specimen of urine. The situation as regards blood, which involves an invasive technique for its provision, is different yet, even here, the criteria for reasonable excuse are very strict: 'no excuse can be adjudged reasonable unless the person from whom the specimen was required was physically or mentally unable to provide it or the provision of the specimen would entail a substantial risk to his health'[14]. If the conditions for reasonable excuse are not met the question can, as a matter of law, be withdrawn from the jury; otherwise, it is a matter of fact for decision. One can imagine certain conditions—for example, a severe skin disease or a horror of injections—that might constitute good reason for not wishing to undergo a needle prick. It has been held that failure to provide a urine specimen even after three unsuccessful attempts had been made by the police surgeon to obtain blood—a thoroughly unpleasant experience—still did not qualify as a reasonable excuse[15].

[12] For a simple exposition of accuracy in analysis, *see* Walls, H. J. and Brownlie, A. R. (1985) *Drink, Drugs and Driving*, 2nd edn., Ch. 7; London; Sweet & Maxwell.
[13] Chapter 4 of Wilkinson's (1980) *Road Traffic Law* 10th edn; London; Oyez Publishing, is indispensable reading in this context.
[14] R. v. Lennard [1973] R.T.R. 252. See Alcock v. Read [1980] R.T.R. 71 as to the discretion of the jury. A medical decision must be taken by a doctor (Chief Constable of West Yorkshire Metropolitan Police v. Johnson (1985) *The Times*, 27 August).
[15] R. v. Harling, [1970] 3 All E.R. 902.

Insistence upon giving a blood specimen from part of the body other than that specified by the police surgeon would be regarded as refusal to provide a specimen[16]. Moreover, one cannot consent to the removal of the specimen by a doctor of one's own choice yet refuse the offices of the police surgeon[16]. But once a specimen has been provided, it is perfectly proper for the accused to refuse to give a second one; neither the police nor the police surgeon can retrieve a technical error made by them[16].

One very common defence to charges under Section 6—that the alcohol shown to be present in the specimen for analysis derived from consumption after the accident—now has the force of law; under Section 10(2) of the amended 1972 Act, the assumption that the proportion of alcohol in the accused's body at the time of the alleged offence was not less than that discovered in the specimen shall not be made if the accused can show that he drank alcohol between the alleged offence and the provision of the specimen and that, if he had not done so, the result of the analysis would not have exceeded the prescribed limit. The former is a matter for credible witnesses; the latter is one for scientific deduction which may be based on the British Medical Association Tables (see footnote 3, page 264). The result extrapolated from the stated amount drunk can be read off and an adjustment made for body weight. This, however, is a maximum theoretical value which is unlikely to be achieved in practice and, to compensate for this, allowance must be made for natural destruction of alcohol in the body—a value of 15 mg alcohol per 100 ml blood per hour reverting to the time of the post-incident drinking is fair to both prosecution and defence; the defence is established if the observed value less the calculated 'post-incident' value is less than the prescribed limit. An alternative is to use prepared nomograms[16a] but it is clear that, whatever method is used, a number of assumptions are made which must be freely admitted.

The determination of alcohol levels in all persons killed or injured accidentally is of further practical importance on two counts. First, virtually all personal accident insurance policies carry an exclusion clause for injuries sustained 'whilst under the influence of intoxicating liquor' and this applies in a temporal sense, no causal relationship being required[17]; the importance to passengers needs no emphasis. Secondly, a realization that the driver is drunk amounts to contributory negligence by a passenger who accepts a lift from him[18]; the blood alcohol concentration must go a long way to establishing the likelihood of such an appreciation.

Charges under the 1972 Act can still be made without the use of a blood or urine test (s. 5) and this will always apply when there is a possibility of driving under the influence of drugs. In this case, a medical examination must be undertaken and the results of this are certainly open to the Court as matters of fact; police surgeons do have, as a point of policy, a standardized form of examination and reporting which eliminates much argument. Fortunately, these cases are now very rare.

[16] Rushton v. Higgins [1972] R.T.R. 456; R. v. Godden [1971] R.T.R. 462. But where both the accused's physician and the police doctor are present together, the general practitioner may take the specimen (Bayliss v. Thames Valley Police Chief Constable [1978] R.T.R. 328, D.C.). In Beck v. Watson [1980] R.T.R. 91, the specimen was dropped; the analysis of a second specimen was considered invalid.

[16a] For example, King, L. A. (1983) Nomograms for relating blood and urine alcohol concentrations with quantity of alcohol consumed. Journal of the Forensic Science Society, 23, 213. For a review of the defence see Mason, J. K. (1984) Section 10 defence to charges of driving with excess alcohol. 128 S.J. 539.

[17] Louden v. British Merchants Insurance Co. Ltd [1961] 1 All E.R. 705, per Lawton, J. 'Influence' was here defined as 'a disturbance of the quiet, calm and intelligent exercise of the faculties' but it is understood that most insurance companies would pragmatically accept a blood level in excess of 80 mg/100 ml as evidence of intoxication.

[18] Owens v. Brimmell [1976] 3 All E.R. 765.

Perhaps the function of the clinical examination that has the greatest medico-legal significance is not so much the detection of drugging as the exclusion of other causes of abnormal behaviour—head injury or disorders of carbohydrate metabolism spring immediately to mind. The distinction is even more important when the subject is being detained in custody on account of apparent drunkenness for reasons unconnected with motoring offences; death of a person in detention dictates a Coroner's Inquiry with jury in England and Wales and will precipitate a Public Inquiry in Scotland (Fatal Accidents and Sudden Deaths Inquiry (Scotland) Act 1976, s. 1(1)(a)(ii)).

Studies of pedestrians killed in road-traffic accidents indicate a very similar pattern of alcohol association to that shown by drivers. *All* persons killed in traffic accidents should be examined *post-mortem* for evidence of alcoholic intoxication; the knowledge that a killed pedestrian was drunk to the state of muscular inco-ordination should be available to the defence of a driver.

Accidental death of other types associated with alcohol

Consumption of sufficient alcohol to remove the constraints of normal care is very often associated with accidental firearm injuries[19]. Theoretically, the level of blood alcohol might be expected to be of diagnostic significance in this connection. Reported results are, however, equivocal, some authors having noted that a high proportion of suicidal gunshot wounds are alcohol associated, and there is no reason why a drunken argument should not end in a shooting. The finding of alcohol in a victim of a gunshot incident is but one piece of evidence to be assessed in conjuction with the findings discussed in Chapter 9.

Other accidental deaths associated with alcohol are directly related to the more severe physiological effects. At a level of about 200 mg alcohol/100 ml blood, a loss of equilibrium will be superimposed on inhibition of the critical faculties. Falls from heights, particularly out of windows, are likely to be precipitated and it may be extremely difficult to establish the total innocence of the death in conditions of group alcoholism; very little force will be required to overbalance an intoxicated person and any minor marks sustained in a mêlée might be obscured by, and would certainly be difficult to differentiate from, the effects of terminal impact. Similarly, drowning is associated with alcohol, particularly in docks or canals beside which the less uninhibited would be wary of walking and where the high sides make escape from the water very difficult. However, I have been impressed by the high incidence of artefactually raised blood alcohol levels (*see* page 274) in cases of drowning and this possibility should be excluded before a firm association is accepted in individual cases.

Stupor is likely at higher blood levels and this is a very common underlying cause of death from burning, a cigarette dropped from the hand setting light to the bedclothes; many such deaths are due to the synergistic effects of alcohol and carbon monoxide poisoning. Other forms of carbon monoxide/alcohol deaths include the situation in which the subject 'passes out' in front of a carboniferous source of heat which burns with decreasing efficiency. Overlaying of small children while in alcoholic stupor is fortunately uncommon now that adequate housing is

[19] Before issuing a Firearms Certificate, the Chief Constable must be assured that the applicant is not of intemperate habits (*see* Chapter 9).

more widely available; it is an offence both in England and Wales and in Scotland for a responsible person to be drunk while in bed with a small child (*see* page 214). At comatose levels, hypothermia constitutes a major hazard, the physiological protection provided against the cold by constriction of the peripheral blood vessels being countered by the pharmacological action of alcohol; the man who lies down in a field on a cold night on the way home after a drinking bout is at great risk. At even higher levels of intoxication, accidental death may be due to no more than the action of the alcohol itself; this may well be the tragic ending to the 'dare' or race to drink an entire bottle of spirits which, if done rapidly, can elevate the blood alcohol level to an order of 600 mg/100 ml.

The problem of asphyxia due to inhalation of aspirated stomach contents has been discussed in Chapter 13; while many experts are sceptical, I believe massive inhalation of vomit to be a genuine cause of death that is particularly associated with intoxication by drugs or alcohol.

Suicidal alcoholism

Deliberate suicide through the use of spirits that are ordinarily consumed must be extremely rare though it has been reported. There are, however, two other aspects that are relevant. First, suicide may well be effected by the consumption of toxic alcohols of which ethylene glycol, available mainly as antifreeze, is the most probable. Secondly, ethanol is most commonly associated with suicide when both alcohol and drugs, particularly barbiturates, have been taken together. An additive effect undoubtedly occurs—indeed, the action of very many drugs is enhanced by alcohol—and some apparent suicides may be accidents that are due to sheer ignorance of the possible consequences. Others have suggested that these deaths are accidental in that the subject, who is accustomed to taking a hypnotic as a routine, fails, in a state of alcoholic confusion, to distinguish the number of capsules he or she is taking; this seems unlikely. Many such deaths are undoubtedly suicidal but, even then, it is doubtful whether the alcohol component is taken with deliberate self-destructive intent; it is more probable that a state of alcoholic depression contributes to the suicidal frame of mind. These distinctions have become of less importance since the passing of the Suicide Act 1961; in addition, a Coroner's verdict of self-killing is now virtually unknown in the absence of confirmatory circumstantial evidence.

One form of alcoholic suicide, which probably occurs more often than is recognized, is the deliberate contrivance of a vehicular crash while under the influence of alcohol. In one case that I have investigated, a man with flying experience and of unstable personality had a series of altercations with his family and, on being left alone, went to an airfield where he borrowed a light aircraft; he crashed after 60 minutes' flying which was observed to be of progressively more dangerous character. A broken half-bottle of spirits was discovered in the wreckage and the post-mortem blood alcohol level was 313 mg/100 ml. Similar cases have been reported by others both in aircraft and in motor vehicles. The function of the alcohol in these tragedies is probably of two types. Either it is consumed in the certainty that it will ultimately precipitate an accident—a type of subconscious guilt transference; or the alcohol consumed merely serves, deliberately or otherwise, to inhibit a normally dominant moral rejection of self-destruction.

Alcohol and serious assaults

The most obvious association of alcohol with serious assaults is the typical 'pub brawl', so liable to end in a fatal stabbing. In English law, drunkenness in itself is no excuse to a criminal charge. However, if the crime charged is one that requires proof of a specific intent (e.g. murder or wounding with intent to do grievous bodily harm, but not manslaughter or unlawful wounding), then, but only then, evidence of drunkenness may be admitted as evidence of lack of that specific intent[20]. The effect of the acceptance of such evidence is to reduce the guilt of murder to that of manslaughter. The legal rules concerning drunkenness are based on policy rather than on logic. In Scotland, a charge of murder cannot be reduced to one of culpable homicide on the basis of self-induced intoxication—the recklessness in getting drunk compensates for any debatable question of intent[21].

The interpretations of the relationship between alcohol and rape that are made in England and Wales and in Scotland are discussed in detail in Chapter 21. Such considerations apply both to the state of the victim and of the rapist.

Rape is an example of a crime that may involve the type of injury likely to cause death from vagal inhibition of the heart. As discussed elsewhere (Chapter 13), an association has been noted between such deaths and a state of alcoholism, generally of moderate degree only, in the victim. There is little doubt that the finding of a level of, say, 150–200 mg alcohol/100 ml blood in a fatality resulting from an assault—particularly one involving the neck—could be taken as supporting a claim by the assailant that the death was unexpected.

Excessive alcoholic intake is positively associated with wife battering. In criminal proceedings, the general principles derived from *Majewski's* case would almost certainly apply and alcoholic intoxication would have to be recognizable as insanity if it was to be used as a successful special defence—the insanity could be either temporary or permanent by reason of alcoholic brain disease; otherwise, any mental or pathological condition short of insanity is relevant only to the question of mitigating circumstances and sentence. The same thinking would apply both in England and in Scotland. In civil law, it is unlikely that even true alcoholism would provide a defence for a husband accused of behaviour such that his wife could not reasonably be expected to live with him.

Alcohols other than ethanol

Alcoholic addiction is not confined to ethanol intended especially for human consumption; unusual preparations containing alcohol—such as cheap eau-de-Cologne—are often used, while hand lotions and rubbing alcohols can be ingested; the alcohol involved is isopropyl alcohol which is more toxic than is ethanol.

The main alcohols other than ethanol that are of medico-legal significance are methanol (methyl alcohol) and ethylene glycol. The latter requires only a brief mention—it is the basic ingredient of many antifreezes and produces much the

[20] D.P.P. v. Beard [1920] A.C. 479; D.P.P. v. Majewski [1976] 2 W.L.R. 623; R. v. Garlick (1980) 72 Cr. App. R. 291 where it was held that the correct question to be put to the jury was whether the drunken man formed the intent rather than was he capable of forming the intent. See also R. v. Caldwell [1981] 1 All E.R. 961.
[21] Brennan v. H.M. Adv. 1977 S.L.T. 151, in which the court overruled previous decisions suggesting that the decision in Beard (fn. 20) was in conformity with Scots law.

same effects as does ethanol but in far more exaggerated form. There is severe involvement of the central nervous system and death in coma is to be expected when more than 100 ml is drunk. There may be severe damage to the kidneys in the event of survival from the immediate effects.

Methyl alcohol is absorbed in the same way as is ethyl alcohol but it is metabolized far more slowly by the liver. As a result there is a cumulative effect in addition to its inherent toxicity. Methanol is used in industry and is a constituent of some antifreezes but it is more generally available as 'methylated spirits'. Industrial methylated spirits, consisting of ethanol with 5 per cent methanol added, is widely used in medicine and can be obtained from pharmacists on a written order by medical practitioners, laboratories and the like; not more than 1 pint can be dispensed to a patient at any one time and the container must be marked 'for external use only'. The ordinary houschold equivalent is known as mineralized methylated spirits which is 9 per cent methanol in ethanol with added disgustants and colouring matter.

A blood level of 80 mg methanol/100 ml is dangerous, the toxic action being twofold—the body is rendered severely acidotic and there is depression of the central nervous system. Methanol almost specifically affects the eyes and, even if a generally toxic dose is survived, visual impairment of permanent or temporary nature, or even complete blindness, may persist. Very occasionally, methanol poisoning is caused by the use of lotions containing the substance but, in general, it results from either involuntary or voluntary ingestion. Involuntary ingestion is associated with drinking ordinary commercial spirits that have been deliberately or accidentally contaminated. I was once confronted in the Second World War by a body of foreign combatants who had visited a 'strip club' the night before—all were suffering from temporary methanol-induced loss of vision. Voluntary 'meths' drinking—often in association with a cheap source of palatable ethanol—is a resort of many impoverished alcoholics; there is no doubt that some habituation to methanol, similar to that seen in ethanol drinkers, must occur. The sale of methylated spirits is controlled in Scotland where it can be retailed only by authorized sellers under similar regulations as apply to Part II poisons[22].

Alcohol and disease

Alcoholism is associated with disease both directly and indirectly.

Direct association is represented by disease of the mind—alcoholic dementia—and by conditions that are primarily centred on the gastrointestinal system.

Alcoholic dementia—of which the most prominent examples are Korsakov's psychosis and delirium tremens—is of little direct medico-legal importance other than as to testamentary capacity. It is sufficient only to emphasize that crime committed while suffering from such conditions is clearly committed within the legal concept of insanity. In addition to causing mental disturbance, alcohol also has a direct toxic effect on the peripheral nerves (alcoholic peripheral neuritis).

Alcohol-associated gastrointestinal disease may be of relatively minor character, such as the so-called alcoholic gastritis which is a degenerative process in the stomach lining rather than a true inflammation. This condition may lead to malabsorption of essential foodstuffs; an unsatisfactory diet may compound a

[22] Methylated Spirits (Sale by Retail) (Scotland) Act 1937.

deficiency of protein and of vitamins. Coincidentally, there is degeneration of the liver of fatty type with, ultimately, fibrous destruction of the liver tissue; the condition of alcoholic cirrhosis is established and this may well be fatal.

Indirect association of disease with alcohol is of little medico-legal significance. Most examples stem from the inhibition of higher critical faculties; thus, sexually transmitted disease is often mediated alcoholically while unwanted pregnancies contracted under the influence of alcohol may pose problems in relation to legal abortion.

There is a distinction in the medico-legal disposition of alcohol-associated deaths in England and Wales on the one hand and in Scotland on the other. In the former, the mere mention of alcohol in the death certificate—e.g. liver failure due to chronic alcoholism—would dictate reference of the case to the Coroner by the Registrar[22a]. There is no such obligation on the Procurator Fiscal in Scotland unless the death were sudden and unexpected—as, for instance, an accidental death associated with acute alcoholism.

Alcohol and the doctor

Alcoholism provides a main reason for disciplinary action against doctors and dentists by the General Medical and Dental Councils.

The subject is discussed in greater detail in Chapter 30. Any court conviction of a medical or dental practitioner will be reported to their respective disciplinary bodies. Proven motoring offences are reportable and convictions relating to alcoholism will certainly result in warning letters if not more serious reaction. Less commonly, but certainly more seriously, professional negligence resulting from alcoholism virtually 'speaks for itself' and will inevitably result in a complaint to the GMC or GDC. In the extreme case, alcohol may be the factor that precipitates a prosecution for manslaughter through criminal negligence. A doctor, above all persons, should be able to appreciate the likely effect of alcohol on his clinical judgment and expertise; in the case of a medical practitioner convicted of delivering an obstetric patient while under the influence of a drug (chloral hydrate), the judge, in passing sentence of 3 months' imprisonment, indicated that a much more severe sentence would have been passed had alcohol been proved to be the cause of the prisoner's condition[23].

A new dimension is introduced by the establishment of a Health Committee of the GMC (*see* page 328). Little experience of the effect of this innovation is available at the time of writing; there can, however, be little doubt that alcoholism will figure prominently in its deliberations.

Particular problems of post-mortem blood alcohol analyses

Many reviews involving post-mortem determinations of ethanol draw attention to the occurrence of certain artefacts. Although the literature is confused, there is fairly widespread evidence that certain bacteria and yeasts can produce alcohol as part of their normal metabolism and that, prominent among these, are bacteria

---

[22a] But the Coroner can no longer attribute death to chronic alcoholism specifically (Coroners Rules 1984, Sched. 4 (S.I. 1984/552)).

[23] R. v. Wight, quoted in Rentoul, E. and Smith, H. (eds.) (1973), *Glaister's Medical Jurisprudence and Toxicology*, 13th edn., p. 13; Edinburgh; Churchill.

responsible for post-mortem putrefaction[24]. Vehicular, and especially aircraft, accidents produce severe open injuries in which micro-organisms can flourish. Post-mortem enzymatic activity may also convert sugar to alcohol. There is, therefore, a potential for falsely raised blood alcohol values to be obtained using post-mortem specimens, and this applies particularly to those derived from accident cases; the possibility of artefact has to be taken into consideration when responsibility for the accident is being considered.

Experience has shown that a urine sample taken *post mortem* may be a more reliable qualitative index of ante-mortem intoxication than is blood but many Courts are reluctant to accept quantitative urine evaluations. It has been recommended that, if a post-mortem blood analysis is to be interpreted with certainty, blood specimens should be obtained from three different sites in the body and that these should be tested by two gas chromatographic techniques; but it is doubtful whether many laboratories abide by such counsels of perfection. These considerations apply only to putrefying blood specimens; *in-vivo* specimens taken from motorists are placed immediately in bactericidal containers and are extremely unlikely to show artefacts due to contamination.

[24] For editorial comment, *see* Post-mortem alcohol; *Lancet* (1975), **ii**, 229. An exhaustive review of the complex subject is to be found in Corry, J. E. L. (1978), Possible sources of ethanol ante- and post-mortem: its relationship to the biochemistry and microbiology of decomposition; *Journal of Applied Bacteriology*, **44**, 1.

26

Forensic toxicology

J. S. Oliver

The role of the forensic toxicologist is the detection, identification and measurement of poisons in human biological materials. This differs from that of the clinical toxicologist, who recognizes poisoning from the symptoms and specializes in the care and maintenance of the poisoned patient. Both require a knowledge of the physiological action of the poison, the latter for the care of the patient and the former to assist either the police surgeon or the pathologist with the interpretation of the results.

The training of the forensic toxicologist is primarily in the field of analytical chemistry. He employs and modifies instruments and techniques available to the analytical chemist to detect, identify and measure poisons that are mostly in trace amounts with respect to the biological material submitted for analysis. In addition, his training must take cognizance of the biochemistry and pharmacology of poisons, elementary human physiology and pathology. This aspect is particularly important when interpreting laboratory results.

Poison

The term poison, through popular usage, indicates a substance that, when ingested in small amounts, destroys life or impairs health. This definition indicates to the lay person a limited range of substances which, by and large, have gained the reputation of being poisons through use throughout history. Such popular or historical poisons would include arsenic, cyanide and strychnine.

A better definition of a poison is a substance that, when taken by any route, has a deleterious action on the body. This definition sets no boundaries on the types of substance involved, the quantities ingested or the route of entry. Far from limiting his field of interest, the toxicologist's ability as an analyst must be comprehensive since practically all substances are poisons when taken into the body in sufficient amounts.

In practice, the type and range of poisons encountered are determined largely by the availability of materials. The poisons available in the United Kingdom are mostly medicinal drugs, alcohol, household and garden chemicals in an industrial environment; in an agricultural environment, industrial pesticides have to be added to the list.

Samples and information

Samples for analysis can be received from either the living or the dead. In the case of the living, the specimens are generally blood and urine and occasionally hair and nail clippings where metallic poisons have been suspected. Samples from the post-mortem will, in addition, normally include liver, stomach and intestine contents, kidney, lung and brain. If an injection site has been found then this should be submitted together with the underlying fat and muscle. Blood and urine specimens should be divided between two clean containers. One set should be preserved with sodium fluoride for blood and phenyl mercuric nitrate for urine, and the other set should be free of preservatives. The preservative is used to prevent formation of ethyl alcohol should the specimens be contaminated with yeasts from the atmosphere. The tissue specimens should be packaged in clean, sealed and properly labelled polythene bags; hair and nail samples should be packaged in clean polythene bags. An entire lung, tied off at the main bronchus, should be submitted if a volatile solvent is suspected as a possible poison. An aliquot of the trapped air can be taken quickly in the laboratory for analysis and a portion of the lung can then be returned to the pathologist for histological investigation. All specimens should be kept cool and transported to the laboratory as quickly as possible. Frozen specimens are not usually required and can cause unnecessary delays.

The information required by the laboratory for record and interpretation comprises name, age, sex, significant post-mortem findings, observed behaviour prior to death and, in the living patient, a report of the symptoms observed by the doctor. In addition, efforts should be made by the reporting officer to ascertain the previous relevant medical history. Where death has occurred, medicine containers that are available should be labelled and submitted with the biological specimens even if they are empty. Drinking vessels found at the locus, again even if they appear to be empty, can reveal rapidly the nature of the toxin when analysed using sensitive laboratory procedures. Where household chemicals have been involved, the remnants must be submitted with the specimens. The information yielded, and the subsequent time saved in the laboratory, is well worth the effort.

Analysis of specimens

The analysis of a biological specimen for a poison has four steps—the drug must be isolated from the complex matrix, detected, identified and the quantity present measured. The first problem is to isolate a poison that may or may not be present in minute amounts in a biological sample. An extraction procedure that recovers most of the poison contaminated with as little co-extractable biological material as possible is required. The analytical steps are designed to make the poison as insoluble as possible in the biological material and as amenable as possible to the extraction procedure. In the case of volatile poisons, such as alcohol and solvents, simply warming aliquots of material in a closed phial causes sufficient solvent to escape into the vapour above the sample for the analysis to be made. The addition of acid to a blood sample will cause any cyanide present to form volatile hydrogen cyanide and, in a closed system, this vapour can be trapped in dilute alkali prior to further analysis.

Most analysis is carried out for drug substances. This is the area where terminology causes the greatest confusion for the non-scientist. The toxicologist is primarily interested in that property of the drug which can be of use in its isolation. As a result, drugs are classified as acids, neutrals, bases, amphoterics (which behave as acid or base) or water soluble (such as quaternary ammonium compounds). The pathologist, for example, may request an analysis for drugs, with a particular interest in analgesics. Such a classification is based on the pharmacological action of the drug and comprises analgesics, narcotics, hypnotics, anticonvulsants, antidepressants, tranquillizers, etc. Each group can contain chemically related drugs but also may contain others that are totally unrelated. For example, both chlorpromazine and meprobamate are tranquillizers but, chemically, the former is a basic and the latter a neutral drug.

The steps in the isolation of the drug are determined by its chemical classification and by knowledge as to whether it becomes linked to protein in the body or is changed biochemically to a water-soluble conjugate. A protein-bound drug can be released prior to extraction by breaking down the protein either by enzyme digestion, warming with acid or by precipitating the protein. Water-soluble conjugates require hydrolysis with a suitable enzyme to release the conjugating group. Thereafter, the chemistry of the drug is the determining guideline. An acid drug will be less soluble and more amenable to solvent extraction in an acid solution; similar principles apply to a basic drug in an alkaline solution. Neutral drugs can be extracted directly into a solvent. Amphoteric drugs can be rendered less soluble in the aqueous medium by careful adjustment of the pH of the solution (see page 26) to the correct narrow range in which the drug changes from being an acid to an alkali. Quaternary ammonium compounds can be extracted after conjunction with 'ion-pair' reagents. These chemicals bind highly water-soluble drugs into complexes that are more soluble in the extraction solvent; after extraction, the complex can be broken easily to permit further analysis.

This guide is by no means comprehensive. It indicates the initial steps necessary to produce an extract of the biological materials which can then be concentrated and used for further analysis. The extracts produced may be impure and contain co-extractable biological materials, such as lipids, from which the drug must be separated.

Analytical techniques

Chromatography

A poison can be separated from the crude extract for the purposes of detection, identification and measurement by using the various forms of chromatography.

For the non-scientist, the technique of chromatography can best be understood by relation to a familiar occurrence—for example, the use of a proprietary dry-cleaning solvent or paraffin to remove a dye stain from a piece of cloth. The technique used is to dab the stain with a tissue soaked in the solvent. Some of the stain transfers to the tissue; some spreads outwards from the stain into the material following the spread of the solvent into the cloth; the solvent, as it spreads through the cloth, has tried to take the dye with it thus causing it to move over the material. In a laboratory, the cloth can be replaced by a sheet of blotting paper about 10 cm^2. The dye stain can be reproduced by making a single dot 1 cm from one edge. The solvent can be applied by dipping that edge into a trough of solvent, keeping the dye spot above the surface. Capillary action will cause the solvent to flow up the paper. As it passes the dye spot, it tries to carry it along while the binding of the dye to the paper tends to hold it back. The rate at which the dye moves over the paper relative to the solvent is determined by its solubility in the solvent and the strength of the binding between the dye and the paper. Thus by the time the solvent has reached the other edge of the paper, the dye will have moved a distance determined by its speed of movement.

A different dye will have a different binding strength and a different solubility in the solvent and will, therefore, move at a different rate. As a result, it moves a different distance in the time taken for the solvent to reach the top of the paper. This means that a mixture of the two dyes would separate if the experiment was repeated in that way.

Since the rate of movement of one of the dyes, say A, would be the same if run alone or in a mixture with dye B, it would be a simple matter to identify dye A in the mixture. This could be achieved by dotting the mixture on to the paper and dotting a known sample of dye A on an imaginary line through the spot and parallel with the edge that will dip into the solvent, the origin line. The mixture will separate into two spots, one of which will be directly opposite the spot formed by dye A which has been run as a reference. This identifies one of the spots as dye A.

Expand this problem to the situation where the unknown dye may be one of several hundred; some other criterion is then required since it will not be practical to spot each dye for reference purposes. This is achieved by making use of what is called the R_f value; this is found by dividing the distance travelled by the spot by the distance travelled by the solvent. Its value is governed by the relative affinity or binding strength of each dye to the paper for a given solvent system.

This system of chromatography can be used to identify dyes by initially chromatographing all the dyes likely to be encountered and tabulating their R_f values. The unknown can then be chromatographed and its R_f value calculated. The dyes with similar values should be listed. The use of a different solvent system will identify another group of dyes with the same R_f values. Comparison of the groups will reveal one dye common to both groups, thus identifying the unknown. Using this dye as a reference, a third system should be chosen with different solvent characteristics to confirm the identity.

This identification procedure using paper chromatography for dyes is identical with that used for drugs except that, whereas dyes can be seen, drugs have to be revealed by spraying or by dipping the chromatogram into a colour-forming reagent. The drug is, thus, revealed as a coloured spot against a uniform background. The colour formed by the drug may, itself, provide an aid to identification that is additional to its R_f value.

The outlined identification procedure shows the limitation of this and all other forms of chromatography—they are constrained as means of identification by the availability and comprehensiveness of reference tables.

The technique of paper chromatography has been superseded by thin-layer chromatography in which glass plates coated with a thin layer of absorbent material are used instead of paper. The major advantages are that separation can be achieved over a movement of 10–15 cm in approximately 30 minutes as opposed to several hours when using paper chromatography. Also, corrosive colour-forming reagents can be used directly on the layer.

Although it is possible to use the procedure for identification purposes, it is difficult to achieve reproducible layers and conditions. The technique is used primarily as a screening method to indicate the presence or absence of a drug. It can then be used to confirm the identity of a drug by chromatographing the extract together with a reference of the suspected drug. The procedure can also be used as a purification step prior to the use of other analytical techniques.

Gas chromatography

A schematic diagram of the apparatus for gas chromatography is shown in *Figure 26.1*. The apparatus is expensive and complex but its function can be understood by direct analogy to paper chromatography. The paper is replaced by a glass or stainless-steel tube packed with a fine granular powder. In gas–solid chromatography, the powder alone is selected for the separation; in gas–liquid chromatography, a selected wax or grease coating on the powder is used. The column is mounted in an oven since separations are achieved in the vapour phase. The liquid solvent of paper chromatography is replaced by a gas called the carrier gas.

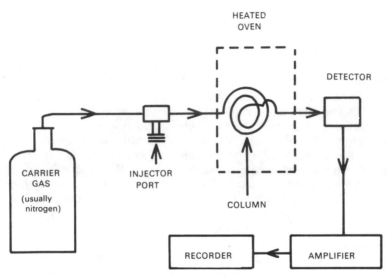

Figure 26.1 Schematic diagram of gas chromatography equipment.

The sample is injected on to the start of the column where it is vaporized. The carrier gas sweeps it through the column, where the packing material retards its progress. As a result, components of samples are retarded to greater or lesser extents and are thereby separated; they emerge from the column at various times after injection, these being determined by their speed of progress through the column. This retention time is the characteristic that will ultimately identify the unknown.

As a component emerges from the column, it passes through a detector which causes an electrical signal to be generated; this signal is amplified and displayed on a strip chart recorder. A typical chromatogram is shown in *Figure 26.2*. The peaks have been formed by the change in detector signal made as each component emerges. The interval from the time of injection to the appearance of the top of the peak is called the retention time of the component. When this is divided by the retention time of a co-chromatographed reference compound, the resultant relative retention time for the system chosen will be constant and will correct for any minor variations in columns and conditions between laboratories. Comprehensive tables of relative retention times for drugs sought under standard conditions have been compiled and are consulted for the initial identification of a drug.

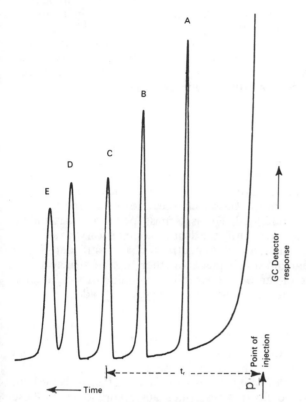

Figure 26.2 Gas chromatogram showing resolution of components of a mixture of substances A−E. t_r = Retention time of substance C.

The size or area of the peak is determined by the amount of component that passes through the detector. This measurement of area can be calibrated to measure the quantity of drug in the extract. Gas chromatography is most commonly used in the laboratory for the detection and measurement of alcohol in blood samples. Other instruments with different columns and detectors are set to measure drugs, solvents, gases and pesticides. The technique is specific in that it will separate a drug from its metabolites and measure each individually but it is constrained by the availability and scope of reference tables of retention data.

The technique of high-performance liquid chromatography produces similar tracings to those resulting from gas chromatography. Instead of a carrier gas, a solvent is pumped at high pressure through a short column of tightly packed absorbent material. The extract may be injected directly into the column although it is better to flush the extract into it using a valve with a sample loop. As before, the passage of the components through the column results in separation. The components are 'seen' by the detector as they emerge and the resultant signal is amplified and recorded. Identification of a component is made by comparing retention times; quantitation is achieved using a measurement of the detector response.

The main advantage of this procedure over gas chromatography lies in its ability to separate components that are not volatile. Sample preparation can be minimal and may involve merely the precipitation of protein while the separated components can be collected for further analyses since the technique is non-destructive. A possible disadvantage of the procedure is that assays tend to be for small groups of structurally related drugs rather than for the large groups that are possible by the use of gas chromatography for chemically related drugs. Otherwise the technique has replaced and improved many of the analyses formerly carried out by gas chromatography.

Mass spectrometry

The mass spectrometer is the most powerful analytical tool available in the forensic science laboratory and can be used either on its own or coupled to a gas chromatograph. The instrument functions by bombarding the unknown drugs with a stream of electrons which causes the drug to break down reproducibly into charged fragments. By separating and measuring the mass to charge ratio of these fragments, a cracking pattern for the drug can be obtained. This is its mass spectrum and is unique for the drug in question. It can be used to identify the drug by comparison with a library of drug spectra. If no matches are found, a skilled spectroscopist can still identify the chemical formula of each fragment and slowly piece together possible structures for the unknown. Comparative spectra can be prepared by obtaining or synthesizing indicated reference materials and, hence, an identification can be made.

Ultraviolet spectrometry

Just as the eye can differentiate between coloured dyes in daylight, the ultraviolet spectrometer can record the 'colour' of the drugs in the ultraviolet region of the spectrum. A rainbow displays the various components, or wavelengths, of visible light and the colour of a dye is formed by the molecules absorbing some of these components. The ultraviolet spectrometer sequentially shines different wavelengths of ultraviolet light through a solution of the drug and measures the amount of light absorbed. This measurement is compared with the amount of incident light and is recorded on a scale of absorbence plotted against wavelength.

This plot is an instrumental look at the 'colour' of the drug in the ultraviolet region. It can be used to indicate the identity of a drug by referring to tables of wavelengths at which absorbence is maximal. It is a useful, non-destructive analytical aid. The presence and possible identity of a drug can be indicated when the crude extract is dissolved in acid, alkali or ethanol. The quantity of drug present may be estimated by measuring the absorption but the identification is not absolute since drugs of similar molecular structure can produce identical spectra. Also, the metabolites of drugs will probably have identical spectra with the parent drug. For this reason, the measurement of drug levels should only be related to the total drug present and be used as a guide for further analysis to determine the amount of individual components.

Immunoassays

Radioimmunoassay and enzyme-multiplied immunoassays are techniques that make use of the body's immune response to foreign proteins (*see* page 17). Antibodies can be obtained from a host animal that has been injected with a foreign protein to which the drug of interest has been linked. The antibody will recognize and bind itself to the drug molecule in a solution and this binding has been used as the basis of both techniques.

The techniques are sensitive, they require small sample volumes and they are relatively rapid. Unfortunately, they are not specific—an antibody raised to recognize morphine will cross-react to a greater or lesser extent with the other opiate drugs while an antibody raised to diazepam will cross-react with other benzodiazepines. As a result, these assays, although useful and highly acceptable in the clinical laboratory, have to be treated with caution for evidential purposes. Without preliminary separations, they are best used in the laboratory as presumptive tests for the presence or absence of a group of drugs.

An acceptable use is to couple immunoassays with high-performance liquid chromatography. For example, this combination forms the only means of proving the presence of lysergic acid diethylamide (LSD) in a biological sample. Standard detectors available have insufficient sensitivity to demonstrate the drug's presence. However, by collecting aliquots from the column and analysing them by radioimmunoassay, it may be possible to obtain positive reactions in those that have been collected at retention times corresponding to LSD and its metabolites. The retention time identifies the drug while it is both detected and quantified by the immunoassay.

Interpretation of results

Analytical techniques for detecting and measuring drugs are similar from laboratory to laboratory, but not always identical. The choice of techniques to solve a particular problem is largely a matter for the personal skill and preference of the analyst. Safeguards must be incorporated to ensure that the chosen procedures will have sufficient sensitivity to detect significant amounts of drug or metabolite, that the identification is beyond doubt and that the measurement techniques employed yield a true estimate of the quantity of drug present.

All measurements have errors. For example, the measurement of alcohol in blood by gas chromatography in the hands of a careful analyst is known to be within 2 per cent of the true value. However, bearing in mind the range of conditions of tissue and blood, from fresh to badly decomposed, that form the work-piece for the analyst, results are more realistically regarded as lying within 10 per cent of the true value. Procedures used should be tested against standards dissolved in whole blood or tissue slurries as appropriate.

The interpretation of the drug level found should be done in consultation with the clinician's or pathologist's findings. The level of the drug should be checked initially against known therapeutic levels and, if available, levels that have been measured in cases of fatal and non-fatal poisonings. A similar procedure must be adopted if a metabolite has been measured since some metabolites are more active pharmacologically than is the parent drug. This approach will solve the majority of cases encountered and will generally explain the clinician's or the pathologist's findings when the known pharmacological effects have been considered.

Approximately 40 per cent of all poisoning cases involving drugs also involve alcohol and this combination is, perhaps, one of the most difficult to interpret. Where sufficient cases of poisoning with a particular drug have been encountered both with and without alcohol, a statistical analysis of the drug levels should reveal the influence of alcohol on the toxicity of the particular drug. Probably the effect will be seen to be additive.

A satisfactory explanation of death is not always possible in cases in which several drugs have been detected at low to therapeutic levels. However, careful sifting of the information available in the medical literature may reveal a recorded adverse reaction when two of the drugs have been used together. Observed symptoms should be considered against those recorded.

The relationship of blood alcohol levels to the alcohol consumed is the most frequent calculation required of the toxicologist in court. Such requests vary in complexity from the estimation of the quantity of beer or spirits that could account for a particular blood alcohol level to the calculation of the contribution of post-accident consumption of alcohol to the subsequent blood alcohol reading.

As a result of laboratory experiments with volunteers of known weight consuming known amounts of alcohol, it is possible to predict a blood alcohol level from a known consumption. However, it must be remembered that variations in the order of plus or minus 20 per cent in the maximum readings are usual after the consumption of the same amount of alcohol by volunteers of the same weight in the laboratory. The consumption of some foodstuffs prior to an experiment can reduce the predicted maximum.

Where alcohol consumption has taken place over a period of time, the effect of metabolism must be taken into account. Alcohol is removed from the body at a constant rate for the individual. This rate averages 15 mg per 100 ml blood per hour but, experimentally, it has been shown to vary within the range of 9–27 mg alcohol per 100 ml blood per hour. It can, thus, be seen that a blood alcohol level resulting from the consumption of a known amount of alcohol must lie within a wide range of possible values.

Analysis time

Popular television series such as 'The Expert' and 'Quincy' give the impression that an analysis for poisons can be almost instantaneous. Unfortunately, this is not true. If adequate specimens and information have been provided and adequate trained staff and equipment are available, results for most routine toxicology cases should be available, on average, within 2 working days. This can be, and often is, short circuited to provide interim verbal reports within a few a hours when the need arises and where the indicated poison falls within a group of readily analysable substances. The written report must be prepared only when the full toxicological investigation has been completed.

While the above statements are true for perhaps 99 per cent of cases, unavoidable delays occur when an obscure poison or a complete unknown is encountered. In such cases it is impossible to predict an analysis time. The solution may take from a few hours to several weeks. Occasionally, the poison may remain undetected despite the best efforts of the analyst using the best available equipment.

27

Radiology in forensic medicine

Radiological techniques have many applications in forensic science. Amongst these may be included the examination of fingerprints and of documents. There is, however, no intention to discuss the purely scientific field in this section which deals only with forensic medicine.

Forensic medical radiology falls into two functional categories—those investigations concerned with identification and those directed to diagnosis.

Radiology and identification

As described in Chapter 3, methods used for the identification of dead bodies may be, first, of a deductive nature. These are designed to indicate the type of person who should be sought in the missing-persons files; this approach is dictated when there is no clue as to identity. But once there is reason to suppose a personal identification, this is proved largely by means of comparative methods. Radiological assistance is invaluable in the former circumstance and has a very special place in the latter; only a few of those benefiting from a National Health Service have not been X-rayed at some time during their lives. However, current United Kingdom regulations require the retention of X-rays for five years only and there is no provision for microfilming.

Deductive identification methods

The age of a cadaver at death is particularly well estimated radiologically. In infancy and early childhood, the presence of centres of ossification can be demonstrated with accuracy and ease; the union of these centres can be observed in childhood and adolescence up to approximately 25 years of age; in later life, degenerative changes may give some indication of maturity, but this is only over a wide range—the chief value of X-rays of adult persons is to distinguish between two or three bodies who are known as a group but are of unknown individual identity. The main ossification details are given in Appendices F and G.

The sex of a mutilated or charred body can also be established with some certainty and without the need for extensive cleaning processes if suitable bones are available for X-ray. The pelvis is by far the most useful bone in this respect (*see* page 40).

Comparative identification

Provided X-rays taken in life are available, any similar radiograph taken after death can be used for comparison. Identification can be based on similarities either in normal or in abnormal structures; the value of the latter in positive identification is proportional to the rarity of the abnormality.

Of the normal structures routinely used for comparison, the skull sinuses—the frontal sinus in particular—are the most satisfactory; the number of variations in shape and size that are potentially available is so diverse as almost to make a radiographic outline unique to the individual; the problem is mainly one of obtaining a view in the cadaver identical with that available in life. If an adequate front view is not available, the general outline of the skull, including the shape of the pituitary fossa, may provide almost equally good evidence.

One particular form of comparison of the normal that should be mentioned is the process whereby a post-mortem X-ray is superimposed on a photograph of the living person. Again, the technical difficulties of obtaining a precisely similar scale and orientation are formidable but the method has been used with success in several classic cases of investigation of homicide[1].

Abnormalities that may be of value are so numerous that only a few illustrations can be given. Congenital abnormalities such as absence of bones, displacement or malformation may be so rare as to be virtually diagnostic of identity. Others, such as fusion of the ribs, are not uncommon and should only be regarded as confirmatory of other circumstantial evidence. Pre-existing disease—in the form of changes in bone density, arthritic deformities and the like—may provide unequivocal evidence of identity of dead persons from whom films taken in life are available for comparison. Such opportunities are not confined to bone; unusual calcification—of tuberculous origin in the lungs or lymph nodes or due to degenerative changes in the uterus and many other organs—may show a pattern as individual as is that of a fingerprint. The presence of healing fractures in sites known to have been broken in life would obviously provide strong confirmatory evidence of identification but, even more useful, is the presence of surgical prostheses or of supportive implants such as plates, pins or orthopaedic screws—not only can the X-rays be compared but the appliance can be removed from the cadaver and superimposed. Surgical implants are of very great use in identification after mass disasters; if, for example, one man is known to have a bone plated, it is simplicity itself to screen that bone radiologically in all unidentified bodies.

The importance of dental identification in both the single unknown body and in the mass has already been stressed. Dental radiography very greatly enhances the contribution of the odontologist. The mere presence of a single or double restoration in one or two commonly filled teeth would be insufficient to prove a positive identification as opposed to an exclusion of identification. The precise shape of the fillings is, however, likely to be unique and it would not be impossible

[1] R. v. Ruxton, 1936, Manchester March Assizes; *see Glaister's Medical Jurisprudence and Toxicology* (1973), 13th edn., p. 90; Edinburgh; Churchill Livingstone.

R. v. Dobkin, 1942, C.C.C.; *see* Simpson, K. (1979), *Forensic Medicine*, 8th edn., p. 40; London; Edward Arnold.

to make a reasonably certain identification from a comparison of post- and ante-mortem radiographs of a single filling. Dental radiography may also show up significant root shapes, socket outlines or abnormalities of tooth eruption, development or decay; it is the policy in the Scandinavian countries, among others, to record the dentition of their commercial aircrew radiographically as a routine.

Another useful adjunct provided by radiology in identification in the mass lies in the occasional localization of significant possessions that have been embedded in charred tissues; generally, this represents no more than a 'fringe benefit' of radiographic examination for other purposes—such as a search for injuries due to explosives—but it is, none the less, often of great value.

Diagnostic radiology

Diagnostic radiological techniques are of value both in accidental and in criminal deaths.

Accidental deaths

Accidental death is a major epidemic of modern times and is attracting increasing interest throughout the medical world; forensic pathology has a great part to play in satisfying this interest since all such deaths are investigated through the medico-legal system. It is doubtful whether a busy forensic pathologist can be expected to demonstrate individually all fractures present after a fatal accident, despite the fact that some of these may be of research significance; routine X-ray coverage of accident cases simplifies the whole procedure. Moreover, some fractures—notably those of the spine—are difficult to demonstrate satisfactorily by post-mortem dissection. The prevention of spinal fracture in vehicular accidents is one of the main objectives of the bio-engineers; in some unusual procedures—such as escape by ejection from high-speed aircraft—it is, perhaps, the main limiting factor to added safety. Ideally, the complete autopsy in vehicular accidental death should include adequate radiography of, at least, the spine. X-rays may be of great assistance in distinguishing ante- from post-mortem fracture, an observation that may have profound significance in the reconstruction both of accidental and of homicidal deaths. Finally, X-ray diagnosis is not confined to the study of bones; very useful information in relation to soft-tissue changes can also be obtained.

Homicidal death

The most obvious use of X-rays in potentially homicidal death lies in the demonstration within the body of bullets and other missiles (*see* Chapter 9). The technical difference between searching for a single bullet in a cadaver with and without the assistance of radiographic localization needs no emphasis; moreover, fragments of bullets or of bomb casings or contents can easily be missed in an unaided dissection; much important information might, thereby, be lost to the ballistics expert.

Hijacking of aircraft is a particular modern use of firearms. The diagnosis of sabotage has been discussed at page 93; the possibility of demonstrating hijacking as a cause of a fatal accident would depend, to a large extent, on the finding of bullets in the crew members, a task that would be physically impossible to discharge with assurance in the absence of X-ray facilities. This particular aspect also highlights the importance of radiography in distinguishing a true shooting from artefact. In one case of historic interest, bullets were found in the arm of a fatality from an aircraft that was carrying an important person and that was believed to have been shot down; the radiographic demonstration of percussion caps and fragments of cartridge case clearly showed that this appearance resulted not from criminal activity but from the explosion, during the post-crash fire, of bullets carried on the person of the VIP's bodyguard[2].

The importance, both to the reconstruction of events and to the subsequent investigation, of localization of shot from smooth-bore weapons and of fragments of explosives has been discussed in Chapter 9. Any radiographs that have been taken for the purpose of investigation can be retained as permanent records and, if necessary, used as exhibits or productions at trial.

Other forms of homicide are also well illustrated in the form of X-rays. Particularly noteworthy is the radiography of the larynx in cases of strangulation; fractures of the thyroid cartilage or hyoid bone are generally well shown, particularly in the aged in whom the cartilages are often calcified. Attention has been drawn at page 113 to the role of post-mortem injection methods particularly in relation to the diagnosis of subarachnoid haemorrhage.

Perhaps, however, radiography and radiology reach their apogee in the examination of suspicious infant deaths. X-ray examination in the non-accidental injury syndrome (discussed in detail in Chapter 20) does more than merely demonstrate the presence of fractures. Its particular value is to prove the infliction of injury at various times—evidence that is essential to the concept of 'battering'. The X-ray picture can clearly demonstrate the difference between healing and fresh fractures and can often differentiate different periods of repair in the former. Attention has also been drawn to the possibility of indicating parental inattention to fractures sustained. Fractures unite by the elaboration of primitive bone known as 'callus'. The deposition of callus is particularly marked when the fracture has not been properly treated by immobilization.

Additionally, the radiologist may be able to demonstrate that a fracture has been caused in an unusual way—as, for example, by severe twisting. Such evidence strongly negates a defence, say, of an accidental fall.

X-ray examination of the living

Industrial diseases

The importance of X-rays in the assessment of dust diseases is discussed in Chapter 15. The diagnosis and assessment of disability due to coal miners' pneumoconiosis, which are based on the distribution and size of pulmonary nodules, are virtually in the hands of the radiologist.

Angiography

Angiography or arteriography—the study of the arteries by means of X-rays—is performed by injecting radio-opaque material into a blood vessel and observing its

[2] Stevens, P. J. (1970). *Fatal Civil Aircraft Accidents*, p. 44. Bristol; Wright.

subsequent movement and distribution. There are two major medico-legal applications of the technique.

First, angiography of the cerebral vessels may be used as a test of brain death. It can be taken that a situation exists that is incompatible with function or revival of the brain if serial observations show the intracranial circulation to have been absent for 15 minutes; the permanence of the films provides lasting evidence of the fact of death and this method of establishing death is increasingly used in Continental Europe in relation to transplantation (*see* Chapter 12).

Secondly, angiography of the coronary arteries is achieving some prominence in relation to the diagnosis of disease of the coronary arteries in persons in whom sudden collapse poses a particular risk to public safety—the most obvious example is the commercial pilot. Although there have been no case decisions at the time of writing, there is the possibility that failure to diagnose arterial inadequacy prior to an accident attributed to such disease might result in a successful negligence suit, and the diagnosis of coronary artery disease—as opposed to frank disease of the heart muscle—is impossible to make with certainty using current standard electrocardiographic techniques. Recourse to more specialized tests is sometimes indicated and the current position of coronary angiography in this situation seems to be as follows. First, while the examination may show the presence of the disease, there is no certainty that the disease will prove fatal—in one series of observations, only 60 per cent of persons with 80 per cent narrowing of all three main vessels and, presumably, symptoms at the time of examination, had died from coronary heart disease 6 years after the test; the 6-year mortality for persons with obstruction of only one artery was 20 per cent. It follows that the test might unnecessarily prevent a competent person being properly employed; the risk would have to be balanced against the many other factors involved[3]. Secondly, the test is not without danger and has some mortality in its own right[4]; it follows that it would be quite unreasonable to suggest its use on a routine basis. In my opinion, coronary angiography has presently no place in the *selection* of persons in high-risk occupations. It might well be useful in the evaluation of cases in which there was doubt of fitness on other criteria; but, if the doubt was sufficient to justify the investigation, common prudence would already have impressed the need for suspension from duty. When the test has been used along these lines, the specificity of results has been found disappointing[5].

Routine X-ray examinations and negligence

Finally, it is noted that failure to make an X-ray examination in a case of head injury or in any other situation in which fracture might reasonably be anticipated might, in the circumstances of modern hospital practice, be difficult to justify no matter how full the clinical examination may have been[6]. The development of

---

[3] It might, for example, be difficult to find an experienced airline pilot without some degree of coronary narrowing; the results of reducing the overall experience of airline pilots might well be worse than the risks involved in well-organized 'double-crewing' by older men.

[4] The overall incidence of complications is in the region of 4–5 per cent and the mortality lies somewhere between 0.3 per cent and 1.0 per cent. This applies to investigations performed on persons with symptoms; certainly, the risk in 'normals' would be expected to be less.

[5] Froelicher, V. F., *et al.* (1973). The correlation of coronary angiography and the electro-cardiographic response to maximal treadmill testing in 76 asymptomatic men. *Circulation*, **48**, 587.

[6] *See* Nathan, H. L. (1957), *Medical Negligence*, p. 45; London; Butterworth.

disability due to a fracture being undiagnosed for this reason would almost certainly result in an action for negligence; many cases would be indefensible. The same might well be so were the presence of a foreign body to remain undiagnosed. The presumption of negligence is, however, by no means certain. Denning M.R.[7] is reported as stating, 'In some of the earlier cases the doctor had been criticized for not having taken X-rays with the result that they had sometimes been taken unnecessarily. This case showed that the Courts did not always find that there had been negligence because a patient had not had an X-ray; it depended upon the circumstances of each case'. The increasing number of radiographic examinations must undoubtedly make a significant contribution to the total dose of radiation delivered to the population and, in general, there should be a genuine medical need to justify such an examination[8].

The hazards of radiation

The dose of X-rays given to an individual during a single diagnostic procedure is well controlled and the earlier complications, such as radiation skin burns, are now unlikely to be seen. Nevertheless, radiation used outside the field of clinical medicine may affect the genetic structures or the blood-forming tissues and represents a hazard which is growing in importance. Radiation injury of all types falls within the ambit of forensic medicine and has potential, even if not current, medico-legal significance.

Electromagnetic radiation (*see Table 27.1*) is of two types—*non-ionizing* and *ionizing*—the precise type and effect of the radiation depending upon the

TABLE 27.1 Types of Electromagnetic Radiation

Very	1 MHz	Radio	
low	1 GHz	Radar or microwave	
	10^3 GHz	Infrared	Non-ionizing
Frequency	10^5 GHz	Light	
	10^7 GHz	Ultraviolet	
	10^9 GHz	X-rays	
Very	10^{10} GHz	Gamma rays	Ionizing
high	10^{12} GHz	Cosmic rays	

N.B. 1 Hz = 1 cycle per second. For an explanation of SI units see Appendix P

frequency of the waves. Non-ionizing radiation is not without danger. In the industrial field, long exposure to microwaves may result in cataract (or opacity of the lens of the eye), while laser workers may develop burns of the retina; such cases are rare but may increase as the devices become increasingly used. Infrared radiation is detected by the skin and is, therefore, only a hazard in unconscious persons. Ultraviolet light, on the other hand, is not detected by the skin; everyone is familiar with resultant burns due to excessive sunbathing while extreme exposure

[7] In Braisher v. Harefield and Northwood Hospital Group Management Committee, C.A., July 13, 1966. This case is quoted by Jellie, H. (1966), *Lancet*, **ii**, 235; I cannot discover the definitive reference. See also an older case—Sabapathi v. Huntley [1938] 1 W.W.R. 817—where a similar view was held.
[8] The medico-legal dilemma is ably discussed by Jennett, B. (1976), Some medico-legal aspects of the management of acute head injury, *British Medical Journal*, **i**, 1383.

undoubtedly predisposes to cancer of the skin (particularly of basal cell or 'rodent ulcer' type). Ionizing radiations are clinically more important and owe their biological effects to their ability to alter the chemical properties of 'ionized' cells. The original unit of X-rays was the roentgen but, from the point of view of their biological effect, it is the energy absorbed that is significant. Ionizing radiations were originally measured in 'rads', one rad closely corresponding to the energy absorbed when one röentgen is received by 1 g of tissue. There are, however, variations in response to radiation and, accordingly, the biological effect on man was measured as 'rems' (rem being the acronym for röentgen equivalent for man); rads and rems are numerically equal for X-rays, gamma rays and beta particles but, for alpha particles and neutrons, 1 rad is equivalent to 10 rems. These units are not used in the International System of Units (SI) which is now in widespread use; they have accordingly been recently replaced by the gray (Gy; 1 Gy = 100 rad) and the sievert (Sv; 1 Sv = 100 rem). The effective unit for man is, therefore, the Sv. The effect of radioactivity is to produce electromagnetic radiation in the tissues. The unit of radioactivity was originally the curie but this is a massive number; the new SI measure is the becquerel (Bq; 1 Bq = 1 disintegration per second)—this is about one 4000 millionth of a curie!

For ease of description it can be taken that rapidly growing and multiplying cells are the most sensitive to ionizing radiation. The organs within the body most easily damaged are the bone marrow, the epithelium of the bowel, the testes or ovaries and the lymphatic glands. Similarly, children, because they are growing faster than adults, are generally more sensitive to radiation. External sources of radiation, other than those of natural origin, act in a relatively transient fashion—most can either be avoided or switched off. But a source of radiation that is bound to the tissues will exert a continuous influence until it decays. Such foci of radiation can come, first, from radioactive substances deliberately introduced into the body, almost invariably for medical diagnostic purposes[9]. It is imperative that such substances decay rapidly, the rate being dependent upon the 'half-life' of the radioactive element; the half-life is defined as the time taken for half the available radioactive atoms to disintegrate. An alternative source of internal radiation is food that has itself been contaminated by external sources of abnormal radio-activity. The half-life of such radioactive elements may be long and in certain cases, notably strontium 90 (which is chemically similar to calcium), the element is stored in the body; this type of radiation therefore constitutes a serious health hazard.

The effects of radiation will vary from person to person but, in general, it can be said that high doses, of the order of 5–10 Sv and above, will kill within a matter of weeks; medium doses may cause malignant disease, particularly of the blood, several years after exposure; and low doses may cause genetic damage to future generations. It is small wonder that radiation hazards are strongly controlled by legislation[10]. In particular, the amount of radiation sustained by workers in

[9] A certification of authorization is now required before a doctor or a dentist can administer radioactive medicinal products for diagnosis, treatment or research (The Medicines (Administration of Radioactive Substances) Regulations 1978, S.I. 1978/1006 and associated regulations).

[10] The EEC directive of 1 June 1976 (76/579/Euratom) on radiological protection is mandatory. The relevant UK legislation includes Factories Act 1961, the Unsealed and Sealed Sources Regulations made under the Act (S.I. 1968/780 and S.I. 1969/808) as amended, Radioactive Substances Acts 1948 and 1960, Radioactive Substances (Carriage by Road) (Great Britain) Regulations (S.I. 1974/1735), Nuclear Installations Acts 1965 and 1969 as amended by the Energy Act 1983 and Radiological Protection Act 1970 which established the now 12-man National Radiological Protection Board, Regulations will be consolidated under the Health and Safety at Work etc. Act 1974.

occupations associated with the hazard is monitored by sensitive devices such as film badges or thermoluminescent dosimeters and by periodic blood tests[11]; the maximum permissible dose for such workers is set by international regulation at 0.05 Sv per year[12]. The corresponding permissible dose for the public at large is 0.005 Sv per year, the difference being accepted as a safe compromise that allows for the use of radiation in an advantageous way, cost and social benefit being taken into account. In practice, very few radiation workers receive a dose above 0.015 Sv in a year. The accepted limits exclude exposure for the purposes of medical diagnosis or treatment.

As indicated above, the ill effects of radiation are of two types. First, there is the production of disease that may result either from the destructive effect of ionizing radiations or from their capacity to stimulate cells into abnormal activity and, thus, predispose to cancer. The tissue most commonly destroyed is the bone marrow, a process that leads to very severe anaemia; the lymphoid tissue is also sensitive to radiation and its destruction results in an increased susceptibility to infection. Manifest acute damage of this type is limited to the levels of exposure sustained in an atomic bomb explosion or in the treatment of cancer; none the less, increasing exposure to radiation carries with it an increased statistical risk of disease of those systems that are most sensitive. Cancer may be provoked in many sites by radiation—particularly in the blood (leukaemia), lungs and thyroid gland. Symptoms of the disease may be delayed for many years after exposure, a fact that may be of very great medico-legal importance in establishing a cause-and-effect relationship, particularly when it is remembered that the annual incidences of leukaemia and other forms of cancer are approximately 5 and 25 per hundred thousand of the general population.

Classic industrial examples include cancer of the lung occurring in miners in radioactive mines, particularly in Central Europe, and the malignancies induced in painters of luminous dials; there is little doubt that a high incidence of malignancy is to be found among those who are employed as uranium miners. Blood dyscrasia—which would include leukaemia—due to ionizing radiation is a prescribed disease when related to exposure to electromagnetic radiations other than radiant heat or to ionizing particles; since anaemia always accompanies leukaemia, the latter could also be held to be notifiable as a form of 'toxic anaemia' (Appendix K).

The second group of adverse effects results from genetic damage; alteration of the chromosomes in the gonads may be caused by direct ionizing damage or by an increase in the rate at which spontaneous changes occur—the process of mutation. The dose of radiation required to produce genetic change is certainly less than that needed to provoke cancer and, for all that is known at present, it may be very small. The effects of abnormal gene changes are also problematical. As discussed in Chapter 18, most harmful genes are eliminated and are certainly recessive. But should there be a sudden widespread increase in altered genes there would follow an increase in homozygous, clinically abnormal persons—the elimination of the harmful genes might then be difficult; it is encouraging that there has been no obvious increase in genetically controlled abnormalities in the cities of Hiroshima and Nagasaki since 1945.

Although there is no certainty that even small doses of radiation are completely harmless, any estimate of the hazard induced by man himself must be measured

[11] Blood tests will identify an exposure of 0.2 Sv delivered rapidly.
[12] Standard set by the International Commission on Radiological Protection.

against a natural background radiation which delivers some 0.0002 Gy per year in chalky soils and up to 0.002 Gy per year in the granite of Aberdeen, a value that far exceeds any effects from artificial sources. About one-quarter of the natural dose results from cosmic radiation which, arising in space, is filtered by the atmosphere. Its effect is, therefore, greatly dependent upon altitude and dictates specific shielding for astronauts; perhaps of more general concern, some form of premonitoring is needed in supersonic transport aircraft, although the risk of significant exposure of crew or passengers is negligible save during the cyclical spasms of solar hyperactivity. Internal radiation constitutes the third most important form of natural exposure and is due to the presence of infinitesimally small amounts of radioactive potassium which are present as a proportion of the total amount of that element in the body.

Of the artificial sources of radiation, the most dramatic is that derived from the detonation above ground of nuclear bombs or test devices. The explosion of a nuclear bomb results in a central zone of massive destruction surrounded by a wide area of lethal heat; beyond this is a circle of radiation which falls off in intensity from an original area in which a rapidly fatal dose is sustained. Additionally, radio-activity is displaced into the upper atmosphere, returning to earth with rainfall over a prolonged period; it is this type of radiation fall-out that gives rise to a persistent hazard as the radioactive elements, being taken up by plant life, become a source of internal radiation to animals and humans—the particular importance of strontium 90, which is stored in bone, has been mentioned.

The possibility of dangerous leaks of radioactivity from nuclear power stations has recently been receiving much publicity. Fortunately, there have been very few accidents and, in these, a significant dose was sustained only by those working close to the plant. The risk from nuclear power plants can, therefore, be looked at in two ways. Either it may be seen as providing a potential disaster situation, or one could compare the total adverse effect of even occasional accidents with the amount of disease and suffering resulting from the production of other sources of power, especially coal and coal burning (*see* page 230). A far more worrying aspect of nuclear power is the ultimate effect on world-wide natural radiation of the disposal of waste products in increasing quantities—a problem that is more one of economics than of technology and one which has achieved far greater safety than is possible with many other solid wastes.

In practice, however, the most significant source of man-made radiation stems from its use in medicine as a diagnostic aid and as a form of treatment. The hazard to the population is proportional to the sophistication of its medical services and, while there is no real danger from this source provided that reasonable pre-cautions have been taken, all radiologists are deeply conscious of their respon-sibilities in this connection. In Britain, the radiation dose to the population result-ing from the use of X-rays in medicine approximates to one-fifth of the natural background exposure.

Exposure to a diagnostic X-ray constitutes very little hazard to the individual patient, particularly when this is balanced against the advantages derived—a chest X-ray, for example, delivers a dose of about 0.001 Sv. Nevertheless, there are certain circumstances in which a decision to make such an examination would be taken only after careful consideration, the absence of which might well constitute negligence. These mainly concern pregnant women and the possible effect on the fetus; diagnostic pelvic X-rays are rarely taken in pregnancy and, during this time, the internal use of radioactive substances for the diagnosis of disease in the mother is contraindicated. Only in emergencies should a radiological examination be made below the waist of a woman more than 10 days after her last menstrual period[13]. In general, a pelvic X-ray taken in error during pregnancy is likely to double the chances of childhood malignancy in the fetus; there is no absolute indication for a therapeutic abortion if the dose has been less than 0.02 Sv but, in the event of a developmental abnormality appearing, a cause-and-effect relationship would be likely to be upheld. Non-essential X-rays of all types are always to be deprecated, perhaps not so much for their possible effect on the patient as for their contribution to the total population exposure.

The hazards of ionizing radiation used for medical purposes are, however, well understood and are controllable; it is the non-medical sources of exposure that are likely to have an increasing medico-legal significance.

At the same time, the possible ill effects of non-ionizing radiation cannot be overlooked, particularly of those in the microwave range. In Britain, the presently advised maximum occupational exposure is 100 watts per square metre, which is the same as in the USA but ten times the permitted dose in Canada. The safety aspects of non-ionizing radiation have been taken over by the National Radiological Protection Board; despite some rather pessimistic reports from the USSR, it is likely that the EEC will adopt the British standard.

[13] *See* The ten day rule, *British Medical Journal* (1975), **iv**, 543.

28

An Introduction to Forensic Psychiatry

A. K. M. Macrae

Identification of the mentally disordered offender

This chapter is not, in the main, concerned with the origins of mental disorder or with details of treatment[1]; rather it seeks to show the way in which people may offend because they are mentally disordered and how they may be most humanely cared for and rehabilitated. It is based on the generally accepted medical model of mental disorder; the legal framework within which the psychiatrist has to operate is also outlined.

Within that framework, the psychiatrist engaged in forensic work has a number of tasks. His first is to identify those who offend because of mental disorder; his second is to advise the Court on the most appropriate disposal; and his third is to treat and rehabilitate the offenders. The treatment and rehabilitation setting may be penal, in hospital, in the community or a combination of all three.

Identification of the mentally disordered offender, particularly the adolescent, can be very difficult. Adolescents are typically rebellious and ranged against authority, questioning the standards and philosophy of their elders. This is normal and healthy. The activities to which this attitude can lead them may depend on their environment. Fifty per cent of all crime is committed by youngsters under the age of 21. Their characteristics are well known. They tend to come from large families, from broken homes, are intellectually under-average, have under-achieved at school and live in a criminogenic area where their only chance of acceptance by their peers—and adolescents are rigid conformists within their own group—is to join them and emulate them in their usually petty criminal activities. These conformist youth groups tend to form themselves into gangs and the end result may be more sinister than is petty crime. Most violent crime is committed by the 17–21 age group, closely followed by the 14–17 age group.

It would be absurd to see all of these youngsters as psychiatric cases in need of treatment. Disturbed, wayward and antisocial they may be, but the solution to their problems and the prevention of repetitious behaviour lies less in the province of psychiatry than in sociopolitical action to counter the effects of ghetto areas (including high-rise flats and housing schemes with no amenities), of labelling and of our present meritocratic society.

[1] An authoritative exposition of psychiatry written in popular terms is to be found in Stafford-Clark, D. (1971), *Psychiatry Today;* London; Penguin.

It would seem reasonable to regard as abnormal only those who do not have this background and yet offend, together with those who show an escalation in the type of crime they commit.

Clearly this is a 'grey' area and there are many others. Since an individual's personality and his reaction to the strains and stresses to which he is subject arise from a combination of his heredity, innate intelligence, parental attitudes and environmental influences, there must be situations where one or other of these factors assumes a dominant role. Most people have flaws in their personality due to failure at some stage in its development during their formative years. Where such failure to adapt has been serious, the resultant personality may be clearly abnormal. Such abnormal personalities include the dependent (always leaning on Mum, demanding attention and unable to come to any independent decision), anxious (seeking reassurance and prone to hypochondriasis), obsessional (parsimonious, punctual, pernickety, pedantic, always double-checking, rigid, methodical and meticulous, obstinate and stubborn), assertive (hectoring and domineering with considerable drive but without consideration for the feelings of others), or hysterical (extroverted, histrionic, manipulative, suggestible and emotionally shallow).

The psychopath, who represents the most extreme example of abnormal personality, deserves further consideration. It has long been recognized that there is a type of person who displays no sign of disorder of thinking, of mood or of intellectual deficit and yet whose actions are inexplicable in ordinary terms. Such people have been termed 'psychopaths' and this term was incorporated in the Mental Health Act 1959. Unfortunately, the term has been used so loosely in the last 50 years that it has lost any precise meaning and has been dropped from the International Classification of Diseases to be replaced by the term 'Personality Disorder'. Yet, provided fairly rigid criteria are used, a group of people is fairly easily identifiable as being, by any reckoning, abnormal and who are some of the most disturbed, disturbing and dangerous members of our society. Let us still call them psychopaths.

Basically, although they have reached adult stature and adult intelligence, they have not progressed beyond childhood in their emotional development. They are still child-like in their impulsive demand for the immediate gratification of their wishes—no matter what the cost. They will tolerate no frustration and will meet any with aggression. They have no capacity to love or be loved and no conscience.

They are, consequently, totally egocentric, they cannot relate to others, they have no remorse or guilt for whatever they do, they act on impulse with no regard for the consequences and they are unable to learn from experience. They will lie, cheat, swindle or defraud, embezzle or thieve to gratify their immediate desires or, if frustrated, they will assault or kill. They can be superficially charming—'flowers without perfume'—but are emotionally cold with no feeling for anyone. Their treatment and rehabilitation has been a recurring disappointment to the extent that the *Report of the Committee on Mentally Abnormal Offenders*[2] has finally come out with the statement that 'the psychopath is, in general, untreatable, at least in medical terms'.

They are a small group, yet among the most destructive and dangerous members of our society. They remain a major challenge in criminology and forensic work.

---

[2] Butler, Lord (Chairman) (1975). *Report of the Committee on Mentally Abnormal Offenders*. Cmnd. 6244. London; HMSO.

In times of stress, neurotic disorders such as hysterical conversion, anxiety and phobic and obsessional states arise from abnormal personalities. Although they are widespread and disabling illnesses, neuroses have few criminal effects. The commonest anxiety states do not lead to criminal actions; neither do obsessional states, although it is not unusual for a defence to claim that some criminal action—e.g. fire-raising, shop-lifting, indecent exposure—has arisen because of an obsessive compulsion and to enhance this with a pseudoclassical term such as pyromania or kleptomania. The true obsessional often has fears of committing some criminal act but rarely does so. Those offenders who claim an irresistible compulsion are usually acting either for material gain or for a generally superficial emotional satisfaction.

Mental handicap

This is the most severe form of developmental defect and combines defect of intellectual development with social maldevelopment. It has a number of synonyms—mental retardation, mental impairment (as in the Mental Health Act 1983) and mental handicap (as in the Mental Health (Scotland) Act 1984). Basically, people thus handicapped, because of a failure of brain development from whatever cause, are unable to learn at the same rate as their fellows and indeed may be unable to learn at all. The most severely afflicted have a multiplicity of developmental defects, physical as well as mental, and do not survive long even with expert nursing and medical care.

Our concern is with those whose handicap is of a more limited nature. The vast majority are genial, law-abiding citizens, doing routine jobs and protected by their families and their community. A few do offend and they are generally those with an emotionally or socially unstable background or those who have additional brain damage. The inability of this minority to learn means that they tend to repeat their wrongdoings; they are also caught more readily. Their crimes are commonly minor and against property—shop-lifting, theft and housebreaking—but more serious crimes, such as arson, sex offences and homicide, are also committed, although rarely, by the handicapped.

Fire-raising is commonly a revengeful act or a source of excitement and may be repeated. Sexual offences are often the result of rejection by girls of their own age, together with immature development. Baulked of a normal sexual outlet they may turn to children, often unappreciative of the abnormality of their actions. Some handicapped females engage in prostitution.

One way of identifying the mentally impaired is to measure his Intelligence Quotient (IQ)—that is, to measure his performance in various tests against that which would normally be expected from a person of his age. If he performs up to the standard of his own chronological age, then his IQ score is 100; his IQ is above or below 100 to the extent that he falls below or exceeds that standard. It would be generally accepted that anyone with an IQ of 75 or lower would be regarded as mentally impaired, although some would put it as high as 80 and others as low as 70. However, this is only one measure of how the individual copes with his social surroundings; many other factors come into account and a measurement of intellectual ability alone cannot be decisive.

Mental illness

So far, we have been considering only those whose disability is the result of developmental failure. We now come to consider those whose development is relatively normal but who are overtaken by an illness. We are entering the sphere of the major psychoses, the serious mental affections where contact with reality is lost. We shall encounter some 'grey areas' here too, but the main syndromes are clear cut. They divide into two groups—those called *organic*, where there is some clearly demonstrable structural or biochemical damage, usually in the brain, and the *functional* where such damage, although suspected, has not yet been conclusively demonstrated.

Organic psychoses

The key disturbance in the organic psychoses is a degree of confusion and clouding of consciousness, either transient (acute) or permanent (chronic). The patient does not know the time or place and misidentifies people (disorientation). His memory, short term or long term, is defective. Such a confusional state may arise from damage to the brain itself (by trauma, tumour, toxins, infection or vascular accident) or from systemic disease in other parts of the body that affects either the quantitative or qualitative supply of blood to the brain (e.g. congestive cardiac failure, hypoglycaemia, liver disease, vitamin or hormone deficiency).

The damage to the brain may be small and discrete and clinically interesting but, criminologically, it is only occasionally important. A lesion in the frontal lobes may totally change the individual's personality, making him asocial, tactless, fond of silly jokes and uncaring for the feelings of others; a lesion in the temporal lobe can produce not only epilepsy but also all the characteristics of the 'epileptic personality' (*see* below); other lesions in the region known as the hippocampus may produce an aggressive, assaultive individual.

These, however, are rare; the most common brain defects are due to diffuse processes occurring in old age including arterial disease, general degeneration or, more rarely, infection and trauma. These are, moreover, of most legal significance.

The normal process of ageing, whether or not complicated by minor arterial accidents (or strokes) leads to changes in the person's ability to grasp new ideas, in his memory (most commonly his recent memory) and in his personality. Personality characteristics tend to be exaggerated so that a person with a life-long suspicious nature believes that objects he cannot find, because he cannot remember where he put them, have been stolen by some malevolent neighbour; he becomes a persistent nuisance to the police, to whom he is always complaining. A person in such a senile paranoid state can be a source of embarrassment to his family, neighbours and local police. Another source of discomfiture is the process of disinhibition that accompanies the ageing process; the elderly man may discover an inhibited sexual drive which may be directed towards children or expressed in exhibitionism.

Two areas where the individual's failing may have legal significance are shop-lifting and testamentary capacity. An elderly person may take something from a shop without realizing that he has not paid for it. Only an expert examination may reveal a disturbance of memory which explains his action. As to testamentary capacity, the testator most understand that he is making a will and have a recollection of the property he means to dispose of, of the persons who are to be the objects of his bounty and the manner in which it is to be distributed between them. Unfortunately these are questions that tend to be asked after the testator is dead; in such circumstances one inclines to the view that such clinical retrospection is not a medical function.

Acute brain damge, either from infection (encephalitis), trauma or deficiency of hormones or vitamins is unlikely to lead to any criminological problem. Long-term effects of infection such as that due to syphilis (general paresis) used to be important but are now very rare.

More important, nowadays, are the effects of trauma. Road-traffic accidents, if not fatal, can lead to a range of disability from the totally disabled to the minimally brain-damaged. We are not concerned here with those who have a clearly demonstrable neurological deficit from actual brain injury but rather with those who have no such deficit and yet show a change of personality which may be attributable to their head injury. First, there are those who complain of the effects of the head injury upon themselves and, secondly, there are those whose behaviour after the accident gives rise to complaints by others.

The first group are variously described as suffering from postconcussional or postcontusional states or from compensation neuroses; they have certain characteristics in common. They have suffered a change from stable, outgoing personalities into nervous, apprehensive individuals, prone to severe headaches, intolerant of noise, emotionally labile and unable to follow their previous occupation. They have suffered a head injury in circumstances in which someone else or some corporation is to blame and they expect compensation. This is a 'grey area' between hysteria and malingering. There is no doubt that their symptoms are genuine and unconscious and, yet, the longer the compensation is delayed, the longer the symptoms will last; moreover, the symptoms will clear up after adequate compensation is paid. Recovery is not immediate as it would be in malingering and may take some years.

In the second group the patient has no complaints and yet those who know him well describe a change in personality. A previously mild and stable person has become unusually aggressive, irritable and liable to be assaultive especially after taking small amounts of alcohol which he could previously tolerate well. Such people can be very dangerous.

The final group of brain-damaged people are the epileptics. The vast majority are perfectly normal people but they do suffer from social disadvantages in that they are barred from certain occupations and certain pastimes. This may not matter if they are socially accepted but, if they are not, they may react in an antisocial way. Prior to the 1939–45 War, it was thought that there was a definite 'epileptic personality'. Affected persons were thought to be impulsive, assaultive, ingratiating, religiose and untrustworthy. It was then realized that the epileptic personalities described were those of seriously disturbed epileptics who were in mental hospitals; the picture was not that seen in the epileptic living in the ordinary community, who was no more assaultive or criminal than was the rest of the population. Recent research has, however, shown that epileptics have a higher expectancy of criminal conviction than have the rest of the population but this, curiously enough, is not for violent crime. It seems likely that, while the majority of epileptics do not differ from the rest of the population, those who are rejected and socially disadvantaged react by committing crime. Those who are impulsively assaultive are very quickly steered into the hospital—and particularly the Special Hospital (see below)—system rather than into the penal system, and they remain there for a long time.

Functional psychoses

These are called 'functional', as opposed to the organic, because although the basis of their abnormality is suspected to be genetic, biochemical or metabolic there is, as yet, no clear evidence that this is so; indeed, many of them appear to be explicable on a psychological basis.

As with the organic psychoses the gross abnormality appears to be determined by a break with reality caused either by pathological variations of mood or by catastrophic disorders of thinking. The two broad groups concerned therefore are the *affective psychoses,* where the disorder is primarily in the sphere of mood, and the *schizophrenic psychoses,* where the disorder is primarily in the thought processes of the individual.

Affective psychoses

We are all subject to changes of mood ranging from deep despair to wild elation. Such changes are usually reality based and depend upon external events; sometimes they appear to arise *sui generis.* Whatever the cause, external pressures and our own resilience usually ensure that we return to an even keel within a short time. In the affective, or manic–depressive, psychosis, however, the change of mood, in either direction, may not appear to have an adequate precipitant or, if it has, its intensity and duration may be quite out of keeping with that precipitant. A bereavement, for example, is a saddening affair which normally lightens as time goes on; but in an affective psychosis the depression deepens and intensifies until all contact with reality is lost.

This loss of contact with reality is demonstrated by the appearance of delusions and hallucinations. A *delusion* is a mistaken belief that is out of character with the individual's background and is unshakeable by reasoned argument. A *hallucination* is a sensory experience without any real sensory stimulus. In this it differs from an *illusion* which is a misinterpretation of a sensory stimulus.

Manic–depressive psychosis derives it name from the fact that sufferers are, at different times in their lives, either profoundly depressed or unduly elated. They tend to come from families whose members show the same tendencies; they incline to a certain body build (short, thick-necked, barrel-chested and prone to vascular disease); and they have cyclothymic personalities—they are subject to unpredictable swings of mood. In the extreme example of this syndrome there are swings from deep depression to exalted elation with only brief spells of normality. It has become fashionable to emphasize that the depressive swing is much the more common and to talk of unipolar and bipolar depression depending on whether or not a manic phase has appeared.

In the manic phase the patient is elated, has considerable pressure of talk and of ideas, is convinced of his own ability to carry out new schemes and of his financial wizardry. He is therefore at risk of being charged with assault and breaches of the peace (due to his intolerance of the fools around him), of road-traffic offences (his judgment being impaired) and of fraud or embezzlement because he has used money that is not yet there.

In the depressed phase he is despondent to the point of despair. It seems that there is no future for him or for his family; not only is he doomed, but everyone connected with him is equally damned. Suicide is, of course, the major risk but when a depressive includes his family in his delusional system there is the danger that he may decide to 'save' them at the same time as himself and thus perpetrate a ghastly family tragedy. One-third of all murder suspects in England and Wales commit suicide; only about 5 per cent do so in Scotland and North America.

The other crime characteristic of the depressive is shop-lifting. The person concerned may not necessarily be of the classic manic–depressive, or 'endogenous', depressive type but may be one of those who are overwhelmed by external circumstances and who have a depressive and anxious personality. Typically, the culprit is a middle-aged woman of hitherto impeccable character and with a full purse who shop-lifts in a state of confusion as a 'cry for help' and as an indication of her depressed state of mind. The shop-lifter who does so because she is depressed may be in need of urgent help, and a significant percentage of women in the age group 40–60 years who are caught shop-lifting are suffering from some degree of depression. Most shop-lifters are psychologically normal and a small percentage are professionals.

Schizophrenia

Schizophrenia is probably a group of conditions that have certain characteristics in common and that may arise in a number of different ways. The key factor is a disorder of thinking; the component from which it derives its name, a split between the affect and the content of thought, is a secondary factor. In essence, schizophrenia can be seen as a disorder of perception; the world the schizophrenic sees around him is one that is distorted by hallucinations, illusions and delusions.

Because of his perceptual distortions, the schizophrenic lives in an environment of fantasy. This may so beguile him that he lacks all drive and ambition—the once-promising pupil fails to fulfil his early promise (schizophrenia simplex). On the other hand, he may be so beset by his fantasies and delusions that his whole thinking becomes too distorted for clear expression; he talks in a confused 'word salad' with numerous *neologisms* (hebephrenic schizophrenia). Thirdly, his perceptual distortion may lead him to a total withdrawal (stupor) or to a wild and impulsive attack on those around him (catatonic schizophrenia). Finally, he may translate his distorted view of the world around him into an aggrieved sense of a hostile environment and, while retaining much of his original personality, he will interpret any action or spoken word in the belief that everyone is against him (paranoid schizophrenia). There is a withdrawal from the real world and a lack of emotional response in all the varieties of schizophrenia. There is also a lack of appropriateness between the thoughts expressed and the emotion accompanying these thoughts, e.g. the expression of a belief that a person is about to be disembowelled may be accompanied by a fatuous smile.

The schizophrenic's delusional ideas are so bizarre and the personality dilapidation is so marked that there is no difficulty in seeing him as insane; he is none the less potentially dangerous. His auditory hallucinations may command him to attack an innocent bystander. Most dangerous of all is the well-preserved paranoid schizophrenic who, convinced of the evil intentions of certain people who are plotting against him, retains enough grasp on reality to counter such plots with deliberate action.

Schizophrenics may commit any sort of crime but, in practice, their crimes are mainly petty. Their lack of drive and persistence leads many of them into a vagrant existence and they steal in order to live. This leads to a well-known vicious circle in which they steal and are apprehended; they are admitted, either informally or through the Courts, to a mental hospital where they are treated with psychotropic drugs; they are discharged, discharge themselves or, most commonly, abscond; they stop taking their medication, they relapse into schizophrenia and, with no job, stable background or support, they steal in order to live.

Occasionally, a series of petty crimes by a previously blameless individual may be the prodromal phase of schizophrenia. More dramatically, the first sign may be a sudden unprovoked homicidal attack on a member of the family, an acquaintance or a stranger, often prompted by hallucinatory voices. A careful history will, however, usually reveal that the young person concerned (schizophrenia most usually begins in the late teens or early twenties) had recently been rather strange and withdrawn and had been falling off in his performance at work, all of which had been ascribed to an 'adolescent phase'.

While a schizophrenic may kill anyone, the very rare crime of matricide is characteristic of the condition and, in general, the more bizarre and unusual a crime, the more likely it is that it was committed by someone mentally disordered.

The very dangerous state of morbid jealousy, sometimes referred to as the 'Othello syndrome', is allied to paranoid schizophrenia but generally occurs without the characteristic thought disorder of true schizophrenia. In the 'Othello syndrome', the person, usually male, has delusions of infidelity about his wife or mistress. The man is usually in his 40s, has been married or associated for 10 or more years and has held his delusional ideas for 4 or 5 years during which time he has often upbraided or physically assaulted his partner. The end result may be murder or attempted murder. In such a situation, divorce is probably the only safe course for the spouse.

Forensic psychiatry in practice

All of the major categories of mental disorder have now been reviewed but clinical cases are seldom as clear cut as are the syndromes that have been described. Many are more complex and there are graduations between one form of illness and another. For example, one may encounter an elderly woman, accused of some crime, who is clearly depressed. Further examination may reveal that she has been subject to episodes of depression throughout her life, that her forebears were similarly affected, that she has always been a dependent personality, that her adult life has been beset with serious problems and that she is now showing signs of early intellectual deterioration. In such a case it is neither easy nor helpful to arrive at a single diagnosis; it is more profitable to state a formulation of her present mental state and relate that to the crime she is accused of committing.

Serious forms of mental disorder are found in a small proportion (1–3 per cent) of offenders but psychological factors may be found in many cases. Reference has already been made to crime in adolescents. Very few of these youngsters have a serious mental disorder other than some degree of personality disorder but many thieve—the commonest form of delinquency—because of psychological factors which range from simple bravado in an attempt to prove themselves to themselves or to their peers, through complex unconscious desires to hurt their parents to a desire to be punished due to a sense of guilt.

Psychological mechanisms also enter into the use and abuse of alcohol, which is an important factor in many crimes. Alcohol is a central nervous system depressant and its apparent stimulant effect is due to its disinhibiting action which releases tendencies that might otherwise be resisted. This effect is so well known that it is common for offenders to plead that they were acting under the influence of alcohol. It is, therefore, difficult to estimate the true part played by alcohol in the commission of crime but it is probable that its influence is related to the extent to which the abuse of alcohol is tolerated in the community. Its role is particularly important in assaultive crime and research has shown that, in such instances, intoxication in the victim is almost as important as it is in the assailant.

Persistent excessive drinking can lead to the disease of alcoholism. Alcoholics are those excessive drinkers who become so psychologically dependent on alcohol that it interferes with their health, social functioning and interpersonal relationships. The development of alcoholism follows a familiar pattern. It begins by the person choosing his social activities according to the amount of alcohol to be expected, then 'doubling up' on his drinks, surreptitious drinking from an ensured supply, increasing tolerance of alcohol, amnesic episodes with no more than the normal amount of alcohol and the experience of general tremulousness and irritability every morning. The tremulousness may lead on to 'the shakes' and eventually to delirium tremens (DTs) with vivid and terrifying hallucinations. The psychological dependence on alcohol may take the form of an inability to abstain (a need for a constant level of alcohol) or an inability to stop (continued drinking until all resources are expended). This progressive dependence may be spread over a number of years during which jobs, driving licence and marriage are lost. The stereotype picture of the skid-row alcoholic, living on meths on a bomb-site or in a model lodging house on social security is, in reality, less common than is the business executive gradually slipping down the socioeconomic scale.

The need for alcohol—and the occurrence of withdrawal symptoms show it to be a physiological as well as a psychological need—may involve alcoholics in many crimes such as breach of the peace, road-traffic offences and dishonesty. Depending on the social level of the alcoholic, offences of dishonesty may take the form of fraud and embezzlement or breaking and entering—in each case in order to acquire money for further drinking. It is only rarely that an alcoholic is involved in major crime such as murder, although alcohol is a potent factor in murder. One must learn to distinguish between those who commit crime after normal drinking and alcohol dependants who commit crime because of their dependence.

Sexual offences are also influenced by psychological abnormality. A distinction must be made between those crimes in which the direction of the sex drive is normal (indecent assault, rape and attempted rape) and those where it is abnormal (homosexuality, paedophilia, incest, bestiality). In the former, there may be either an unconscious resentment of women, stemming from a poor mother–child relationship, or an immature inability to make proper heterosexual contacts; but the majority stem from a combination of strong normal sexual drive in a compromising situation, lubricated by alcohol and with an aggressive component. There is an aggressive factor in most rapes and it is interesting that, while convictions for abnormal sexual crimes have remained steady, those for rape have tended to rise, *pari passu*, with the increasing occurrence of crimes of violence.

Abnormal sexual drives result from developmental failure or from immaturity. The offences arising are best understood as an attempt to achieve sexual expression in one who has not attained full sexuality. Many homosexuals enrich our lives in cultural and artistic fields while others spell misery for themselves and others. The majority of sex offenders are pathetic people trying to find their own solution and most offend only once. Those whose offences escalate are very dangerous. Child sex murders are very rare and usually the result of panic in the offender.

The electroencephalogram

We have already talked of those who are brain-damaged in various ways. Some of these—particularly the epileptics—may be identified with the electroencephalogram (EEG).

An EEG abnormality is not pathognomic of brain damage since non-specific abnormalities occur in about 12 per cent of the adult population and in a much higher proportion of adolescents in whom the brain takes a variable time to mature. Significantly, there is a very high incidence of abnormal EEGs in those who are recidivist criminals and particularly in those who are repeatedly convicted of assaultive crime. It would seem that a considerable number of these individuals have some form of non-specific brain damage.

Criminal responsibility

It has long been accepted in all civilized countries that children and those who are seriously mentally disordered are not responsible in law for any crime that they may commit. This is enshrined in the old doctrine of 'actus non facit reum nisi sit mens rea' which means that there cannot be a criminal act without criminal intent.

When it is proven that the accused was insane at the time of committing the act, the Court returns a special verdict of 'not guilty by reason of insanity'. The difficulty has always been in determining what degree of mental disorder is necessary to absolve the person from responsibility. Until relatively recent times, the test applied was whether his or her powers of reasoning were impaired and, indeed, this was the basis of the McNaghten Rules. Daniel McNaghten was a paranoid schizophrenic who held the delusional belief that he was being persecuted and that this could only be stopped by shooting the Prime Minister of the day—Sir Robert Peel. He attempted to do so but, by mistake, shot and killed the Prime Minister's Private Secretary—Mr William Drummond. He was acquitted on grounds of insanity but his acquittal raised such public concern that the House of Lords put a series of questions to the Judges. The Judges' answers are contained in what are known as the McNaghten Rules, the most relevant portion of which reads:

'The Jurors ought to be told in all cases that every man is to be presumed to be sane and to possess a sufficient degree of reason to be responsible for his crimes until the contrary be proved to their satisfaction; and that to establish a defence on the ground of insanity it must be clearly proved that at the time of the committing of the act the party accused was labouring under such a defect of reason from disease of the mind as not to know the nature and quality of the act he was doing or, if he did know it, that he did not know he was doing wrong.'

The Rules would have very limited application if they were strictly interpreted and they have been criticized ever since their introduction in 1843. Nevertheless, they have been followed in most English-speaking countries although their application has been, generally, liberal.

The main criticisms of the Rules stem from their emphasis on reason as the main factor in determining an individual's behaviour while ignoring the potent effects of emotion, delusional beliefs and hallucinations.

Several attempts have been made to find an alternative, particularly in the United States. The first of these was the New Hampshire formula in 1865:

'So far as a person acts under the influence of mental disease, he is not accountable.' The second was the so-called Durham formula in 1954:

'The accused is not criminally responsible if his unlawful act was the product of
   mental disease or mental defect.'
The most recent is the proposal in the American Law Institute's model penal code
of 1959 that:
   'The question be whether the defendant as a result of mental disease or defect
   lacked substantial capacity either to appreciate the criminality of his conduct or
   to conform his conduct to the requirements of law.'
   The difficulties of these formulae lie in the fact that mental disease or defect is
not defined in any of them and, in giving evidence, psychiatrists are apt to be drawn
into stating a conclusion about the nature of the accused's mental disorder and its
relationship to his responsibility rather than concentrating on the facts indicating
mental disorder and leaving the question of responsibility to the jury.
   The McNaghten Rules have never been part of Scots law although their spirit has
influenced many judgments. In 1867, Lord Deas first propounded what became
known as the doctrine of 'diminished responsibility' in the case of *Dingwall*[3]. This
doctrine has been developed over the years and has for a long time been a
well-established part of Scottish law. It recognizes that there are differing degrees of
mental disorder and, in general, a defence of diminished responsibility requires
evidence of 'a state of mind bordering upon but not amounting to insanity'. This would
cover certain organic states, depressions, obsessional states and some paranoid states.
   This doctrine of diminished responsibility, which is limited in its application both
in English and Scottish law, to cases of murder, was incorporated in English law in
the Homicide Act 1957, s. 2(1) which provides that: 'where a person kills or is party
to the killing of another he shall not be convicted of murder if he was suffering from
such abnormality of mind (whether arising from a condition of arrested or retarded
development of mind or any inherent causes or induced by disease or injury) as
substantially impaired his mental responsibility for his acts and omissions in doing
or being a party to the killing'. The effect of a successful plea of diminished responsibility is to reduce the charge from one of murder to one of culpable homicide in
Scotland or manslaughter in England. This reduction of the charge gives a wide
discretion to the Court in disposing of the offender and includes the use of the provisions of Part III of the Mental Health Act 1983 and its Scottish equivalent (*see*
below) to provide a hospital disposal if the condition of the accused so warrants.
Originally, psychopaths were not regarded as falling into the category of those
whose responsibility was diminished but severely abnormal psychopaths may now be
dealt with in this way.
   Just as it has been accepted that it is inhuman to punish someone who is not
responsible for his actions, so it has been accepted that it is inhuman to subject to
trial someone who by reason of mental disorder is unable properly to defend
himself; such a person is judged to be unfit to plead. The generally accepted criteria
for fitness to plead are that the accused should be able to:

1. Understand the nature of the charge and the possible consequences to himself.
2. Follow the proceedings in court.
3. Challenge the jurors.
4. Properly instruct his defence.

If the accused is unable to fulfil these requirements and is found to be unfit to
plead, the trial does not proceed and he is committed on a Hospital Order. In

[3] Alex. Dingwall (1867)5 Irv. 466.

serious cases, this Hospital Order will be to a Special Hospital with a restriction order without limit of time. It is possible for the prosecution to reopen the case if the accused recovers quickly from his mental disorder and thereby becomes fit to plead, but this seldom happens since the degree of disorder leading to unfitness to plead is usually of a very serious nature. The disposal may seem an unsatisfactory one from the point of view of the accused since he sees himself as being confined to and restricted in hospital by reason of a crime that has never been proved against him. Because of this it is important that unfitness to plead should be used only very sparingly and, indeed, there are some authorities, particularly in the United States, who would abolish the concept and insist that everyone be tried no matter what his mental state.

The Home Secretary also has power (under the Mental Health Act 1983, s. 48) to order the detention in a mental hospital without trial of a person committed in custody for trial whom the Home Secretary is satisfied is suffering from mental illness or severe subnormality that warrants his detention for treatment.

The Butler Committee[4] considered the question of fitness to plead and of insanity at the time of the the crime in considerable detail. They recommended that the term 'Unfit to plead' should be replaced by the phrase 'Under disability in relation to the trial' which could be shortened colloquially to 'Under disability'. They also recommended the introduction of an 'Interim Hospital Order'[4a] which would have the effect of postponing the trial until such time as hospital treatment might enable the accused to become fit to stand trial. This Order would have a limit of 6 months. Such an Interim Hospital Order would also be useful where the defendant required medical care during a custodial remand and where a period in hospital was required to determine whether a Hospital Order was appropriate. The Interim Hospital Order would have the effect of ensuring that only those who were likely to be permanently unfit to plead would be denied the opportunity of defending themselves.

In relation to insanity at the time, the Butler Committee recommended a new formulation of the Special Verdict, namely 'not guilty on evidence of mental disorder', the grounds for which should comprise two elements:

1. a *mens rea* element approximating to the first limb of the McNaghten Rules (did he know what he was doing?); and
2. specific exemption from conviction for defendants suffering from severe mental illness or severe subnormality at the time of the act or omission charged. They propose a definition of severe mental illness which details the clinical features that would have to be present in order to justify such a finding. The clinical features are those that would only be present in someone who is seriously psychotic. It would be for the examining psychiatrist to show clearly that they were present in the accused and for the jury then to determine whether the defendant was 'not guilty on evidence of mental disorder'.

The legal framework

The vast majority of people suffering from mental disorder are treated informally, i.e. without any legal compulsion on either an out-patient or in-patient basis. Even about 90 per cent of those admitted to mental hospitals are admitted informally. The

[4] Butler, Lord (Chairman) (1975). *Report of the Committee on Mentally Abnormal Offenders*. Cmnd. 6244. London; HMSO. The recommendations of the Committee were concerned with England and Wales only.
[4a] Now in operation (Mental Health Act 1983, s. 38).

prosecution will sometimes drop minor charges in the case of a mentally abnormal offender if he or she agrees to enter hospital for treatment as an informal patient. One quasi-informal disposal available to the Courts is a probation order with a condition of treatment, either as an out-patient or in-patient. In such a case, the patient is free to discontinue treatment at any time but in doing so runs the risk of being held in breach of this probation order. Such orders have only a limited usefulness.

The provisions of Part II of the Mental Health Act 1983 or the Mental Health (Scotland) Act 1984 may be invoked in those few instances in which a mentally disordered person does not recognize that his mental state may constitute a danger to the health or safety of himself or others. Sections 4, 2 and 3 of the 1983 Act and Sections 24 and 18 of the 1984 Act provide that a mentally disordered person may be compulsorily detained for 3 days (s. 4 of the 1983 Act and s. 24 of the 1984 Act) as an emergency on the certificate of one doctor. He may be detained for assessment for 28 days (s. 2 of the 1983 Act) or, for treatment, initially for 6 months (1983, s. 3; 1984, s. 18) on the agreed recommendations of two doctors—preferably the one who knows him best (his family doctor) and the one who knows most about his condition (the hospital consultant). In all of these cases, the test is that he must be in such a state of mental disorder that either his own health or safety or that of others is at risk and that no other form of treatment will be effective.

A detained patient must have the authority for his detention renewed, on the recommendations of two doctors, after 6 months' detention, after a further 6 months and thereafter after every year[5a]. He is automatically discharged if the doctors do not find grounds for detaining him further. He can be discharged at any time by his doctor if he no longer suffers from mental disorder or no longer requires to be compulsorily detained. He can appeal each time his detention is renewed, in Scotland to the Sheriff, in England to the Mental Health Review Tribunal, a regional body which continues to exist by s. 65 of the 1983 Act and consisting of a lawyer, a doctor and someone knowledgeable in social services. In Scotland, in addition, he can appeal to the Mental Welfare Commission, an independent body set up under the Mental Health (Scotland) Act 1960, responsible directly to the Secretary of State and charged with exercising generally protective functions on behalf of mentally disordered patients[5]. The managers of the hospital and the nearest relative may also demand the patient's discharge but this may be refused if the responsible medical officer issues a report that the patient is dangerous. The patient is automatically discharged if he absconds and remains at liberty for 28 days (3 months if he is mentally handicapped). The only avenue for discharge available to a patient under a restriction order alternative to the discretion of the Home Secretary is through the Mental Health Review Tribunal (see page 310).

In recent years it has been argued that to take compulsory powers over someone whose own health or safety only is at risk is paternalistic and an infringment of the individual's liberty to dispose of his own life as he thinks fit; such compulsory powers should only operate where the health and safety of others are compromised. This argument might have some force were it always possible to separate the two hazards but, as we have seen with the depressive and schizophrenic

---

[5] The Mental Welfare Commission has wide powers including a duty to visit hospitals regularly and to investigate complaints of any kind; in the course of such investigations it is empowered to compel attendance of witnesses and to take evidence on oath. The chairman is a High Court judge.

[5a] Mental Health Act 1983, s. 20; Mental Health (Scotland) Act 1984, s. 30.

murderers, it may be a matter of chance whether the afflicted person kills himself or others or both. Furthermore, the argument rests on the assumption that the individual is making a rational choice, whereas the people catered for in the Acts are those whose actions are determined by totally irrational forces.

Up to 1982, certain classes of mental disorder were excluded from compulsory admission to hospital by virtue of age restriction; age now has no significance. Those suffering from mental illness, severe mental impairment, psychopathic disorder and mental impairment may all be admitted when medical treatment in hospital is appropriate, but it is a condition of admission of those suffering from psychotic disorder or mental impairment that treatment is likely to alleviate or prevent a deterioration in their condition[6].

Special provision is made for those mentally disordered individuals who have committed crimes. Under s. 37 of the 1983 Act, where someone has committed a crime normally punishable with imprisonment and where the Court is satisfied on the evidence of two doctors, one of whom must be approved for the purpose, that the offender is suffering from mental disorder, the Court may impose a hospital order instead of a penal disposal[6a]. The effect of such a hospital order is virtually the same as a committal under Part II of the Act; the practical difference is that the responsible medical officer may be more chary of discharging someone who has committed a crime than one who has not.

An extension of this caution in discharging those who have committed crimes is exemplified in s. 45 of the 1983 Act which empowers the Court, having regard to the seriousness of the crime and the likelihood of its repetition because of mental disorder in the offender if he were prematurely discharged, to impose a restriction order on his discharge. Such restriction orders mean that the patient cannot have parole, be transferred from one hospital to another or be liberated either conditionally or unconditionally without the express and personal consent of the Secretary of State. It is increasingly the custom to make such orders without limit of time; this not only means that a person who does not recover can be held indefinitely but also allows for someone who makes a rapid recovery to be disposed of more readily than if he were subject to a fixed term of restriction. It is thus more flexible. Furthermore, a fixed term implies a prognostic skill that neither the judge nor his psychiatric advisers are likely to possess.

The whole question of compulsory committal is at present controversial. There are those who would argue that the mentally disordered commit no more crimes than do their fellow citizens. This is statistically true but it ignores the fact that most of those who are mentally disordered and likely to commit crimes are safely tucked away in hospital. In recent years the liberalization of mental hospitals has led to the presence in the community of many more patients than before and recent research has suggested that, under this policy, more crimes are committed by the mentally disordered. Emphasis is placed on the common-sense view that a mentally disordered individual who is prone to antisocial acts should be prevented from perpetuating them by being contained.

Mental hospitals currently adopt a very liberal policy with open doors and a minimum of compulsion and supervision; this has greatly increased the dignity of

[6] Mental Health Act 1983, s. 3 (2)(6).
[6a] The Court must be assured that admission within 28 days will be possible.

the individual patient and the therapeutic relationship between patient and staff at the expense of making it more difficult to control those few who may be disruptive, destructive and dangerous. Modern methods of management in mental hospitals have been a great advantage to the majority of patients but have posed dangers to the public because of the unrealistic actions of the few really dangerous patients. In consequence, an increasing burden has been thrust on the Special Hospitals set up by the Government for the treatment of those patients with violent and dangerous propensities who require treatment under conditions of special security. These hospitals—Broadmoor, Rampton, Moss Side, Carstairs and, now, Park Lane— were originally established to care for those patients who could not be dealt with by the ordinary locked mental hospital and, in the main, took their cases from the Courts where the individual had been convicted of a serious crime and had been found to be mentally disordered. They must now deal, as well, with those who are unmanageable within the open-door policies of ordinary mental hospitals.

Because they have special skills in the management of these patients, they are also expected to have special skills in the prediction of the future behaviour of those patients they discharge. They tend to be over-cautious because the safety of the public may seem to be more important than is individual liberty. Hence, their problems are exacerbated by overcrowding. It was because of this that the Butler Committee recommended the setting up of regional secure units to deal with the lesser degrees of dangerousness. The Butler Committee recognized that too great a gap existed between the open units dealing with non-dangerously persons within their own area and the Special Hospitals dealing with the dangerously mentally disordered on a country-wide basis. There has been some difficulty in establishing regional secure units due to resistance by the local public.

It is difficult to strike a balance between the right of the individual to lead—and end—his own life and the right of the community to be protected from the irrational acts of those whose perceptions of the world about them are distorted by mental disorder. On the whole, our Mental Health Acts are fair. They put no obstacle in the way of those who wish to be treated for their distress on an informal basis and yet provide that persons without insight who might be a danger to themselves or to others can be contained and treated. At the same time, they ensure that the latter are safeguarded not only by the knowledge and qualifications of those who commit and treat them but by the number of people who can demand their discharge.

New legislation

The law relating to mental health has changed dramatically during the existence of the second edition of this book; it now lays more emphasis on patients' rights. Because some patients seldom or never appeal, all cases now have to be referred to a tribunal if they have not done so within the first 6 months or if it has been 3 years since their last appeal[6b]. The age limits on the detention of psychopaths and the mentally subnormal (to be renamed mentally impaired) are removed and instead the test for their detention, even by a Court, is whether treatment is likely to alleviate or prevent deterioration of the patient's condition—a 'treatability' test. A Mental Health Act Commission is set up under Part V of the 1983 Act, with the remit of exercising generally protective functions on behalf of detained patients, similar to the Scottish

[6b] Mental Health Act 1983, s. 68.

Mental Welfare Commission. Restriction orders may only be made so as to protect the public from 'serious harm'. Interim Hospital Orders, as recommended by the Butler Committee, are introduced by s. 38 of the 1983 Act.

The most contentious part of the Act is likely to be that concerned with treatment. It is generally accepted that an informal patient cannot be given treatment without his free and fully informed consent. The detained patient is in a different category and very difficult medical and ethical problems arise from his situation where, because of his detention and, by inference, of his severely disturbed and insightless mental state, he is unlikely to be able to give a free and fully informed consent and yet may require treatment in order to recover. Two questions have to be answered—is he in a fit state of mind to give or refuse consent and is the proposed treatment so likely to be efficacious as to justify its administration without his consent? These matters have been under anxious consideration for some years by psychiatrists, lawyers and other interested bodies and guidelines have been promulgated by the Royal College of Psychiatrists and by the Butler Committee. The Act lays down a legal framework, separating treatments into different groups. These are described, sometimes by implication, as irreversible (s. 57), hazardous (s. 58) and non-consensual (s. 63). The first requires the consent of the patient and certification from a registered medical practitioner and from two other persons—all appointed for the purpose by the Secretary of State—that the patient can understand the procedure and has consented to it; before giving the certificate, the doctor must have consulted a nurse and another person who has been concerned with the patient's treatment. Hazardous treatments include electroconvulsive therapy, and the section also deals with any treatment which extends beyond three months. In these cases, either the patient must consent and an appointed medical practitioner must certify his ability to understand or an appointed doctor must certify that the patient cannot understand and that the treatment should be given; in the latter circumstance, the doctor must, again, consult with two concerned persons, one being a nurse. These conditions do not apply in an emergency when treatment is necessary to save the patient's life; treatment other than that which is irreversible may be given urgently to prevent serious deterioration while treatment other than irreversible or hazardous may be given in an emergency and without consent when it is medically necessary and is the minimum needed to prevent the patient from behaving violently or being a danger to himself or to others (s. 62)[6c]. There is comparable legislation in Scotland by virtue of the Mental Health (Scotland) Act 1984.

An important amendment was necessitated by a decision of the European Court of Human Rights[7]. In 1974, a Mr X, a restricted patient on conditional liberation, was recalled to Broadmoor because of a deterioration in his mental state and was further detained there on the sole authority of the Home Secretary, as was perfectly legal under the 1959 Act. The patient appealed to the European Convention of Human Rights. The Commission upheld his appeal on the grounds that such patients should have a right of access to a Court to challenge their detention. The European Court of Human Rights endorsed the Commission's decision a few days before the Bill was presented to Parliament. As a result, the Government introduced amendments which enable restricted patients to appeal to a Mental Health Review Tribunal 6 months after committal and yearly thereafter. In such instances the Tribunal is chaired by a lawyer with substantial judicial experience in the criminal courts, normally a circuit judge or a recorder. The Tribunal has powers of absolute discharge and conditional discharge. Conditionally discharged patients have the same right of appeal and a recalled patient may appeal within a month of recall to hospital. The Home Secretary retains his power to discharge, to remove restrictions or to recall patients to hospital if necessary.

[6c] *See* Mental Health (Hospital, Guardianship and Consent to Treatment) Regulations 1983, S.I. 1983/893.
[7] X v. The United Kingdom (1982) 7 E.L. Rev. 435.

Mental disorder and civil actions

Aside from criminal acts, the mentally disordered person is at risk in civil actions. In making a contract, for example, one who is mentally defective or mentally ill may be held to be incompetent. While this is generally true, the law recognizes that such a person may have a lucid interval and, if his medical attendant is prepared to certify that at the relevant time the patient was capable of understanding what he was doing in making the contract, that contract may be valid.

Marriage is a special form of contract which was previously considered separately under the Matrimonial Causes Act whereby it was possible for a person to petition for divorce on the grounds that the spouse had been continuously under care and treatment for 5 years and was incurably insane. Under the new divorce laws, however, irretrievable breakdown of a marriage can be shown, for example, by the fact that the couple had lived apart for 5 years[8].

Reference had already been made to testamentary capacity in which the testator needs to know not only the extent of his estate but also those who would normally be expected to benefit from his bounty. Evidence that his dispositions are distorted by delusions may go to show lack of testamentary capacity. The will of mentally disordered persons may be shown to be invalid, either because their knowledge is wrong—by organic mental disorder—or because their dispositions are unfair—by paranoid ideation, of schizophrenic or depressive type, or by hypomanic overvaluation.

Similarly, a mentally disordered person may be incapable of managing his affairs. In such a case it may be necessary to appoint someone else to manage his affairs, either through the Court of Protection in England and Wales or by the appointment of a Curator Bonis in Scotland.

Automatism

Although not of great importance in the context of psychiatry as a whole, automatism is a topic of abiding interest to the criminal lawyer.* The defence of automatism is firmly established in the criminal law of most Commonwealth jurisdictions and continues to test the lines of communication between psychiatrists and lawyers.

Automatic behaviour is conduct that is performed by an actor whose consciousness is impaired to the extent that he is not fully aware of his actions. There may be no consciousness at all of the actions in question or there may be awareness that falls below the level of consciousness that accompanies normal behaviour. This alteration of consciousness may be produced by a variety of organic factors or, in the case of dissociative states, by non-organic factors such as stress or shock.

The main factors productive of automatism recognized by the criminal courts are[9]:

1. Concussion or cerebral disease: In *R. v. Charlson* [1955] 1 All ER 859 the accused was acquitted of assault after medical evidence was produced to the effect that he may have been suffering from a cerebral tumour.

---

* Accordingly, this section has been kindly contributed by Dr R. A. McCall Smith, PhD, LLB.

[8] Matrimonial Causes Act 1973, s. 1.(2).

[9] Some medical writers treat acts performed in a state of acute intoxication as being examples of automatic behaviour, but the law usually treats such behaviour as coming within a separate category.

2. Hypoglycaemia: *R. v. Quick* [1973] QB 910 where it was alleged by the defence that the accused, a diabetic, had acted automatically in a hypoglycaemic state[9a].
3. Epilepsy: In *R. v. O'Brien* (1966) 56 DLR (2d) 65 psychomotor epilepsy was considered a possible explanation of an unprovoked violent attack[9b].
4. Somnambulism: In the well-known Scottish case of *Simon Fraser* (1878) 4 Couper 70, Fraser was acquitted of the murder of his son whom he killed somnambulistically.

If automatism is satisfactorily established the criminal law accepts that there is no voluntary act and that, therefore, there can be no criminal liability. Complete acquittal, however, does not necessarily ensue, as the Courts have developed a significant distinction between non-insane automatism and insane automatism. This distinction, developed in the case of *Bratty v. Attorney General for Northern Ireland* [1963] AC 386 and endorsed in subsequent decisions, leads to the description of insane automatism as those states that are, first, caused by a disease of the mind and that are, secondly, likely to recur. In such cases, the convicted offender will be treated in the same way as other insane offenders, while those who successfully plead non-insane automatism will be completely acquitted.

Acts performed during an epileptic seizure have been classified in some cases as insane and in others as non-insane automatism. The approach favoured by Courts will depend, in the final analysis, on the social danger presented by the accused. Automatism produced by non-organic factors, such as severe emotional stress, has been discussed in a number of Canadian cases. Automatic behaviour in the disassociative state resulting from such stress has not been sympathetically viewed by the Courts and has tended to be categorized as insane automatism.

It may be difficult to succeed in a defence of automatism both because of judicial scepticism and because of the problem of establishing a medical explanation for the behaviour in question. For example, although there may be evidence of a history of epileptic seizures in a case where epileptic automatism is suspected, medical witnesses will be able to do no more than postulate that epileptic automatism may have been involved in the case in question.

In Scotland, judicial scepticism over this defence reached its high-watermark in the case of *H.M.Adv. v. Cunningham* (1963) JC 80. As a result of this decision the defence of non-insane automatism is now, strictly speaking, unavailable in Scotland[9c].

[9a] *See also* R. v. Bailey [1983] 1 W.L.R. 760.

[9b] But for English law *see* R. v. Sullivan [1983] 2 All E.R. 673.

[9c] Although it was widely criticized, this doctrine has been reinforced (Carmichael v. Boyd 1985 SLT 399).

29

Forensic odontology

Human dentition

Human dentition is of two types—the deciduous of infancy and the permanent; the former consists of 20 and the latter of 32 teeth. The permanent dentition comprises 4 symmetrical quadrants each containing 2 incisors, 1 canine, 2 premolar and 3 molar teeth. Although the differentiation of individual molars, premolars and lower incisors presents some complications, it is generally not difficult for a dental practitioner to identify an individual tooth on the basis of its size and shape; for Court purposes, however, the opinion of a specialist dental anatomist may well be sought.

Several systems for recording the dentition are current but that attributed to Zsigmondy and used in the National Health Service can be regarded as the standard method in Great Britain. In this, the teeth in each quadrant are numbered consecutively from the midline in the front; the second molar tooth in the right lower jaw thus becomes lower right 7 or, in common dental notation, 7⌋. The five deciduous teeth are annotated A–E in a similar fashion. An alternative system, which is being lobbied at an international level, substitutes the prefix 1 for right upper, 2 for left upper, 3 for left lower and 4 for right lower quadrants; using this notation the second molar in the right lower jaw would be designated 47[1]. The deciduous teeth are prefixed 5–8 according to quadrant. This is known as Viohl's Two Digit System.

If one considers a tooth for descriptive purposes as a cube projecting from the jaw, it has five surfaces. The surface that is opposed to its fellow in the other jaw is called the occlusal surface (O in shorthand); except in unusual circumstances, such as the loss of rear teeth, there is no occlusal surface on the incisor and canine teeth which are sharp. The surface nearest the anterior midline is called the mesial surface (M), and that furthest away the distal (D). The surface contacting the cheek is called buccal (B), and the inner surface is designated palatal (P) in the upper and lingual (L) in the lower jaw. Thus, the common massive filling that involves the biting surface and the mesial and distal walls of a tooth would be noted as MOD.

[1] The commonest notation in the USA numbers the upper right third (back) molar tooth as 1. Each tooth is then numbered consecutively, the upper back molar on the left side being 16. The lower left back molar is then numbered 17 and the process continued to 32 which represents the lower right back molar.

Any tooth may be unerupted, it may be normal, it may contain a cavity caused by caries or a lost filling or a cavity may have been restored. The restoration may be by synthetic porcelain or epoxy resin complexes, by a silver/tin amalgam or by gold; the tooth may have been capped or crowned. A tooth may have been extracted and, if so, been replaced by a partial denture, or bridge, or there may be a complete denture; the dentures may be made of plastic or of metal, they may be deliberately coloured, marked or even numbered and national practices lead to characteristic designs. Add to all these variables the possibilities of removable or fixed mechanical devices to straighten the teeth (orthodontic appliances) or of obvious deformities together with characteristics associated with race or with occupation, not forgetting changes due to age, and it will be appreciated that the potential variations in the mouth are so great in number that the dentition may provide as personal a method of identification as can fingerprints.

The relative merits of odontology and dactylography as identification methods have been mentioned in Chapter 3 and need amplification here. Odontology scores in two main areas. First, in a country provided with a National Health Service, it is at least probable that a record of the dentition of a missing person will be available somewhere—either in the files of a practitioner or at the Dental Estimates Boards where records of treatment are maintained for up to 4 years. By contrast, permanent records of fingerprints are maintained in the United Kingdom only rarely (*see* page 44); there is no way of tracing a *completely* unknown body through its fingerprints although, given some clue to identity, a match may be made with impressions obtained from selected personal possessions. It should be noted, however, that these considerations would not apply in the United States where filed fingerprints are commonplace throughout the population. Secondly, the teeth are very resistant to fire. Odontology therefore becomes the method of choice for identification of that major group of bodies that is unsuitable for visual recognition.

On the other hand, although developmental differences between two persons are almost always demonstrable by X-rays etc., the dentition can only become 'personalized' if abnormalities have arisen or have been induced. The fewer the deviations from the normal, the less precise can be the identification and it is difficult to identify, with certainty, from the mouth someone who has had no treatment or dental investigations; it may be hard even to distinguish between two persons of similar age and race with such an unblemished dental history. Fingerprints, on the other hand, are personalized from birth and remain so until death. It follows that odontological identification finds its greatest use either in confirming or denying an identification suspected in an individual on other grounds or in discriminating between the bodies of a large number of known but individually unrecognizable persons. The reasons why dental identification of, say, a completely unknown skeleton discovered in a wood is generally disappointing will become clear later.

Estimation of age from the teeth

Four observations can be made on the teeth with relative ease. In chronological order of appearance these are: mineralization, formation of the crown, eruption of the tooth and completion of the root of the tooth[2]. These are applicable both to the

---

[2] For full discussion of estimating age from the teeth, *see* Gustafson, G. (1966), *Forensic Odontology;* London; Staples Press.

deciduous and to the permanent dentition and observations may be made on two or more changes at the same time; one can, for example, estimate the eruption of the deciduous teeth and their degree of root development at the same time as assessing the state of completion of the crowns of the following permanent teeth embedded in the jaw.

These variables are shown in diagrammatic form in *Figure 29.1*. There is considerable variation in the appearance of each characteristic. For example, the range of eruption of the first lower deciduous incisors is from 4 to 10 months and, although the remaining deciduous teeth behave more regularly than this, the 'scatter' in the permanent teeth is far greater; in addition, the teeth generally develop rather earlier in girls than in boys. The more characteristics that are examined and taken into consideration, the more accurate will be the final assessment of age. In brief, the dental practitioner will utilize X-ray or microscopic evidence of early tooth development in the fetus or neonate; up to the age of 1 year the eruption of the deciduous teeth combined with an evaluation of the oncoming permanent teeth will give a most useful assessment of age. Following this—up to the age of about 2½ years—age can be estimated from the state of tooth eruption, always accepting the proviso in each case of a 'bracket of probability'. Eruption of the permanent teeth generally begins between 6 and 7 years. Eruption proceeds in a fairly standard order in each individual but the range among different persons may be up to ± 2 years; it is of some interest that Gustafson's *average* ages for eruption are, in many cases, rather higher than those given in standard works on forensic medicine—much depends on the phase of eruption intended. The development of the third molar or wisdom tooth is not shown in *Figure 29.1*; its eruption is variable but its roots are important in the young adult—if its roots are incompletely formed it can at least be said that the body is aged less than 25 years.

After eruption of the permanent teeth there are still characteristics that may lead to a reasonably accurate estimate of age. These are attrition, or wearing down of the teeth; paradentosis, or loosening of the teeth; infilling of the normal root cavity (secondary dentine formation); increase in the tissue holding the root in place (cementum apposition); resorption of the root; and transparency of the root. All but the first two of these six changes need careful laboratory preparation of the material and their assessment is certainly a process requiring previous experience. Gustafson has evolved a mathematical formula that attempts to arrive at a nominal age on the basis of all six characteristics and this gives promising results in *specialized hands*; the current order of accuracy, using computer techniques, is about ± 5 years. It is my experience that a dental practitioner interested in the subject can give a very fair estimate of age—in the region of a decade—from the simple estimation of attrition, paradontosis, mouth hygiene and the like; certainly the odontologist's assessment tends to be more accurate than that of the pathologist in the face of burning or severe mutilation.

Perhaps it is fair to say that odontology as an aid to ageing is most valuable in the comparative context, a further reflection of the importance of the dentist at the major disaster.

Racial and occupational characteristics

The assessment of race or occupation may be of help in the identification of the single unknown body. A few traits approach diagnostic value but most are, again,

316

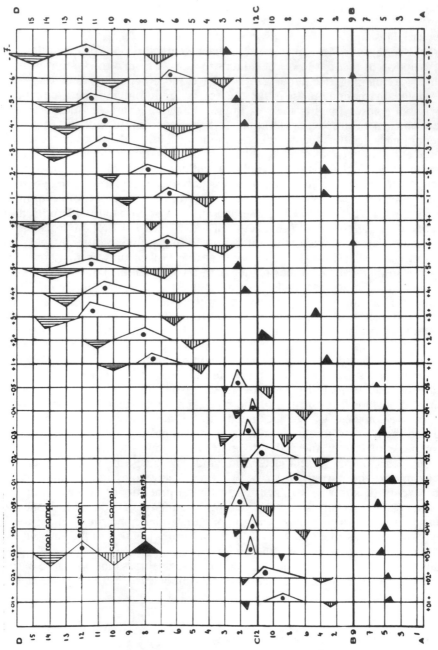

Figure 29.1 Schematic representation of tooth formation and eruption. A–B = intrauterine life; B–C = first year of life; C–D = 2–16 years. Upper and lower teeth are represented by + and − signs, respectively. Deciduous tooth numbers are prefixed by 'O'. The apex of each triangle indicates the average value and the spread of the base the earliest and the latest occurrence of the several features. (Reproduced by kind permission of Dr Gosta Gustafson from his book *Forensic Odontology* (1966); London; Staples Press.)

of greatest use in a comparative role; racial characteristics may be very useful in a preliminary sorting of multiple casualties from, say, an air accident. Except in such a circumstance, when the tentative isolation of a *known* group of negroids from a *known* group of caucasoids may be relatively easy, the problem is essentially one for the specialist anthropologist and little will be said here save to draw attention to the evidence that he might obtain. Three lines of observation might be followed—the size and shape of the teeth themselves, the extent and nature of any restorations and the quality of prostheses (bridges or dentures).

The size of the teeth, which are generally large in primitive peoples, is so variable as to be virtually useless save at extremes of the scale. Mention may be made of the high incidence of so-called shovel-shaped upper incisors in mongoloid and eskimo races. Subtle differences in the premolar and molar teeth are also to be found in these groups. The arch of the jaw is wide in negroid persons and the teeth are usually in good alignment and occlusion; this is in general contrast to the European caucasoid, in whom a narrow arch predisposes to crowding and misplacement of teeth—the wisdom teeth are very commonly unerupted or are extracted.

As to the recognition of restorations and prostheses, it has been pointed out that it is far easier to say that a given piece of work was unlikely to have been done in a certain place rather than to identify the area in which it was performed; moreover, the place of treatment is not necessarily the same as the homeland of the person treated. There are, nevertheless, some interesting geographical variations in dental restoration. Certain nationals, in particular Africans, have remarkably good teeth requiring virtually no restorative treatment; they are therefore very difficult to identify individually from their dentition. The use of gold is far less common in the United Kingdom than elsewhere; it is particularly prevalent in southern Europe and in the mongoloid races. Silver alloys for fashioning false tooth crowns are common in eastern Europe and, while silica and epoxy resin is generally used in Great Britain for restoring front teeth, porcelain is rather more likely to be used in the United States.

Such findings are, however, no more than guides to identification and the same is true of bridges and dentures. Certain types of work may be more common in one country than another but to make an 'exclusion' type of identification solely on this basis would be a hazardous undertaking.

Occupational stigmas can arise from mechanical or chemical injury. Classic mechanical injuries are said to be found in the form of notches in the incisors of those who grasp nails or twine in the mouth—shoemakers, upholsterers and seamstresses. Gustafson has also described changes in the front teeth of musicians, those working in dusty environments and in miners; most of these changes can now be relegated to historical interest. Chemical stains are most often due to the use of tobacco which, in pipe smokers, may also produce highly personalized mechanical injury, but chemical injury due to occupation is most common in those whose work involves the use of strong acids; this last effect is more commonly due to drinking fluids containing a high concentration of citric acid. Such observations must, however, be of forensic interest only very rarely.

Identification

Dental identification of the dead at the personal rather than exclusion level depends upon the availability of ante-mortem records. *Figure 29.2* shows how this

318

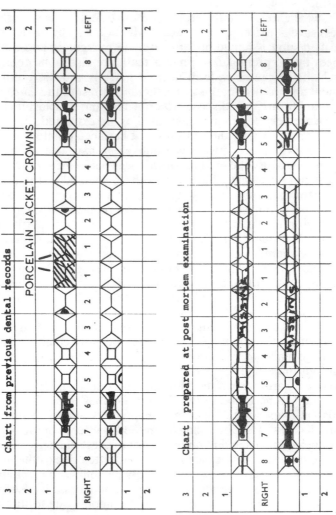

Figure 29.2 Dental identification in practice. The lower chart shows the teeth as recorded in the cadaver; the upper is prepared from previous dental records. Note that the lower 6 is charted as missing at post-mortem examination with a drift of lower 7 and 8 on each side to close the spaces; the lower 8 on each side is charted as missing in the dental records. The cavity recorded in the dental records in the lower right 5 was found to have been filled at post-mortem. A new cavity, not previously recorded, was found in the lower left 5 at post-mortem. Such inconsistencies are compatible with a positive indentification which can be made despite the loss of much of the anterior jaw during the accident. (The example has been kindly contributed by Group Captain Keith Ashley, RAF.)

operates in practice. It follows that nothing can be done in the absence of a retrieval service for these records and it is this which so severely limits the value of the method in the case of the wholly unknown body. It is certainly true that, in cases of major importance, a description of a cadaver's teeth can be sent to every practising dentist and hospital, but the process is time consuming and expensive. An identification service has been set up in Scotland under the aegis of the Home and Health Department utilizing the Regional Dental Officers through whom dental charts, with X-rays when available, are distributed on a scale commensurate with the information available; but success generally attends only when there is *some* indication as to identity.

This is largely because dental charts are seldom absolutely correct even when they are available. Some dentists record only the work that they have done, others are not so thorough as perfection would demand, while a large number of persons undergo emergency treatment which may not appear in their records until noted at a later date. The Dental Estimates Board keeps records only of extractions or major work. For all of these reasons, dental identification is at its most useful in a comparative or exclusive role and has been most used in the mass disaster, in particular the aircraft accident in which an especially good indication of the group identity of the dead is available through the list of passengers. Effectively, then, one is searching for the best-fitting charts among a known population.

The essence of rapid dental identification in the mass lies in the speed of retrieval of the records of the missing persons—the conventional methods of the International Police Organization are generally too slow to satisfy public demand for rapid restitution of the dead. British airlines are given service by a firm of funeral directors who maintain a control room for this purpose and whose facilities are at the disposal of the police wherever the accident occurs; the use of the telex system is an essential element in the rapid provision of information.

Dental identification then depends mainly upon comparison between the records of the missing persons and the findings in the bodies in relation to:

1. *Restorative work*: Teeth may require treatment, have been filled, have been extracted or replaced by prostheses.
2. *Unusual features*: Important features may include absence, persistence, malformation or discoloration of teeth; malocclusion of the jaws; and abnormalities of the mouth or lips.
3. *X-rays*: if ante-mortem X-rays are available, matching radiographs taken post mortem may provide unequivocal evidence of identification.

Comparison in any form may be affected by trauma—the possibility of fillings having been dislodged, and the like, must always be considered. A comparison of restorations may result in inconsistencies which can be either compatible or incompatible with a positive identification.

In general, a compatible inconsistency is one that can be explained either by the failure of the dental practitioner to record what he has done or by the treatment having been given subsequent to the last recording. Thus, a filling discovered in a tooth of a cadaver that is not shown in the chart of a missing person need not necessarily exclude a match. An incompatible inconsistency is one that involves negation of a recorded treatment. Thus, the discovery of a single filling in a tooth said to have had three treatments would normally exclude identification. Even so, very occasionally an identification is so certain on other grounds that it must be accepted despite the presence of an incompatible inconsistency. Usually such a

situation is attributed to clerical error or slipshod record keeping. The phenomenon of tooth migration, which occurs particularly in the molar region, may pose
real problems both for the recorder and observer. Identifications allowing for such
anomalies must, however, be accepted only after careful analyses by competent
authorities of all the relevant factors.

Strong confirmatory evidence of identification can also be provided by dentures.
As discussed previously, many of these may have national characteristics. Different
colours are used and the majority of laboratories incorporate some mark by which
they can identify their work. Such observations are particularly useful, say, in
separating the last three bodies from a large number of casualties. There is also a
growing habit of including a number in the denture; once the laboratory
performing the work for the deceased has been identified, this number may be as
certain evidence of identification as is the use of identification discs. Occasionally,
the patient's name is incorporated.

Accident reconstruction

A large proportion of persons killed in automobile or aircraft accidents sustain
maxillofacial injuries. The precise distribution of these when correlated with the
crash environment and the safety harness in use may give invaluable information as
to the direction and strength of the deceleration forces; the observations made may
also have a profound influence on the design of equipment, instrument panels and
the like.

This aspect of forensic odontology has not received the attention it deserves.

Bite marks

Animals may bite humans either in life or after death. However, such injuries are
not the concern of this chapter[3], which will deal solely with human/human bites
and bites in food.

The value of bite-mark evidence lies predominantly in two fields of examination:

1. Of the skin of a person assaulted, a prime objective being to identify or exclude
   the assailant.
2. Of food and other inanimate objects in an attempt to prove the presence of
   someone at the locus at some time.

In either case, the evidence must be of a comparative nature—the dentition of a
person must be examined and compared with the mark before he or she can be
identified or excluded as a suspect.

Human/human bites are most commonly associated with sexually motivated
assault and with non-accidental injury inflicted on children. The examinations may,
therefore, be required in both the living and the dead and, while the majority of
evidence is likely to be derived from an examination of the victim, the reverse
might hold if biting has formed part of a defence reaction to assault.

The comparison of records falls into two phases. The first, recording the bite

---

[3] The general medico-legal associations of vaccine therapy that might arise in the prevention of rabies
are discussed in Chapter 6.

mark, is a matter of urgency in the living person as the mark may alter in intensity and definition with time; indeed, such alterations may also occur in the dead body even before putrefaction intervenes.

In instances of recent biting, say within 5 hours, the first stage of the examination should be to swab the mark for saliva; previous physical examination, or interference by other investigators or mortuary technicians, may remove a large proportion of the saliva available and may contaminate the area with the examiner's own secretions. Approximately 76 per cent of people secrete readily recognizable amounts of either A, B or O ('H') antigens in their saliva and these antigens correspond to the blood group (see Chapter 18). The typing of saliva, which is obtained by swabbing the area with damp cigarette papers[4], may, therefore, positively exclude a suspect as having inflicted a bite—always provided that the group of the suspect is known. Alternatively, a match of antigens may add further to the evidence giving rise to suspicion. Failure to identify antigens may be due to the absence of saliva, to the saliva coming from a 'non-secretor' or to poor collection technique.

Following this, the bite is photographed both in black and white and in colour. Both sets of prints must incorporate a suitable linear scale following the natural curves of the part bitten, and the latter should also show a colour comparison chart; this has special importance in that repetitive colour photography is useful to follow the changes in the appearance of a bite mark and it is important to ensure a standard colour balance. The photographs should be supported by a sketch or tracing showing the actual measurements between landmarks. Useful landmarks are variable but would normally include such items as the distance between the canine teeth and the width of or between any clear individual tooth marks. Obvious abnormalities of size or position will be of major importance. Removal of post-mortem specimens in toto may be found useful but it must be remembered that tissues shrink in preserving fluids even if pinned on a board.

Recognizable marks on the skin may not be due only to direct pressure by the teeth. Scrape marks may provide valuable information in demonstrating characteristic contours of the cutting surface of the front teeth. The combination of suction and pressure by the tongue may result in bruises derived from parts of the mouth other than the teeth or from the surfaces of the teeth in contact with the tongue. It is probably true that no two persons have exactly the same tooth characteristics when these are expressed as a bite impression; in fact, it is difficult to reproduce perfectly a bite mark even when made under experimental conditions by the same participant. Nevertheless, it is a general rule that the more unusual is an abnormality, the more useful it is as evidence of positive identification.

Consideration should be given during this part of the investigation to the possibility of self-infliction—the rapist may force a woman's arm into her mouth or the child may deliberately stifle its cries in order to avoid further punishment. If there is any doubt, evidence that might be needed—i.e. models of the victim's teeth—should be made available.

The second phase of comparison requires the recording of, and obtaining impressions from, the teeth of a suspect and it is here that important considerations as to the legal admissibility of bite-mark evidence arise. The police have clear

---

[4] The subject's own sweat may contain her or his own water-soluble antigens. Control specimens taken from elsewhere (ideally from the same area on the opposite side of the body) are, therefore, essential. For the same reason, the examiner's hands should be gloved.

power to fingerprint, to have physically examined, to take rubbings from the hand and even from the orifices of an arrested person and it would be a logical extension to suppose that they also have authority to examine the mouth of an accused in order to establish whether there is evidence that bears on his/her guilt or innocence. So far as is known, the law of England has never been tested in this respect but it is certainly possible that the dental officer who attempted to take impressions from the teeth of a person under arrest without his written permission—and after full explanation of the purpose of the examination—might be held guilty of an assault[5]. The position in Scotland is rather less certain because, once a person is no more than under suspicion, he is protected by traditional rights based on the principle that he should not be placed in the position of self-incrimination. Certainly an examination should not be made after arrest without the consent of the accused and, ideally, this should be backed by advice from his legal adviser[5a]. On the other hand, it is noticeable that the Scottish Courts, in balancing the interests of the public against the rights of the accused, are tending to give rather more weight to the former in disclosing evidence with a view to securing conviction than to the interests of the latter in preventing disclosure so as to avoid conviction[6]. In these days, evidence derived from findings of a transient nature might well be accepted in serious cases even if it was obtained in the face of an arguable technical irregularity. This tendency was particularly expressed in relation to forensic odontology in the greatly publicized case of *H.M.Adv. v. Hay*[7], where a warrant obtained to make impressions from the mouth of a close suspect, who happened to be detained in an approved school, was held to be valid or, at least, granted in accordance with the overriding public interest.

Having obtained impressions of a suspect's dentition, the next step is that of comparison with the bite mark and, if a match be obtained, the presentation of the case in an acceptable fashion. There is no 'minimum number of points of conformity' required to prove the identity of a biter—it is simply a matter of the skill of the advocate and of the credibility and weight to be attached to the evidence of the expert witness. This is primarily because, in contrast to fingerprinting, the possible configurations in bite marks are less systematized. Similarly, there is no standard system of notation or presentation of the results, various experts having their own chosen methods. Certainly, photography must play an important part; superimposition techniques involving the use of transparencies are very convincing when they can be used but, unfortunately, the elasticity of the skin and the distortion introduced by contours often makes the method self-defeating. The criteria to be met are that the deductive processes should be easily demonstrable to and understandable by a jury and that the method should be free from attack on the grounds of unwitting distortion of the evidence. It is again emphasized that individual, distinctive abnormalities are of greater evidential value than is the general configuration of the mouth.

Compared with those in flesh, bite marks in food are stable evidence and, while it

[5] The procedure is laid down in the Police and Criminal Evidence Act 1984, under which dental impressions are regarded as non-intimate samples. It is not easy to see why saliva is, at the same time, classified as an intimate sample.

[5a] The taking of dental impressions may or may not be covered by Criminal Justice (Scotland) Act 1980, s. 2 (5)(c).

[6] *See*, for example, the opinions of Lord Cameron in Brown v. H.M.Adv. 1966 S.L.T. 105, and Lord Wheatley in Miln v. Cullen 1967 J.C. 21.

[7] 1968 J.C. 40. The case is very fully reported from the odontological aspect in *Journal of the Forensic Science Society* (1968), **8**, 156–217.

is possible to take impressions from marks in the former, they are not nearly so satisfactory as those that can be obtained from apples, cheese and the like. Nevertheless, all foodstuffs lose moisture and become deformed as they decay and this process must involve any tooth marks present. From the evidential aspect, therefore, impressions must either be taken with a reasonable sense of urgency or it must be established that the specimen was preserved in a solution known to preserve the original size and shape of the material. Within these limitations there is no doubt that models made from foodstuffs can provide positive comparisons with those made from the teeth which are easily understood by juries. What seems less credible is the likelihood of criminals leaving such evidence at the locus in any but extraordinary circumstances—but it does occur.

The science of bite-mark investigation is only emerging from the developmental stage[8], largely because practical research presents obvious difficulties. Few dentists can claim to be experts and, as a result, it may be difficult for the police to obtain the essential expertise at short notice. The present situation is that bite-mark evidence is of firmer value in excluding suspects when there are several rather than in confirming the identity of an assailant.

[8] A further extension of forensic odontology—identification by lip prints—has also been introduced recently, particularly in Japan. It has interesting theoretical possibilities but must, for the present, be regarded as mainly an experimental procedure.

30

Legal aspects of medical practice

Medical registration

A registered medical practitioner is one who is registered with the General Medical Council. While anyone may practice his 'healing art', it is an offence to pretend in so doing to be properly registered. A person who has passed the necessary examination and who has received the relevant diploma (Appendix N) may be duly qualified but, without registration, he is denied certain privileges and protection and he is disqualified from holding medical office under the Crown, from holding medical appointments in the public services and from practising under the National Health Service Acts. An unregistered practitioner cannot prescribe or supply certain poisons (*see* Chapter 23), he cannot treat venereal disease, he cannot attend a maternity case without supervision except in emergency[1] and he cannot sign valid medical certificates required under many statutes.

This supervision is based on the various Medical Acts of which the first was passed in 1858 and the most recent is dated 1983. The principal cumulative effect of these has been to establish the General Medical Council[2] with the following major functions:

1. To maintain the official list of medical practitioners.
2. To supervise standards of medical education.
3. To exercise discipline over the medical profession and to lay down standards of fitness to practise.

In addition, the old system of reciprocal recognition of medical qualifications between countries has been abandoned and the Council has taken over responsibility for supervising the employment and registration of overseas doctors.

The official register

The Register contains the names of all fully and provisionally registered practitioners on 1 January of the year in question. Entries in the main Register for those practitioners

---

[1] Veneral Disease Act 1917, s. 1; Nurses, Midwives and Health Visitors Act 1979, s. 17.
[2] The General Medical Council must now contain a majority of elected members. There are 50 of these (39 elected in England, the Channel Islands and the Isle of Man, three in Wales, six in Scotland and two in Northern Ireland); 34 members are appointed by the Universities having medical schools and by the Royal Colleges and Faculties; up to 11 members are nominated by the Queen in Council and the majority of these must be laymen (General Medical Council (Constitution) Order 1979, S.I. 1979/112). Dentists are controlled by the General Dental Council maintained in being by the Dentists Act 1984.

undergoing a compulsory year of postgraduate training are marked by an asterisk; during this time of provisional registration their practice is limited to their appointment.

An annual retention fee of £20 is currently levied and it is within the powers of the registrar to erase a practitioners's name by reason of non-payment of this fee; there is a £20 charge for reinstatement. Erasure may otherwise follow due to loss of contact with the practitioner or as a result of disciplinary action. Reinstatement involves a charge of £20 in the former case; in the latter, provision is made for suspension as an alternative to erasure.

Doctors who have qualified overseas may obtain full British registration if they have qualifications approved for the purpose by the General Medical Council[3], if they have held a year's appointment as a resident house officer in an approved hospital or institution and if they have an adequate command of English. Provisional registration can be granted to overseas practitioners with recognized qualifications on the same basis as it is available to United Kingdom graduates— that is, their practice is limited to resident posts in hospitals or institutions approved for the purpose of pre-registration service. Limited registration, for which a separate Register is kept, is granted in respect of practice only under the supervision of a fully registered practitioner. It is available for a maximum of 5 years to doctors with a wide range of qualifications outwith the United Kingdom who have already been offered an appointment. To be registered, the practitioners must have undertaken an internship of at least 1 year and have passed a test in English. Before proceeding to full registration they must either pass a test of professional knowledge and competence or satisfy the General Medical Council in another way. In the event of refusal of full registration or of extension of limited registration, there is a right of appeal to a review board for Overseas Qualified Practitioners[4]. Doctors qualified in continental countries of the European Economic Community are entitled to full registration as of right[4a].

Supervision of educational standards

The Education Committee which, alone of the Council's Committees, contains a majority of appointed members, can look into the courses given by, and the methods of examination practice of, the universities and other bodies empowered to grant qualification for registration. The Committee oversees the training given in the pre-registration year and has the power to visit any approved hospital or institution to assess the tuition provided. There is also a responsibility for advising on continuing postgraduate education.

Professional conduct

Although the General Medical Council may itself instigate actions against doctors on information received, it most commonly acts only in the event of an allegation

[3] Medical Act 1983, s. 19. Currently, the qualifications relate to Australia, New Zealand, South Africa, Hong Kong, Singapore, Malaysia and the West Indies.
[4] General Medical Council (Review Board for Overseas Qualified Practitioners Rules) Order of Council 1979, S.I. 1979/29.
[4a] Medical Qualifications (EEC Recognition) Order 1977, S.I. 1977/827, as amended.

being made. The disciplinary charge that can be brought before the Council against the doctor is that he was guilty of 'serious professional misconduct', which is to say that his conduct was such 'as would reasonably be regarded as disgraceful or dishonourable by his professional brethren of good repute and competency'. Thus, to some extent, serious professional misconduct is judged on current public attitudes, although professional men are, perhaps, rather less liberal in their views than are the majority.

There are two main ways in which the General Medical Council may become aware of matters needing their attention in a disciplinary role:

1. On a doctor's conviction of a criminal offence by a Court in Great Britain and Ireland (including Eire) or in the Isle of Man or the Channel Islands, the Clerk of the Court will inform the Council of the fact. This applies also to courts martial. Although such cases have greatly reduced since the enactment of the Divorce Reform Act 1969, a doctor justifiably cited as co-respondent in the Family Division of the High Court in a case involving a patient would also be reported.
2. Complaints against a doctor's conduct may be made by members of the public, including other doctors acting in a private capacity, or by such bodies as a Family Practitioner Committee of the NHS, a Hospital Authority or the relevant Department of Health. An individual complaint must be supported by one or more statutory declarations which must include the name and description of the declarant.

Information is first laid by the Registrar before the Preliminary Screener, who rejects complaints that are obviously insignificant and passes the remainder to the Preliminary Proceedings Committee, who may invite the doctor to explain his conduct. Four options are then open. The first discretion is that, in an emergency, the Preliminary Proceedings Committee may itself order an interim suspension or conditional registration for a period not exceeding 2 months. Otherwise, the case may be dismissed, the doctor may be sent a warning letter or the case is referred to the Professional Conduct Committee consisting of the President and 18 members (12 of whom must be elected and 2 must be laymen); five members constitute a quorum and not more than ten may hear an individual case[5].

It is at this point that the lawyer becomes actively involved as the Committee is advised on questions of law by an Assessor and the hearings conform to the practices of a court of law. The respondent may be represented, usually through his protection or defence society, and there is provision in all parts of the United Kingdom for appeal to the Privy Council against suspensions or erasure (*see* below). A similar right of appeal applies to a dentist appearing before the General Dental Council. Findings in a previous court are accepted as factual and may not be argued. The hearings are public, this being a source of justifiable complaint—no matter what his innocence in relation to professional conduct, a doctor's standing in a community can seldom be unaffected by sensational reportage of his private life. S.I. 1980/858 (*see* footnote 5), r.54 allows the Committee discretion to hear parts of the evidence *in camera* if so requested by any party to the case; the Committee can itself make such a direction in the absence of a request. The Professional Conduct

[5] General Medical Council Preliminary Proceedings Committee and Professional Conduct Committee (Procedure) Rules Order of Council 1980, S.I. 1980/858.

Committee has only two courses open to it—to dismiss the complaint or to find the allegations proved and amounting to serious professional misconduct.

There is no delimiting definition of serious professional misconduct but, in general, the Committee is likely to regard as most serious any misconduct that implies that the doctor has taken advantage of his privileges and of his special training and position as a professional man. Thus, false certification and the improper prescription of—or self-indulgence in—drugs are bound to be censured; in the latter case, further action may be taken by the Secretary of State under the Misuse of Drugs Act 1971 (*see* Chapter 23).

Use of his training to procure an illegal abortion will certainly not go unpunished and such cases still occur occasionally despite the wide compass of the Abortion Act 1967. The most publicized abuse of the doctor's professional position relates to adultery with a person with whom he or she is in a professional relationship. Such accusations may often be made in a spirit of revenge and much of the case may depend upon the definition of a professional relationship; recent cases indicate that the Committee's interpretation is generally strict. Other manifest abuses of position, such as indecent assault or attempted rape, will usually reach the Committee by virtue of notification from a Criminal Court and are, therefore, irrebuttable.

Advertising is one aspect of professional misconduct that illustrates how the climate of public opinion may influence professional ethics. The age of 'instant television' and the widespread interest in medical matters have dictated a relaxation of the old rule of professional anonymity in public. The current view seems to be that, as long as a doctor is already a recognized authority in the field under discussion, the public have a reasonable right to know his name and its publication would not constitute an offence; such an attitude would not be held, however, were the doctor using a television interview to raise his professional reputation or to attract patients. An equally dangerous source of potential misconduct in the course of an interview lies in the unwitting criticism of a fellow practitioner.

The most frequent cause for notification is conviction for the abuse of alcohol, particularly in association with with Road Traffic Acts. Most first offences are dealt with by warning letter, but repeated convictions not only bring the profession into disrepute but also indicate that the doctor may be a danger to his patients; more serious action is likely in the end.

The somewhat aloof attitude of the General Medical Council in its refusal to define professional misconduct has always been subject to criticism. Since 1978, the Council has assumed a duty of providing advice for members of the medical profession on standards of professional conduct or on medical ethics.

After a finding of proven 'serious professional misconduct', the Professional Conduct Committee may postpone sentence, in which case the practitioner is, in effect, put on probation, or it may suspend the doctor's registration for a period not exceeding 12 months. In addition, the Committee may now make a doctor's registration conditional upon compliance with such requirements as the Committee may impose for the protection of members of the public or in his own interest. The most severe penalty is that of erasure from the Register. Apart from the general right to appeal to the Privy Council, applications for restoration to the Register may, in this case, be made at any time after 10 months have elapsed and thereafter at intervals of 11 months.

It will be seen that the disciplinary function of the General Medical Council is directed to misconduct. Except in unusual circumstances, it is not concerned to establish negligence. Professional negligence is a matter of civil litigation, as is any other tort or delict, and is discussed later in this chapter.

Fitness to practise

The Medical Act 1978 established a Health Committee of the General Medical Council. A doctor's fitness to practise may be questioned by individuals or official bodies. Such doubts as appear to have substance are referred to the Preliminary Proceedings Committee who, again, have the authority to order an interim suspension or conditional registration for up to 2 months. The Preliminary Proceedings Committee may take expert medical opinion before deciding whether to refer the case to the Health Committee, which consists of a Chairman with six elected, three appointed and one lay members[6]. The question to be put to the Health Committee is whether the practitioner is seriously impaired by reason of his or her physical or mental condition. The Committee must arrange for an examination by two independent practitioners and the subject under review may have an examination by a doctor of his own choice. The hearings are in private and legal representation is allowed. The Health Committee may, if they find the case proved, order conditional registration or suspension for not more than 12 months. The President must confer with two other Council members before taking action. An appeal to the Privy Council against the ruling of the Health Committee can be made only on a point of law.

Medical ethics

Much of the ethics of medical practice represents a purely intraprofessional code of conduct and is better described as medical etiquette. The maintenance of good relations often devolves on the professional associations, for example the British Medical Association, and seldom involves the lawyer. Ethics in relation to the patient are, however, another matter and may well result in litigation. Since much of this is based on common or case law, complex arguments may arise. Little more will be attempted than to mention some of the typical problems that may occur.

The medical code

It is doubtful whether any universities now require the recitation of the 'Hippocratic Oath' at graduation. None the less, it is a reasonable assumption that the act of qualifying for registration implies acceptance of a code that has been fashioned over centuries of development and it is worth reiterating the main components of what is held to be the original work[7].

The primary consideration is the welfare of the patient; not only is a general affirmation given to apply one's skills to his or her benefit but it is positively declared to be improper to do anything that might harm the patient. Euthanasia and abortion are specifically condemned and, by implication, so is exceeding one's

---

[6] General Medical Council Health Committee (Procedure) Rules Order of Council 1980, SI 1980/859.
[7] *See The Handbook of Medical Ethics* (1984); London; British Medical Association, for these and other ethical definitions.

skill in undertaking specialist treatment. Improper association with patients or their families is barred and, finally, much importance is attached to what is now known as professional confidence.

These principles, together with those arising from the barbarities peculiar to the twentieth century, are restated in the Declaration of Geneva approved by the World Medical Association, which was reaffirmed in Sydney in 1968.

Consent to examination and treatment

The examination or treatment of a patient without his consent may constitute assault unless an emergency situation exists. The form of consent is, however, not uniform, and special difficulties may arise in relation to medico-legal examinations that may be positively to the subject's detriment.

Consent may be taken as implied when the patient presents himself or herself for examination and treatment[8]. Even so, the implication only pertains to what the patient would reasonably expect—a patient does not expect a vaginal examination if she complains of a cough, although a really dedicated physician might contend that a *full* examination of every patient is necessary for accurate diagnosis. In this case, he should obtain specific consent of unusual clinical methods and it is well to have such consent given in front of a witness. Examinations of the opposite sex, particularly of women patients by male doctors, should ideally always be chaperoned; unfortunately, the current shortage of nursing staff makes this a counsel of perfection which it is almost impossible to observe.

Minor invasive investigations—such as withdrawal of blood from a vein—which might cause pain and have a very small morbidity can, as a matter of practicality, be undertaken on the basis of oral consent; they are no more than part of the normal practice of patient care. Yet the fact remains that any invasion of the patient's privacy is technically an assault which is actionable both in the criminal and civil courts; it is equally clear that valid consent to medical procedures intended for the benefit of the patient absolves the doctor from blame. It is well established in America, that, to be valid, consent must be in the nature of what is popularly known as 'informed consent'. To achieve this, there must be understandable communication between the doctor and the patient. The underlying principle is that a patient must be free to make a choice or decision when such a choice exists; it follows that the wider the choice or the greater the risks involved in one or other course, the greater must be the communication[8a]. For these reasons, the problems of 'informed consent' are discussed in Chapter 31 in relation to major surgical procedures.

The legal age above which valid consent can be given is now 16 in England[9] and may be the same in Scotland[10]. Any consent to examination or treatment of a person below that age must be obtained from a parent or guardian. The doctor is in

[8] This interpretation has been criticized (McLean, S.A.M. and McKay, A.J. (1981). Consent in medical practice. In *Legal Issues in Medicine*, Ed. by S.A.M. McLean, p. 96. Aldershot; Gower Publishing.) but it nevertheless seems common sense.

[8a] In the United Kingdom, the test of adequacy is that of a responsible body of medical opinion (Sidaway v. Bethlem Royal Hospital and others [1985] 2 W.L.R. 480 H.L.).

[9] Family Law Reform Act 1969 (s. 8).

[10] I am unable to find an authority for this generally accepted practice. It was recommended by the Report of the Committee on the Age of Majority, 1967 (Cmnd. 3342, London, HMSO), but the recommendation was not included in the Age of Majority (Scotland) Act 1969. There seems no absolute reason why a Scottish minor (a female over the age of 12 or a male over 14) should not give consent of this type, but prudence would dictate that, up to the age of 16, supplementary consent should be obtained from a parent or guardian.

a dilemma if this is not forthcoming, say on religious grounds, and each such case must be decided, first, on the doctor's assessment of the importance of the matter and, secondly, on the chance of mishap; any decision to override parental opposition must be made on the basis of adequate justification[10a]. Such situations can stem from parental resistance to blood transfusion. The legalistic escape of applying for transfer of the child to the care of the local authority[11] has been advocated but is seldom needed, or now recommended, in the present climate of public opinion.

Unconscious patients or those incapable of understanding for other reasons cannot give consent. In such cases, the consent of a relative should ideally be obtained but is not needed when treatment is immediately necessary to protect life or health. In dire circumstances, such as a road-traffic accident, it is reasonable for a doctor to give treatment that he knows to be inadequate—for example, in the absence of sterile gauze, it would be quite proper to use unsterile material to stop lethal bleeding. Such treatment, must, however, be confined to the actual emergency; any that could be postponed pending admission to hospital should be left aside. The doctor at the roadside is really only justified so far as the doctrine of necessity allows; in Scotland, the concept of *negotiorum gestio*—that is, the management of the affairs of someone who cannot do so on the assumption that he would, if aware of the circumstances, have mandated such interference—would certainly apply to emergency treatment. It is difficult to believe that opprobrium would attach to the roadside doctor save in very exceptional circumstances[12]. The problems of consent to procedures that bear upon others, especially a husband or wife, are considered elsewhere (*see* Chapter 17).

Examinations for legal purposes, the results of which may be damaging to the patient, constitute a special category but, again, a general rule is that, with a few well-defined exceptions, consent is necessary to eliminate any suspicion of assault. The most obvious examples of such examinations are those requested by the police, the conditions for which are codified in England and Wales in the Police and Criminal Evidence Act 1984[12a]. In Scotland, a Sheriff's Warrant might be acceptable to the Courts in the absence of consent. These problems have been specifically argued elsewhere (*see* page 225).

Professional secrecy

It is accepted as a principle that the patient, in confiding in the medical practitioner, can expect that confidence to be sustained. The moral obligation is clear and extends, save in exceptional circumstances, to include the rights of maturing children to secrecy in relation to their parents; it would be difficult today to claim that a person aged less than 16 was not protected from such disclosure[10a] and, in some sections of society, the critical age might even be placed lower. Parental rights are not, however, to be lightly undermined and decisions in such cases must rest with

---

[10a] *See* Gillick v. West Norfolk and Wisbech AHA and the DHSS [1985] 3 W.L.R. 830 H.L. But it is uncertain whether this decision, which related to the issue of contraceptive advice, is more widely applicable.

[11] Children and Young Persons Act 1969, s. 23; Social Work (Scotland) Act 1968, s. 16.

[12] By contrast, it is noteworthy that it is an offence in France for a doctor *not* to stop at an accident (Decree 79–506 of 28th June 1979, Art. 4). Several American States have passed 'Good Samaritan' laws to regularize the position.

[12a] But evidence which is obtained without consent may still be admissible (R. v. Apicella (1985) *The Times*, 5 December).

the individual doctor—aided by his protection society. The results of any subsequent action based on a breach of professional secrecy will be decided largely on the qualification of the party to whom the information was given[13].

Legally, the doctrine of medical confidentiality is founded on the law of contract and of equity. There is surprisingly little case law[14] but the duty of confidence is certainly not absolute. The fact that some qualification exists has been recognized for a long time, the classic reference being Lord Riddell[15] who, describing the necessity and importance of medical confidence, was of the opinion that 'We must recognize also that the rules regarding them exist for the welfare of the community. . . . We must recognize also that they must be modified to meet the inevitable changes that occur in the necessities of various generations'.

This adaptation to changing circumstances has gained momentum in recent years, particularly in relation to the prevention of road-traffic accidents. Thus, it now seems perfectly clear that a doctor who is aware that a driver is subject to epilepsy has a right, if not a duty, to report the case to the licensing authority. Such an ethical duty certainly exists when the patient is in a position to injure many people as, for example, in the case of a driver of public transport; moreover 'it is not out of the question that a doctor who knew an unsafe patient of his was continuing to drive and yet did nothing about it might be liable in damages for negligence to anyone harmed by his patient on the roads.'[16] The important principles lie in the 'right to know' of the person informed and the degree of public risk; nearly half the instances of unconsciousness at the wheel are due to epilepsy and the condition is undisclosed in over three-quarters of these—the public need is clear.

The position of the doctor is uncertain even in situations involving criminality. There is no problem if only the doctor and his patient are concerned, as in a case of self-induced abortion. But what if third parties are involved? Should the doctor provide or offer information disclosed in consultation that he knows will lead to the arrest of a multiple rapist? In failing to do so, he is no longer guilty of 'misprision of felony' (Criminal Law Act 1967) but this merely places the burden of disclosure more firmly upon his own conscience.

In general, such difficulties arise only when the doctor is providing care for his patient. A person submitting to examination for, say, life insurance purposes or for obtaining a pilot's licence is not 'in care' and consents to disclosure of the result of his examination to the appropriate body by virtue of his signature on the document. It would seem, however, that, in default of such consent, insurance companies are not entitled to medical information as of right; the results of a post-mortem examination, for example, would not necessarily be privileged without the consent of the next-of-kin. It is also doubtful whether such consent is implied when the

[13] In General Medical Council v. Browne (1971) *The Times*, 6th and 8th March, a doctor who reported to her parents that a minor had been prescribed contraception was found not guilty of serious professional misconduct. The outcome would be far less certain today (*see* footnote 10a above).

[14] Kitson v. Playfair (1896), *British Medical Journal*, i, 882 is a doubtful authority. Smith, S. and Fiddes, F. S. (*Forensic Medicine* (1955), 10th edn., p. 366. London; Churchill) cite McCardie, J. as referring, in 1927, to the medical profession's duty of keeping inviolate the secret knowledge that they might gain from treating their patients and as stating that a medical man who, without lawful excuse, broke the duty of confidence would be liable to a civil action for damages. A general, but certainly indirect, statement of the position rests in the judgment of Lord Denning M.R. in Att.Gen. v. Mulholland and Att.Gen. v. Foster [1963] 2 Q.B.477.

[15] *Medico Legal Problems* (1929). London; Lewis.

[16] *British Medical Journal* (1974). Doctors, drivers, and confidentiality, i, 399. The proposition seems very doubtful. The doctor is indemnified in Australia against a patient taking action for such disclosure (e.g. Motor Car Act 1958 (Victoria)).

examination is carried out at the request of an employer; if the doctor fails to persuade the person examined either to report an abnormality himself or to change his occupation, the need for breach of confidence must be carefully balanced against any public hazard.

Many such cases are covered by statutes, generally related to public health, e.g. the notification of infectious disease or of abortion. The Misuse of Drugs (Notification of and Supply to Addicts) Regulations 1973 extend this principle to conditions that, strictly speaking, do not necessarily involve others than the individual concerned; there is little doubt that legislation will continue to recognize the rights of the community as often transcending those of the individual. *Pari passu*, the important principle of the need for transmission of medical information only from doctor to *doctor* is gaining ground.

Of the other circumstances in which a doctor is certainly privileged to break his contract in confidence, major importance attaches to statements made in courts of law.

There is no doubt that, in English and Scots law, the doctor cannot refuse to give evidence in Court simply because such evidence is based on information received in the course of a professional relationship. The Courts normally exercise great care in enforcing this doctrine and devices for satisfying the ends of justice and the doctor's conscience—such as passing information on paper—may be used; in the end, however, the implications of Lord Denning's opinion must apply—that judges have the power to direct a doctor to answer a question that is not only relevant but is also a proper and necessary question to be put in the course of justice[17]. Absolute immunity from allegations of breach of contract then follows and this applies also to statements made to lawyers during preparation of a case prior to hearings; Scottish precognitions are equally privileged. A doctor is not excluded when there is a statutory obligation for 'any other person' to disclose information to the police[18].

The provision of confidential medical records is closely bound up with this problem and, again, only the order of a Court can give absolute justification for their publication in advance of trial. This is a statutory right[19]. A potential plaintiff or pursuer can now obtain medical records from a defendant at an early stage—even before proceedings have been started. Furthermore, in cases in which a claim in respect of personal injuries is made, either party can demand a sight of a doctor's or hospital's records once proceedings have started, even if the doctor or institution is not concerned in the action. The Court Order may stipulate that the documents must be produced either to the applicant, his legal advisers or his medical advisers. Beyond this, while there is no doubt that some parties—for example, insurance companies—have a legitimate interest in medical records in certain circumstances, it seems that such records should not be disclosed without

[17] In Att. Gen. v. Mulholland and Att. Gen. v. Foster [1963] 2 Q.B. 377. Relevance is the only consideration in Scots Law (H. M. Adv. v. Airs 1975 S.L.T. 177) except where it is a matter of disclosing an informant (Contempt of Court Act 1981, s. 10).

[18] Road Traffic Act 1972, s. 168; see Hunter v. Mann [1974] 1 Q.B. 767; Prevention of Terrorism (Temporary Provisions) Act 1984, s. 11. *See also* Road Traffic Regulation Act 1984, s. 112 (2)(b).

[19] Supreme Court Act 1981, ss. 33 & 34; Administration of Justice (Scotland) Act 1972, s. 1. The wording of the 1981 Act now eliminates doubts as to whom should the records be disclosed (Dunning v. Board of Governors of United Liverpool Hospitals [1973] 2 All E.R. 454; Davidson v. Lloyd Aircraft Services Ltd., [1974] 1 W.L.R. 1042; McIvor v. Southern Health and Social Services Board, Northern Ireland [1978] 2 All E.R. 625).

the specific consent of the patient or of his guardians or next-of-kin. Good sense must, however, prevail—consent unreasonably withheld can only provoke an adverse reaction and there are now clear indications that reports on medical examinations made for the purpose of litigation should be exchanged if so requested[20].

The doctor and the National Health Service

Up till the passing of the National Health Service (Scotland) Act 1972 and the National Health Service Reorganization Act 1973, doctors involved in the National Health Service were administratively divided. Those practising in hospitals did so through Regional Hospital Boards; those in general practice were contracted through Executive Councils.

The reorganization of all aspects of the service[20a] has modified the administrative and disciplinary procedures within the service although the contrasting concepts of servants to the hospital and contractors in general practice have, if anything, sharpened. There is now no doubt that Hospital Authorities are liable for the actions of all their staff irrespective of their seniority and their consequent freedom to adopt working methods of their own choice. The liability of a master (i.e. the hospital) for the wrongful or negligent acts of his servants extends throughout the hospital hierarchy from non-medical staff to senior consultants[21]. Whether it be *post hoc* or *propter hoc*, all hospital medical staff in the National Health Service are now required to belong to a defence society.

The general practitioner is in no sense a servant of the Health Authority or Board, but, in providing his services, he accepts certain terms of contract which have been drawn up in the interests of the patients dependent upon the service. Breach of responsibility in relation to contracts may be the subject of complaint either by the administration itself or by the patient, or by the patient's spouse or (if the patient is deceased, ill or young) by any person; in this respect, the practitioner is liable for lapses by his nursing or secretarial staff and by any registered medical practitioner acting as his deputy, though he may, at the discretion of the Chairman of the Medical Service Committee, be released from the investigation if his deputy is a principal on the list of the same Family Practitioner Committee (Primary Care Committee in Scotland).

The terms of contract accepted by a practitioner in the Health Service include that he is obliged to take medical responsibility for patients on his list and for certain other relatively minor categories which include any person in need of emergency treatment. A patient may leave the list of a doctor immediately if he obtains that doctor's signature on his medical card and another practitioner accepts him; without the doctor's signature, he must give notice to the Family Practitioner

---

[20] Civil Evidence Act 1972, s. 2(3) (not applicable in Scotland).

[20a] The law is now contained in the National Health Service Act 1977, amended by the Health Service Act 1980 and the Health and Social Security Act 1984, and in the National Health Service (Scotland) Act 1978.

[21] The law on vicarious liability has shown a logical progression from hospital responsibility for staff but not visiting consultants (Collins v. Hertfordshire County Council [1947] 1 All E.R. 633) through no possibility of delegation of responsibility (Cassidy v. Minister of Health [1951] 2 K.B. 343), then including responsibility for the whole staff including those temporary or part time (Roe v. Minister of Health, Woolley v. same [1954] 2 Q.B. 66; Razzell v. Snowball [1954] 1 W.L.R. 1382) and including visiting consultants (Higgins v. North West Metropolitan Hospital Board and Bach [1954] 1 W.L.R. 411). Scots practice was brought into line with that of England in McDonald v. Glasgow Western Hospitals and Hayward v. Board of Management of Royal Infirmary Edinburgh 1954 S.C. 453, the reason for changing policy being the introduction of the National Health Service.

or Primary Care Committee and must wait 14 days before he can register with another doctor; the practitioner can ask the relevant Committee to remove the name of a patient from his list and removal takes effect on the eighth day after the request is received or upon the patient's acceptance by another doctor—whichever is the earlier. If the doctor who wishes the patient to be removed from his list is treating him once a week or more often, he must so inform the Committee. Transfer can still take place immediately upon acceptance by another doctor but, in the absence of such acceptance, the doctor must inform the Committee when he ceases to treat the patient at intervals of 7 days or less; removal takes effect 8 days after the Committee has been so informed.

Inevitably, conflict must occasionally arise as to the interpretation of the terms of contract, the commonest source of complaint being from those patients who believe they have received inadequate consideration. A system of investigation of such complaints exists and has not been significantly affected by the implementation of the 1977 and 1978 Health Service Acts.

Discipline is vested in Service Committees consisting of three professionals—doctors, dentists, pharmacists, etc., as applicable—three lay members and a nominated Chairman. Complaints are originally screened by the Chairman who, with or without consultation with the practitioner concerned, may decide that no hearing is necessary; he will then take it to the Service Committee, who may decide the issue without a hearing. Hearings are of little significance to the legal profession as they are private, and paid legal representatives may not address the Committee; only occasionally are solicitors present to advise. The Committee can make various recommendations to the Family Practitioner or Primary Care Committee, including one to take no further action. The Health Authority or Board can, should they so wish, modify the recommendations. In the event of a decision to withhold remuneration from the practitioner, there is provision for appeal to the appropriate Minister who, if he does not dismiss the appeal on documentary evidence, can call for an oral hearing by the Appeal Body. Evidence at this point is taken on oath and legal representation is permitted on both sides. If it is suggested that the inclusion of a practitioner's name in the appropriate List is prejudicial to the welfare of the Service, the Family Practitioner or Primary Care Committee may refer the matter for consideration by a statutory Tribunal. The practitioner may be represented before the Tribunal, against whose findings he has a further right of appeal.

There is, therefore, a remarkable contrast between the publicity afforded to hearings before the General Medical Council and the privacy of investigations under the National Health Service Acts. The latter process is, however, cumbersome and some of the functions of investigation—particularly in relation to what are loosely termed 'patients' rights'—may be undertaken by the Health Service Commissioner.

The Health Service Commissioner is specifically excluded from action in any case in which the complainant has a remedy through a court of law (National Health Service Act 1977, s. 116). Having assured himself that the body complained of has had a reasonable opportunity to investigate and reply on its own accord, the Health Commissioner can instigate further investigation by his department. Again, it is considered that, in view of the informal nature of the investigation, legal representation should not normally be necessary. Individuals under investigation may be accompanied by a friend, trades union representative or member of a staff association.

Outwith the health service

Doctors working wholly in private practice clearly have no contract with the Health Service but nevertheless have similar duties to their patients which are based on medical ethics. However, in the event of treatment being considered to be of inadequate quality as, for example, by failure to make a home visit when asked, the patient would probably need to show that damage had resulted before legal action could be taken against the doctor; a complaint might, however, be laid before the General Medical Council. Such conditions must be rare in private practice, in which economic laws operate as effectively as do the statutory rules of the Health Service.

Employment in industry carries some ethical difficulties. If employed as a Health Officer, the doctor still must base his professional conduct on a doctor/patient relationship; the acceptance of a contract involving disclosure of confidential information to employers against the wishes of the persons in medical care would certainly lead to a charge of unethical conduct against which there would be no defence. It is generally advised that the factory doctor should firmly dissociate his function from that of an employee's regular medical attendant. Other problems in industry—for example, those associated with experimentation, advertising and the like—might arise and are dealt with below.

On the face of things, the position of Medical Officers in the armed forces is equivocal in that they are the regular medical practitioners of the service personnel and yet at the same time are paid by and clearly owe an allegiance to the Crown which also employs their patients. The principle governing medical practice in relation to servicemen—but not their dependants—must be modified to some extent in favour of the need to benefit the specialized 'community' as a whole. Two main factors work to minimize difficulties which are often the subject of ill-informed exaggeration. In the first place, by accepting service in the armed forces, the patients have accepted—and appreciate that they have accepted—both the advantages and disadvantages of a corporate system while, secondly, the service authorities themselves are only too anxious to preserve a normal doctor/patient relationship in all matters that do not directly and adversely affect the efficiency of a fighting unit. The relevant Service Acts and Queen's Regulations will normally cover any situation in which a service doctor, or a service patient, is in a position of professional uncertainty.

Medical experimentation

A discussion of the ethics of experiments in medicine need only be brief as the lawyer will seldom be involved.

Some form of human experimentation is essential if medical knowledge is to advance to the good of the community; much preliminary work can be done on animals, but, ultimately, it is the effect of the procedure upon human beings in controlled circumstances that will determine its use in practice.

Experiments can be intended as treatment in an experimental fashion, they may be designed to increase academic knowledge with little prospect of immediate practical application or they may be needed to test the efficacy of an accepted treatment or to study the spread of disease. The subjects may be the researchers themselves, healthy volunteers or sick patients. Internationally accepted guidelines are detailed in the Declaration of Helsinki (1975) which emphasizes the distinction to be made between therapeutic and non-therapeutic experimentation (*see* footnote 7, page 328).

Uncontrolled experimental treatment of the individual is ethical only provided that there is no recognized alternative or that the recognized treatments have failed and the patient is seriously ill; the situation should always be explained and consent obtained—certainly if the treatment is painful or possibly liable to shorten life still further; in this case, the additional consent of a spouse or a close relative would be desirable. The principles defining informed consent (*see* below) will obtain most especially in these cases.

The introduction of new treatments for widespread use is ethically more complicated because a controlled experiment dictates that one group of patients must be maintained on the old, and potentially less useful, regimen; if the untried treatment is quite novel, it may be necessary to include a 'placebo group'—that is, one that is effectively being deluded as to therapy. Again, the lawyer's only concern lies in the importance of fully informed consent in an experiment involving patients. In practice, all such investigations now have to be approved by Ethical Committees which include lay and paramedical members.

Experiments designed mainly for academic advancement of knowledge are inapplicable to patients and are the prerogative of dedicated research workers and their assistants; much heroic work of this type is undertaken by physiologists—it is doubtful, for example, whether modern air travel would have been possible in its absence. Two points of medico-legal importance arise. First, the head of department must ensure that the risks taken are calculated to eliminate so far as is possible any serious danger to health. Secondly, the problem of the use of students as volunteer subjects often arises; such students will be of adult status but, while 'paternalism' is currently deprecated, most teaching organizations are conscious of some responsibility *in loco parentis* and formulate very stringent rules.

Much interest centres around the use of disinterested groups who are easily controlled—prisoners, soldiers, etc. Such experiments can only be justified provided that they do no significant harm to the subjects and that the results are likely to be generally beneficial. Yet again, valid consent is at issue. It must be freely given and not associated with unreasonable reward—it is at least arguable whether prisoners can ever meet these requirements; the exact nature of and the discomfort associated with the experiment must be explained; withdrawal must be possible at any time; and the subjects must be capable of consent—a matter of mental capability and of age. The use of children for medical experiments is a particularly emotive subject and one that has medico-legal implications in that it is doubtful whether a parent or guardian has the right to consent to a technical assault on a child unless the procedure is of positive benefit to that individual child. It should be noted that, whereas minors above the age of 16 are empowered to consent to medical treatment or examination, they have no similar statutory authority in relation to research investigations[22]. Nevertheless, advances in paediatric medicine must be made despite the evident difficulties. Clearly there can be no 'blanket' approach to a subject that is governed, in the end, by humane pragmatism.

Medical negligence

The lawyer may well become involved in cases of medical negligence, which is a subject so wide that it cannot possibly be covered fully. Only an outline of the principles involved will be attempted.

Criminal negligence can be dismissed rapidly. It is virtually confined to situations in which the patient has died, and it then implies negligence involving such a degree

[22] Family Law Reform Act 1969, s. 8(3) (not applicable in Scotland).

of recklessness as to amount to manslaughter or culpable homicide—unlawful killing 'not amounting to murder'. The great majority of such cases are associated with drunkenness or with impaired efficiency due to the use of drugs by doctors. The museum of Forensic Pathology in Edinburgh contains a specimen of some 2.4 m (8 ft) of small intestine removed by a drunken obstetrician in mistake for an umbilical cord. Such cases are indefensible; as Simpson has said, since a professional man should be more able than most to appreciate his impairment of function due to alcoholism, the fact that he was drunk at the time of a negligent act merely aggravates the offence[23].

The vast majority of actions for negligence are civil actions for tort or delict and certain well-known facts must be proved for the action to succeed.

First, the doctor must have owed a duty of care to the complainer or plaintiff. This, as has been seen, may not always exist despite the fact that an examination has taken place as, for example, in relation to fitness for employment. On the other hand, no bilateral agreement is needed to establish a duty of care. The essential feature is the intention of the doctor to treat or to heal; once the intent is established, the duty continues until the need for care is past or until alternative arrangements have been willingly made.

Secondly, it must be shown that the doctor failed in his duty of care. Failure is a relative term; its degree must be measured against the skill that might reasonably be expected of the individual doctor. Much will depend upon the diagnostic and therapeutic aids available at the time; a doctor would be expected to be more efficient in an intensive care unit than by the roadside. The acceptance of such common-sense principles in British law makes it unnecessary to pass 'Good Samaritan' protective legislation as has been required under many other jurisdictions. Provided he has executed reasonable skill and care, a doctor cannot be held negligent for a mistake in diagnosis or treatment. The classic authority for this is Lord Clyde who, when Lord President, stated, 'In the realm of diagnosis and treatment, there is ample scope for genuine difference of opinion, and one man clearly is not negligent merely because his conclusion differs from that of other professional men, nor because he has displayed less skill or knowledge than others would have shown'[24]. The principle remains but the test—the standard of the ordinary skilled man exercising and professing to have that special skill[25]—is now different. It is clear that, while an error of clinical judgment need not necessarily be negligence, it can be so if it is reached in a manner falling below the test standard[26].

In the same judgment, Lord Clyde introduced the concept of 'accepted medical practice', giving his opinion that, having shown that there was an accepted practice and that the doctor failed to follow that practice, the plaintiff in an action for medical negligence must further show that the course the doctor adopted was one that no professional man of ordinary skill would have taken had he been acting with ordinary care. Accepted practice may differ from hospital to hospital; the important point is whether an approach to diagnosis and therapy was or was not reasonable[26a]. In *Hucks v. Cole*[27] a doctor was found negligent in his use of antibiotics despite the evidence of witnesses for the defendant to the effect that the treatment was

---

[23] In *Forensic Medicine* (1979), 8th edn., p. 53. London; Edward Arnold.
[24] In Hunter v. Hanley 1955 S.L.T. 213 at p. 217.
[25] Chin Keow v. Government of Malaysia [1967] 1 W.L.R. 813.
[26] Whitehouse v. Jordan [1981] 1 All E.R. 267 per Lord Edmund-Davies at p. 276.
[26a] Maynard v. West Midlands Regional HA [1984] 1 W.L.R. 634.
[27] 1968 112 S.J. 483.

acceptable; the case did, however, have unusual features and the general principle was restated. On the other hand, it has been reiterated that allegations of negligence against medical practitioners should be regarded as serious and the standard of proof is, therefore, a high degree of probability[28]. In practice, medical negligence may be more difficult to establish than is negligence in other fields.

Thirdly, the patient must have suffered damage. The definition of 'damage' is certainly widening, and, when extended to mental distress, is almost all-embracing. It is, however, a function of the Court to measure the loss or damage in terms of money and, while this may deter the frivolous action, it also leads to very large sums being paid—this being in part because compensation must be paid in a lump sum and because the Courts cannot take into account the free medical attention available under the National Health Service[29].

Damages resulting from death due to negligence have recently altered in their application. It is now possible for a casualty to obtain damages not only in respect of lost earnings for his years of life expectancy after injury but also for the lost years that would have accrued to him had his life not been shortened by injury[30]; a negligently injured man can, therefore, now make provision for his family as if he were of normal constitution. With less justification, it has been decided that the dependants of a person who is killed negligently can claim both for monetary loss under the Fatal Accidents Act 1976 (or Damages (Scotland) Act 1976) and also as the estate for, among other things, loss of expectation of life under the Law Reform (Miscellaneous Provisions) Act 1934—not alternatively as was the prior case[31]. The result must be to increase the burden on Medical Protection Societies.

A doctor may be liable for the negligence of his subordinates, stand-ins and other members of staff—including, particularly, receptionists who are sometimes forced into making medical decisions[32]. The vicarious responsibility of hospitals for members of staff has been discussed earlier in the chapter.

In certain circumstances, negligence as defined above is self-evident. For example, there has clearly been negligence if a pair of forceps is left in the abdomen and the patient is thereby subjected to a second operation. The doctrine of *res ipsa loquitur* might then operate and it would be for the doctor to prove that he was not responsible or to demonstrate extenuating factors; Denning, L.J. has summarized it: ' . . . that should not have happened if due care had been used. Explain it if you can'[33].

Such cases are commonly settled but, in the event of their being contested, it would seem that this plea is rarely accepted by the Court[34]—in *O'Malley–Williams*, the plea failed because the outcome (injury to the nerves of the arm) was a recognized risk of an aortogram; interestingly, in that case, an additional plea of

[28] Lawton, L.J. in Whitehouse v. Jordan [1980] 1 All E.R. 650 at p. 659. But *see* the contrary view in Ashcroft v. Mersey Regional HA [1983] 2 All E.R. 245, at p. 247.

[29] Lim Poh Choo v. Camden and Islington Area Health Authority [1979] 2 All E.R. 910 per Lord Scarman at p 914, commenting on Denning, M.R. in the Court of Appeal [1979] 1 All E.R. 332 at p. 341, 344.

[30] Pickett v. British Rail Engineering Limited [1979] 1 All E.R. 774.

[31] Kandalla v. British Airways Board [1980] 1 All E.R. 341. *See* 'Damages for the 'lost years', *British Medical Journal* (1980), **280**, 1235 where the trial Judge's reluctance to accept the fact is well précied.

[32] The doctor may, of course be liable in his obligations as a citizen—e.g. to keep his surgery in a safe condition (Occupier's Liability Act 1957).

[33] In Cassidy v. Ministry of Health [1951] 2 K.B. 343, at p. 365.

[34] *See*, for example, Fletcher v. Bench (1973), *British Medical Journal* (1973), **iv**, 118 or O'Malley–Williams v. Board of Governors of the National Hospital for Nervous Diseases (1974), *British Medical Journal* (1975), **i**, 636.

negligence by virtue of not having informed the patient of the risk failed by virtue of the remoteness of that risk (*see* p. 345). Almost invariably, it is for the plaintiff or pursuer to prove the fact of negligence. The doctor, generally in concert with the hospital or other employing authority, may claim that no negligence existed in the true sense; he may defend himself on the grounds that his course of action carried well-known risks that were fully explained to the patient and which the patient accepted; or he may assert that the patient himself contributed to his own disability[35]. It is apparent that two patients can leave hospital each with a disability of comparable gravity and each deriving from the treatment received; yet one may receive substantial damages while the other is not compensated, depending on whether 'fault' was proved. There is much to be said for the introduction of a 'no fault' scheme of compensation operated by some form of compulsory insurance. As Lawton, L.J. has said[36]: 'As long as liability in this type of case rests on proof of fault Judges will have to go on making decisions which they would prefer not to make. The victims of medical mishaps should, in my opinion, be cared for by the community not by the hazards of litigation'. Unfortunately, there is a great deal of practical difficulty in the application of such a policy and it has been rejected in the case of medical mishaps by the Pearson Commission[37]. Perhaps there will be a change of heart if the 'no-fault' system operating in New Zealand[38] is shown to be a success.

Euthanasia

It is arguable that, of all the problems in medical jurisprudence, those concerning the termination of life have escalated most in the last decade. The medical ethos of 'the sanctity of life', implying the unqualified duty to preserve life at all costs, has come under increasing challenge. Modern technology introduces its own economic concerns—the diversion of resources to the treatment of the incurably comatose must compromise other competing causes. Such considerations are beyond discussion here. But an assessment of the legal and medical implications of 'allowing to die' must now be an essential feature of forensic medicine. The problem presents at three main points in time—at the beginning and at the end of natural life, and during life when the person may be severely impaired as a result of brain damage.

The last situation has been partly discussed in Chapter 12 and needs little further consideration. It is enough to emphasize again the essential difference between brain-stem death on the one hand and irreversible brain damage on the other. Understanding is not helped by semantic confusion such as derives from the use of the phrase 'irreversible coma' in the United States[39] which is synonymous with brain-stem death and not, as might be expected, with the persistent vegetative

[35] The acceptance of contributory negligence would not affect the fact of negligence but only the damages awarded.

[36] In Whitehouse v. Jordan [1980] 1 All E.R., p. 661.

[37] Pearson, Lord (Chairman) (1978). *Royal Commission on Civil Liability and Compensation for Personal Injury*, Cmnd. 7054–1, 2, 3. London; HMSO.

[38] Accident Compensation Act 1972. In fact, problems over the definition of the word 'accident' led to supplementary legislation 2 years later.

[39] Beecher, H.K. (Chairman) (1968). A definition of irreversible coma. Report of the ad hoc Committee of the Harvard Medical School to examine the definition of brain death. *Journal of the American Medical Association*, **205**, 337.

state. There is a perceptibly growing movement to do away with a distinction between the two conditions as is exemplified by questioning the value to *Homo sapiens* of *homo* who is no longer *sapiens*[40]. The groundswell cannot simply be ignored.

The problems at the end of life are summed up in the current phrase 'death with dignity', the present mood being to move away from the obligation to preserve life—as propounded in the International Code of Medical Ethics—to the concept of a duty to prevent suffering. Terminal illness is considered best treated by providing the optimum conditions for death rather than by the use of increasingly invasive techniques to prolong some sort of existence. The unconscious patient is presumed to agree to this and many persons now affect what is curiously known as a 'living will' in which this course is specifically directed. The conscious dying patient can, of course, make his own decision; patients' autonomy is now a corner-stone of ethical medical practice and to continue to treat in the face of contrary instructions would be tortious. But the position is not completely clear cut. The doctor has a duty to his patient; if he pleads necessity in dereliction of that duty, he must show that the evil avoided is greater than the evil performed—and it is at least arguable that death is the greatest of all evils. Moreover, abnegating one's duty is to neglect and neglect is within the compass of manslaughter. Failure to treat, thus argued, is indistinguishable from passive euthanasia for which the moral justification is commonly based on the doctrine of 'ordinary' and 'extraordinary' means of treatment. This doctrine, which attempts to distinguish what treatment a doctor *need* or need not give is accepted within the Anglican[41] and the Roman Catholic ethos[42]. The terms extraordinary and ordinary are not, however, to be construed as relating to particular techniques. In making a decision, the distinction must rather be between productive and non-productive means, the condition of the individual patient being the ultimate determinant of the definition. Thus, there is no moral obligation on the doctor to preserve life at the expense of suffering and, if, in the course of good terminal care, the use use of drugs actually hastens death, this is ethically acceptable within the concept of 'double effect'; this, basically, states that an ill effect is morally acceptable as long as there is a greater, and intended, good effect from an action. If this is agreed, it is reasonable to ask why passive euthanasia as a means of alleviating an otherwise intolerable condition should be any less objectionable than would be the active ending of life—something which, in current conditions, is indefensible. Justification can only lie on the grounds that the former is allowing nature to take its course; the latter implies a positive, extraneous intervention.

These considerations are more complex when applied to the beginning of life. Here the problem is whether to assist or obstruct the physically or mentally defective infant in its struggle for life. Such choices are undoubtedly made as a matter of routine. The grounds on which they are based depend on anticipating the 'quality of life'.

[40] Scarman, Lord (1981). Legal liability and medicine. *Journal of the Royal Society of Medicine*, **74**, 11–15. But Lord Scarman clearly says he does not support euthanasia—'There are implications in the right to terminate another's existence of which it is well to be fearful in the absence of a more profound analysis of the problem than that which it has yet received'.

[41] Coggan, D. (1977). On dying and dying well. *Proceedings of the Royal Society of Medicine*, **70**, 75.

[42] Sacred Congregation for the Doctrine of the Faith (1980). *Declaration on Euthanasia*. Catholic Truth Society.

The situation here is different from the end of life in so far as the person most intimately concerned, the infant, is never able to make an autonomous decision—this must be surrogate and made by the parents and the doctor aided, or confused, by the law[43]. While some support an absolute adherence to the 'sanctity of life', most would now agree that a case exists for balancing the possible blessing of an early, painless death against the probable sufferings of a 'fruitless' life—suffering not being measured solely from the point of view of the principal but also of the parents and, indeed, of society[44]. Even so, two problems remain: first, do we really want a society where the 'fruitfulness of life' determines the worth of the individual or his right to live—even more so if that is to be decided in conformity to a materialistic norm; and, secondly, who is to make such a decision? Here, opinion is divided. The medical establishment[45] firmly believes that the decision is for the parents aided by the doctor and this is supported by informed legal opinion[46]. Others, however, demand that such decisions should be in the hands of society[47] and, presumably, society is represented by the Courts. What, then, is the legal, as opposed to the moral, attitude to the 'letting die' debate?

There can be no doubt as to the law relating to active euthanasia. To kill someone deliberately is murder. But the position is less clear when considering passive euthanasia: 'killing both pain and patient may be good morals but it is far from certain it is good law'[48]. When the result of an action is foreseen and certain it is the same as if it was desired or intended and this must apply to an omission—such as to feed an infant—if that omission is a breach of duty. The criminal Courts have, world-wide, been tolerant of doctors in this respect. It is said that only two doctors have been tried for 'mercy killings' in the USA; both were acquitted[49]. In the United Kingdom, there has been a great reluctance to prosecute paediatricians and, quite clearly, the policy is to uphold the principle of medical 'good faith'. In the first apposite case to come to trial—albeit concerned with adult euthanasia[50]—the defendant was acquitted with Devlin, J remarking: 'The doctor is entitled to relieve pain and suffering even if the measures he takes may incidentally shorten life'. Clearly it is the primary intention that is paramount because, at the same time, the Judge's basic premise was to consider whether the acts done were 'intended to kill and did in fact kill'; in which case 'it did not matter . . . if her life were cut short by weeks or months, it was just as much murder as if it was cut short by years'. A second verdict, this time referring to a Downsian infant, has recently found a doctor not guilty of attempted murder; but the case also had unusual features and is of little value as a precedent[51]. The decision in the less contentious case,

---

[43] There is even an indication of confrontation in Havard, J.D.J. (1982), The legal threat to medicine, *British Medical Journal*, **284**, 612.

[44] *See,* for example, Slater, E. (1973), Severely malformed children: Wanted—a new basic approach, *British Medical Journal*, **i**, 285 for an early exposition.

[45] *British Medical Journal* (1981). The right to live and the right to die. **283**, 569.

[46] Williams, G. (1981). Life of a child. *The Times*, Correspondence, 13th Aug.

[47] Kennedy, I. (1981). *The Unmasking of Medicine* Chapter 4.

[48] Edmund-Davies, Lord (1977), On dying and dying well, *Proceedings of the Royal Society of Medicine*, **70**, 73; where Lord Hailsham is quoted as saying 'if you have got a living body you have to keep it alive if you can'.

[49] Jacobson, S. (1979). The right to life. *Journal of the Forensic Science Society*, **19**, 87.

[50] Palmer, H. Dr. Adams' trial for murder [1957] Crim L.R. 365. The defendant did not give evidence and the act of murder itself had to be proved by expert medical evidence.

[51] R. v. Arthur (1981). *The Times*, 6th Nov., p. 1.

in Re B[52], implies that no surgical operation on an infant would have been authorized had there been a likelihood of a life of suffering; the trial judge was considered to have erred in being influenced by the views of the parents instead of deciding what was in the best interests of the child.

Is there any need for specific legislation within this general societal movement? While many of the United States have enacted laws, it may well be that they are counterproductive[53]: 'We think that the State's interest (in the preservation of life) weakens and the individual's right of privacy grows as the degree of invasion increases and the prognosis dims'[54]. This is surely so at the end of life but a 'domino effect' is so probable a result of allowing rejection at its beginning that some enabling—and, consequentially, restrictive—legislation seems needed in respect of selective non-treatment of neonates[55].

[52] Re 'B' (a minor) [1981] 1 W.L.R. 1421 C.A. The parents of a mongol child refused permission for an operation to relieve intestinal obstruction. The child was made a Ward of Court and the operation was ordered.

[53] Lappé, M. (1978). Dying while living: a critique of allowing to die legislation. *Journal of Medical Ethics*, **4**, 195.

[54] Hughes, C.J. in Re Quinlan (1976) 70 N.J. 10, 355 A. 2d 647.

[55] Mason. J. K. and Meyers. D. W. (1986). Parental choice and selective non-treatment of deformed newborns: a view from mid-Atlantic. *Journal of Medical Ethics*, **12**, 67.

31

Deaths associated with surgery and anaesthesia

Medico-legal procedure

Medico-legal interest focuses on deaths occurring during or as a result of surgical operations for several reasons. First, a thorough investigation of fatalities is one means by which surgical treatment can be improved and unsatisfactory techniques can be eliminated. Secondly, such deaths cause considerable concern among those directly and indirectly affected, and actions for negligence may result. Related to both these considerations is the availability of major surgical procedures to patients in increasingly 'high-risk' categories; forensic medicine has a part to play in maintaining a balance in advances in treatment.

Deaths of this type are often loosely referred to as 'anaesthetic deaths'. This is a misnomer which, apart from its undeserved professional implications, may, by limiting the field of investigation, be positively detrimental to progress. The term should be confined to those deaths that, *after full investigation,* can properly be attributed to the anaesthetic; phrases that presuppose this conclusion should be avoided.

Notification of deaths associated with surgery varies between England and Scotland. In the latter, 'anaesthetic deaths'[1] are reportable as a statutory duty and a particular procedure is followed in their investigation. This involves, first, the completion of a standard questionnaire (Appendix O) which is signed both by the surgeon and by the anaesthetist and is forwarded to the Fiscal[2]. The case is then referred to the Police Surgeon who may or may not advise the need for a post-mortem dissection. The Fiscal will then report the facts to the Crown Office, who will dispose of the case according to the findings. The anachronism of isolating death associated with anaesthesia is now appreciated and new regulations as to the investigation of death due to 'medical mishap' are in preparation. The Brodrick Committee has also deprecated the unique attention given to anaesthesia in England where the Registrar is required to report to the Coroner any death appearing to have occurred during an operation or before recovery from the effects

---

[1] Defined as deaths occurring during the administration of an anaesthetic or before recovery from the effects of an anaesthetic.

[2] The Association of Anaesthetists of Great Britain and Ireland clearly approved this practice in their evidence to the Brodrick Committee (*Report of the Committee on Death Certification and Coroners,* 1971, para. 17.12).

of an anaesthetic[3]; many coroners, acting on a purely local basis, insist that deaths occurring within 24 hours of the administration of an anaesthetic should be reported by the hospital authority. In the event of non-fatal mishap, area health authorities or boards may set up an inquiry[4] and evidence will normally be privileged. In the event of a complaint, an inquiry is carried out either by a member of the health authority's staff or by an independent body; both the complainant and the person complained about have access to such proceedings. In very serious cases, the Minister may order a public inquiry under the National Health Service Act 1977, s. 84. It is worth reiterating that many modern techniques of a purely investigative nature and which could not be regarded as surgical operations carry an in-built risk.

Hazards of surgical operations

All surgical operations, whether accompanied by local or general anaesthesia, or when performed without anaesthesia, have some morbidity and mortality. Efficient surgical practice is based on accurate clinical judgment as to whether the risks outweigh the dangers or discomfort to the patient of withholding operation.

Proper consent to operation is mandatory and must now be of 'informed' type—this implying that the patient must be given sufficient information to enable him or her to make an autonomous decision as to an assumption of risk. There are, however, differences as to the extent of disclosure that is required. In the United States, where the principle of informed consent is heavily based on the patient's 'rights', there is an undoubted move to a 'disclose all' policy, the patient being entitled to any information he wants and to any that the doctor is capable of imparting[5]. In the United Kingdom, the emphasis is more on maintaining the trusting relationship between doctor and patient and the test is rather that the latter should have such information as will enable him to make a rational decision[5a]. Thus, the extent of necessary disclosure is proportional to the understanding of the patient, the questions he or she asks, the extent of the risk, the availability of alternatives and any element of experimentation; the effect on the patient can be considered but it is important that any clinical reasons for withholding any information should be adequately recorded. This last concession allows for a somewhat reduced obligation on the doctor if the treatment is necessary and is the only one available[6]. Competence of the surgeon can be assumed and there is no obligation on him to discuss complications that might result from any lack of skill[7].

The patient's consent is, in general, specific to a stated intended course of action; whether an operation can be extended beyond that consented to depends on the urgency and relevance to the primary treatment and on the additional effects of the secondary procedure[8]. It seems now certain that a signature on a 'blanket consent' form would not be regarded by the Courts as adequate[7].

[3] Registration of Births, Deaths and Marriages Regulations 1968 (S.I. 1968/2049) reg. 51.

[4] See British Medical Journal (1982), Hospital inquiries: evidence and privilege, **284,** 591.

[5] Note the change from Natanson v. Kline (1960) 186 Kan 383, 350P, 2d, 1093 in which the discretionary standard of the reasonable physician was upheld, to Canterbury v. Spence (1972) 464F, 2d 772 (DC Cir) where it was considered that the patient's right of self-determination demanded a standard set by law rather than by the physicians themselves; a full disclosure rule was imposed.

[5a] Sidaway v. Bethlem Royal Hospital and Maudsley Hospital HA and others [1985] 2 W.L.R. 480.

[6] Bolam v. Friern Barnet Hospital Management Committee [1957] 1 W.L.R. 583. This case is fundamental to the issues of negligence and consent.

[7] Chatterton v. Gerson [1981] 1 All E.R. 257.

[8] Compare, for example, Marshall v. Curry (1933) 3 D.L.R. 260 where a hernia operation could not be completed without removal of a testis, with Murray v. McMurchy (1949) 2 D.L.R. 442 where a sterilization coincidental to Caesarean section was regarded as beyond the surgeon's discretion.

As indicated on page 329, an operation without consent can be pursued as a battery. While this has the advantage that a battery is actionable *per se*, it is more likely that a 'consent related' action will be based on negligence[8a]. In this case, success depends on the failure of communication being such that the patient would not have consented to an operation had the doctor not failed in his duty to inform as to the risks involved[9]. One million dollars have been awarded in the United States in an action based solely on lack of informed consent[10].

Consent is of special importance when it is being given on behalf of another— e.g. a minor or an unconscious relative—or when an operation attended by some risk, such as the examination of an organ by biopsy, is performed mainly or partly as a research procedure. Consent after full explanation implies acceptance of the risks and, provided that the operation has been carried out in accordance with the principles of good practice (*see* page 337), there can be no question of negligence.

The decision to operate

The correctness of the decision to operate has to be considered whenever a death occurs during or is obviously referable to an operation.

No one would question the validity of an operation of even heroic proportions undertaken to save a life that would otherwise undoubtedly be lost. Very few would dispute the need for an admittedly palliative procedure designed to alleviate the pain of a terminal illness. But what if the risks to life of operation can be assessed as greater than those of inaction? Or what if the disease underlying severe pain has a negligible mortality in relation to suppressive surgery?

Obviously, no general ruling can be given and each case must be assessed by the surgeon and the anaesthetist acting together. Balanced decisions must be based on full preoperative information and must take into account what measures are available to counteract difficulties that are reasonably foreseeable. It might, for example, be justifiable to perform an operation that would be expected to result in severe blood loss; it would be unjustifiable to do so without previously arranging for a readily available supply of replacement blood known to be compatible with the recipient (*see* below, page 354).

The choice of patient

Recent advances in anaesthesia, particularly the introduction of muscle relaxants, allow for a level of narcosis in major surgery that is far less deep than was possible, say, 20 years ago. As a result, patients in an older age group and less physically fit can be anaesthetized with increasing confidence. But, although surgical techniques are continually improving, the physical damage resulting from a given surgical operation remains the same and must affect the old and infirm more adversely than the young and healthy. Paradoxically, therefore, the effect of improvements in

---

[8a] Hills v. Potter and another [1984] 1 W.L.R. 641.

[9] The importance of true answers to specific question put by patients is shown by a comparison of Smith v. Auckland Hospital [1965] NZ L.R. 191 and O'Malley-Williams v. Board of Governors of the National Hospital for Nervous Diseases, *The Times* (1974), 7 Oct.

[10] Jones v. Regents of the University of California (1977) Sup. Ct. San Francisco Co, Calif.

anaesthesia may be to increase marginally the statistical mortality of a particular operation, but this merely reflects the widening availability of complex surgery. An implication of negligence based on the death of a patient in a suspect category might well have the effect of depriving elderly patients of a potentially fuller remaining life simply because of apprehension of the consequences of failure. There are, therefore, very good reasons for dispensing with public inquest in all cases in which there is no evidence of avoidable mishap[11].

The problems facing the investigating pathologist are often formidable and are certainly greatest in relation to the hazards specific to anaesthetics. These must, therefore, be considered separately—but still without prejudice to the thesis that they are only one aspect of the whole spectrum of major surgery. It is convenient to discuss individually local, spinal and general anaesthesia.

Local anaesthetics

These agents, which may be given by infiltration of the area or by blocking specific nerve bundles, act by paralysing the sensory nerves with which they come in contact. Thus, a localized area can be made pain free without narcotizing the whole organism, an obvious advantage when only minor surgery is to be performed or when the subject is unfit for a general anaesthetic.

All these drugs are absorbed to some extent and a maximum therapeutic dose is established for each agent on the assumption that absorption and detoxication will be normal. The old and debilitated may destroy the drug less efficiently but, young or old, the major hazard lies in rapid absorption through widely dilated vessels in the part injected. Absorption is notoriously rapid from some areas—e.g. the nose and throat—and these are well known to anaesthetists. In order to reduce the size of the available vessels, it is common practice to inject a vasoconstrictive agent such as adrenaline at the same time as the anaesthetic. The dilemma then raised is that adrenaline, of itself, may produce adverse reactions. Moreover, the possibility of accidental injection of the drug directly into a major vessel—which will result in the sudden absorption of the whole dose—still remains.

The hazards of local anaesthesia can, therefore, be summarized as:

1. Overdosage of either the anaesthetic or vasoconstrictive agent, the total quantity and concentration of which must be related to the age, stature and fitness of the patient.
2. Rapid absorption from highly absorptive areas or as a result of local vaso-dilatation.
3. Accidental injection of a vessel.
4. Hypersensitivity reactions which most authorities now regard as being, in fact, due to overdosage.

In the event of serious error, there may be a general effect on the central nervous system which is either excitory—in which case convulsions may occur—or depressive—when the danger to life is from respiratory paralysis. Far less commonly, the heart may be directly affected.

---

[11] While the Brodrick Committee could not agree with this entirely, there is a clear indication from their report that they favoured some form of selection in relation to the type of inquiry (*Report of the Committee on Death Certification and Coroners*, (1971), p. 57, p. 207). Such a situation does, of course, obtain in Scotland.

Very occasionally, there may be local residua that result in long-term damage to the patient. Thus, an abnormally high concentration injected directly into a nerve may lead to a permanent loss of function. As with any injection, there is the possibility of needle breakage.

The incidence of severe reactions to local anaesthesia is very low—in the region of 0.05 per cent—but the risks certainly increase with infirmity—so much so that many anaesthetists may prefer to use a modern, relatively non-toxic general anaesthetic in 'high-risk' patients.

Spinal anaesthesia

Whole areas of the body can be rendered insensitive if a local anaesthethic is applied to the spinal cord through the cerebrospinal fluid (CSF). Since the nerves that supply the life-support functions are placed high in the cord, the dangers of spinal anaesthesia increase as the anaesthetic is allowed to rise in the CSF. Some diffusion is inevitable and spinal anaesthesia has a definite mortality which is probably slightly higher than that of even relatively primitive general anaesthetics, particularly when the risks of introducing infection are included. Accordingly, the more difficult technique of epidural anaesthesia, in which the nerve roots are involved but the agent is separated from the central nervous tissue by the thick dura mater, has been introduced. While this method is far safer in theory, a greater dose of anaesthetic must be given; serious complications may, therefore, arise if the agent is inadvertently injected into the CSF—all anaesthetists are aware of this and suitable precautions can be taken.

The problems of the standard method of spinal anaesthesia through the CSF in the subarachnoid space can be summarized as:

1. Those due to unwanted action on the nerves.
2. Those due to alteration in the volume of fluid protecting the brain and spinal cord.

As to undesirable action on the nerves, the difficulty is that in addition to paralysing the sensory nerves there is an action on the sympathetic nerves that control the strength or tone of the blood vessels; a fall in blood pressure is the almost invariable result. A moderate fall in a healthy person is of little significance; but the effect may be very severe if it occurs in the elderly, in those with pre-existing heart disease or in association with haemorrhage. The results may be disastrous if some degree of respiratory hypoxia is added; true coronary insufficiency may be precipitated and there may be either cardiac or respiratory arrest due to the impossibility of maintaining the the circulation. In addition, the vagus nerve is commonly left unaffected. Death may, therefore, occur suddenly and quite unexpectedly due to cardiac inhibition following an unnatural stimulation of the nerve.

The hazards related to the changes in the volume of cerebrospinal fluid are less dramatic but may cause appreciable disability.

Lumbar puncture headache occurs in about a quarter of those recovering from spinal anaesthesia. It is probably due to continuing leakage through the hole made by the needle, so much so that the incidence and severity of the condition is almost proportional to the size of needle used. In addition to headache, the patient may complain of vomiting, dizziness and abnormal hearing. The condition is usually transient but may on occasions last for months.

More significant is the occasional double vision that occurs as a marked complication once in some 1000 cases treated. The probable cause is movement of the brain following removal of protective fluid. Recovery within a month is usual but a few cases sustain permanent paralysis of the muscles of one eye.

Permanent nerve damage associated with the actual agent used may occur in a very small proportion—of the order of 1:10 000—of spinal anaesthetics, while the possibility of haemorrhage after puncture of a vessel also exists. The introduction of sepsis into the spinal canal is a hazard peculiar to the method and one that must almost always be attributable to some form of negligence.

General anaesthesia

General anaesthetics may be given by inhalation or intravenously.

Anaesthetics entering the body by inhalation combine with the body tissues in order to produce a narcotic effect. By any definition, they are toxic substances and it is remarkable that pharmacological and medical skills have combined to limit to miniscule proportions the mortaility from a deliberate interference with the patient's physiological balance.

Children and the very aged are rather more susceptible to general inhalation anaesthetics than are adults in the middle age range; there is some suggestion that negroes are more susceptible to their ill effects, particularly those with sickle-cell trait (see page 9). The general mortality rate is probably in the order of 1:1500 and the causes can be summarized as being due to:

1. The technique of administration.
2. The anaesthetic agent.
3. Hazards associated with unconsciousness.
4. External problems—e.g. explosion.

Death due to inadequate techniques are of two main kinds—vagal stimulatory and hypoxic. Cardiac inhibition due to vagal stimulation is a real threat because the autonomic system is relatively spared in the process of nervous supression; the patient is susceptible to abnormal stimuli despite apparent unconsciousness. Thus, stimulation of the respiratory lining by a high concentration of irritant gas or the passing of a tube through an inadequately anaesthetized larynx may result in sudden arrest of the heart. Vagal inhibition of the heart is much more likely in the presence of oxygen deficit. Cardiac failure of a rather different type (ventricular fibrillation) can result from excessive secretion of adrenaline by patients who have been inadequately sedated; dental patients are particularly susceptible by reason of their generally ambulant treatment, while the use of adrenaline during the induction of anaesthesia obviously increases the risk.

By far the greatest risk in relation to technique is the provocation of tissue hypoxia due to true oxygen deprivation. The skill of anaesthesia lies in reducing hypoxia to a minimum while achieving an unconscious patient; this is done by the addition of oxygen to the anaesthetic mixture supplemented, if necessary, by forced ventilation of the lungs. An inadequate oxygen supply may derive, first, from the apparatus itself. Murder mysteries have been written around mistaken colouring or filling of gas cylinders—and it can happen accidentally. Cylinders may run dry or taps may be inadvertently turned off—or may not turn on in an emergency. Responsibility for the apparatus is clearly vested in the anaesthetist and the prevention of catastrophe due to malfunction depends on his vigilance.

Anaesthesia and hypoxia—which are quite distinct processes—each result in unconsciousness and it is the experience of the anaesthetist that guards the patient; warning signs may be missed by the inexperienced or even by the consultant if he is required to supervise more than one operating theatre. An apparently satisfactory induction may be due not so much to the presence of anaesthetic as to the absence of adequate oxygen, and, unless this is corrected, the patient may suffer any of the long-term effects of hypoxia on being released to the normal atmosphere. Such confusion may result even from the use of the more simple agents such as nitrous oxide; there are particular hazards in dental practice in which, although anaesthesia is generally of short duration, cerebral hypoxia may be exaggerated by the sitting position. Severe shortage of oxygen during deep anaesthesia may be due to inadequate ventilation and can result in sudden death on the table due to heart failure. Again, conditions such as anaemia, haemorrhage or lung disease may have an important synergistic action.

Ill effects from the actual anaesthetics depend upon their toxicity; this may be selective as to organ and some agents—e.g. the almost obsolete chloroform and cyclopropane—are particularly cardiotoxic. This, however, is not to say that such drugs should not be used by competent practitioners if they have other advantages; the delicate balance upon which good medical practice depends is well illustrated in this context.

Severe long-term effects may be seen in the lungs after general inhalation anaesthesia of any type—generally in the form of collapse of portions of the lung or of pneumonia. Fatal disease of the liver may also be attributed to the anaesthetic agent. Chloroform was especially implicated in the past but it is probable that its reputation was ill founded; any toxic effect of an anaesthetic on the liver is greatly potentiated by associated hypoxia and this was especially true of that old agent. Therapeutic dilemmas also arise using modern drugs. Halothane is judged by most practitioners to be the best 'general' anaesthetic agent available. But it seems possible that repeated administration of anaesthetics of this group may load the liver with problems of metabolism to which it may succumb—particularly if the anaesthetics were repeated at very short intervals and the liver was previously unhealthy, for example, due to the effects of alcoholism[12]. The doctor must balance the advantage to the patient of a good anaesthetic agent against the possibility of subsequent liver damage; the important point is that this is a legitimate decision that becomes unacceptable only if the judgment is unconsidered.

Some patients are unduly susceptible to anaesthetics and may react abnormally. Malignant hyperpyrexia—or rapid and severe rise in body temperature—is one such example which can be associated even with such simple agents as nitrous oxide. Susceptibility to malignant hyperpyrexia, and probably to other forms of hypersensitivity, is genetically controlled; the importance of taking a good preoperative history is emphasized.

The unconscious patient poses special problems because he is unable to take correcting reflex action if an adverse situation arises. The commonest danger lies in failure to protect the air passages against inhalation of foreign material. Stomach

[12] There is very great controversy over this question. *See* for example Inman, W. H. W. and Mushin, W. W. (1974), Jaundice after repeated exposure to halothane; an analysis of reports to the Committee on Safety of Medicine, *British Medical Journal*, **i**, 5. The views expressed in this paper were contested in the USA by McPeek, B. and Gilbert, J. P. (1974), Onset of postoperative jaundice related to anaesthetic history, *British Medical Journal*, **iii**, 615.

contents may flow back into the mouth and air passages of a supine patient or the patient may vomit—particularly if there had been no preoperative sedation. Blood, swabs or even teeth may be inhaled without reflex coughing—there is an obvious potential association with dental surgery. Even without aspiration, the patient's tongue may fall back and cause suffocation. An acute asphyxial death may follow aspiration but survival can also be accompanied by an inflammatory process in the lungs of great severity associated with the acidity of the inhaled stomach contents; the aspiration of a solid object will cause collapse of a part of or the whole of the lung which will then be particularly susceptible to infection.

Occasionally, patients who have been operated upon may appear well for several days, until quite unheralded sudden death occurs. The cause is nearly always pulmonary embolism—a clot of blood, usually forming in a leg vein, detaches and lodges in the pulmonary artery. The formation of such clots is naturally associated with immobility in bed and, while every prophylactic care may be taken, occasional instances are inevitable; death is effectively due to natural causes.

The spectacular nature of fires and explosions probably leads to exaggeration of their frequency; nevertheless, very considerable effort must be put into their prevention. Cyclopropane and ether are highly inflammable, especially when combined with oxygen; it would be desirable to use gases that will not burn and this is one reason for the preference of halothane. If explosive gases are used, the concurrent use of electric tools or operation by diathermy must be severely limited and all equipment for lighting the inside of the body must be battery-powered. The main danger, however, lies in the static spark which cannot be anticipated; preventive measures include the use of conducting rubber equipment, the use of conducting materials for the floor and the maintenance of a relatively humid atmosphere.

Special factors relating to intravenous anaesthesia

Anaesthesia is often induced by the injection of ultra-short-acting barbiturates of which methohexitone is the most commonly used. Occasionally, the whole surgical procedure may be covered by this method.

Barbiturates have a profound effect on the blood pressure and on the action of the heart; as a result, they must be used with particular care in the elderly and unfit. There is no physiological control over the absorption of a substance injected into a vein; the whole dose is instantly available for transmission to the tissues and it cannot be removed; everything depends, therefore, on the skill of the injector.

Intravenous barbiturates also act on the respiratory centre which is affected by overdose so that the breathing becomes ineffective. Moreover, a tendency to uncontrolled reflex spasm is especially marked under barbiturate anaesthesia and any irritation of the throat may result in spasm of the glottis and suffocation of the patient. A lengthy intravenous anaesthetic can, therefore, be dangerous, as the anaesthetist's attention may be unduly taken up with the locus of injection at the expense of the airway.

The hazards of intravenous anaesthesia are most dramatically illustrated in the field of dental surgery where, despite recommendations to the contrary[13], the single-handed anaesthetist/surgeon is not uncommon. Although the practice has

[13] Ministry of Health (1967). *Dental Anaesthesia, Report of Joint Sub-Committee of the Standing Medical and Dental Advisory Committee on Dental Anaesthesia.* London; HMSO.

been defended by experts, several deaths have been reported which make very clear the difficulty of performing two expert functions at the same time; coincidental complications with resuscitative apparatus have also been described[14]. Coroners' inquests have revealed some dramatic examples of hazards related to the maintenance of apparatus or the training of assistants, including unnoticed breakage of the tap on the oxygen cylinder or lack of oxygen, dictating the summoning of help from the fire brigade; one assistant is reported as stating that she 'had not been on any course but had trained by watching others'[14]. From the medico-legal aspect, such circumstances arc of far greater significance than are the physiological problems of anaesthesia.

Hazards associated with relaxant drugs

The use of relaxant drugs, which has opened up major surgery to a wide group of patients who might well have died under a comparably effective unassisted general anaesthetic, is not without hazard—mainly because of concurrent paralysis of the respiratory muscles. This is immaterial during the operation as the anaesthetist will be using, or have available, artificial respiration; nevertheless, persistent failure to breathe after the operation is not uncommon. Although this can be treated, the danger lies in relapse after the patient has left the expert care of the anaesthetist. Paralysis of the throat muscles may also occur and the danger of inhalation of regurgitated stomach contents is increased by using muscle relaxants.

The expert witness

The pathologist's evidence in a case of death during an operation may well be limited. There will be little difficulty if death has resulted from a frank surgical mishap—the result, say, of failing to secure adequately an artery of moderate size is very obvious. Beyond this, the findings and interpretations become progressively less dogmatic. Thus, the presence of a tooth or a swab in the main air passages may be simple to demonstrate, but to state with certainty that death resulted from vagal stimulation as a result of their presence is very much harder. Vomit may be found in the trachea but it may be extremely difficult to decide whether this was the cause of, or the result of, a hypoxic death.

The pathologist will seek and demonstrate any pre-existing disease. But having done so, the standard dilemma in the interrelationship of disease with any accident remains to be solved—was it causative, contributory to or incidental to the death? It is seldom easy to make the choice with certainty and a cautious approach by the witness may be a sign of experience rather than of indecisiveness. If disease discovered is considered significant, further consideration must be given as to whether it was noted or, if not, should have been noted before the operation.

The real problem lies in the fact that the majority of operation deaths, and certainly most of those correctly regarded as 'anaesthetic deaths', will be of a physiological nature. There will be no anatomical evidence available to the pathologist and much of his opinion must be based on exclusion and reasoning. One cannot do better than quote Simpson[15]: 'The pathologist is bound to rely in

---

[14] *British Medical Journal:* (1974) Another death during dentistry, **iv**, 352; (1975) Death in the dental chair, **i**, 293. Erasure from the register may result from such practice (Abrol v. General Dental Council (1984) *British Dental Journal*, **156**, 369).

[15] In *Forensic Medicine*, 8th edn., p. 155; London; Edward Arnold.

part on what he is told of the events leading to death, for functional lapses like fall in blood pressure, cardiac arrhythmia, spasm of the glottis, or vagal inhibition leave no trace at autopsy.'

The post-mortem in such cases is incomplete without toxicological analyses designed to disclose a positive overdose of anaesthetic or other therapeutic agent, and it is important that both the pathologist and the analyst be properly informed as to the drugs that have been administered. Specimens should also be taken to assess any biochemical or enzymatic abnormalities that may have caused the catastrophe or that may indicate its mechanism; due regard, must, however, be paid to post-mortem changes which may affect the analytical result. But even with maximum investigation, the pathologist is often able to do little more than decide 'death was due to anaesthesia but there is no [or, and there is] evidence that the anaesthetic was given incorrectly'.

It is inescapable that the true answer will probably not be reached in the absence of full and frank discussion between surgeon, anaesthetist and pathologist. This is most likely to be attained in an atmosphere in which all parties are working together for the good of future patients; such a state is more easily achieved under the Scottish system of investigation and was clearly the objective of the Brodrick Committee.

In eliciting expert evidence, the advocate should remember that the pathologist is seldom an expert clinician. He is often pressed to state whether an operation or anaesthetic procedure was good or proper; his correct attitude is to refuse to be drawn unless he has a special knowledge or unless the matter is of great simplicity.

Responsibility for the patient at operation

It is almost impossible to lay down dividing lines of responsibility between the surgeon and the anaesthetist that can be applied as a generalization. Decisions taken can only be assessed in the light of the particular circumstances. The operating theatre in some ways resembles the flight deck of an aircraft—the captain is undoubtedly in command and takes ultimate decisions but it would be an unusual man who disregarded the advice of his navigator without careful consideration.

On this analogy, the surgeon is the captain and is ultimately responsible for the decision to operate, the extent of the operation and for any decisions as to whether to complete or abort his intended routine. But in making these, he will be advised by the anaesthetist as to the patient's preoperative physical state and his condition during the operation. The anaesthetist is responsible for the functioning of the anaesthetic apparatus, for maintaining adequate anaesthesia and adequate respiratory function during the operation and for ensuring that the patient is fit to be returned to the ward.

The most 'twilight' area of authority lies in the maintenance or resuscitation of the patient by means of intravenous fluid replacement therapy. Generally, this would be regarded as a function of a member of the surgical team, but during the operation it may be so much a part of maintaining the patient's physical state that the anaesthetist assumes responsibility.

Fluid replacement therapy

The body subjected to operation may be deficient in fluid for any of three reasons:

1. The condition requiring treatment may have precipitated fluid loss—e.g. haemorrhage from a ruptured vessel in a stomach ulcer.
2. The operation itself may lead to significant loss of fluid. All operations incur some blood loss and it is the mark of the good surgical team to reduce this to a minimum. But fluid loss is to be anticipated even in the best of hands in many procedures.
3. The condition of hypovolaemic shock may be present before, or arise during or after, the operation.

Hypovolaemic shock may result from active blood loss, from severe pain, from burning, from crushing, from circulating toxins or, indeed, from any condition in which the body's physiological defences are overstretched. Whatever the precipitating cause, fluid is removed from the circulation and is either lost to the exterior or left stagnant in the tissues; the effective volume of the blood is reduced. If whole blood is lost, there is reduction in the number of oxygen-carrying cells; if only plasma is lost, the blood thickens and the red cells circulate inadequately. In either case, oxygenation of the tissues is impaired and fluid loss from the consequently damaged capillaries is accentuated. This vicious cycle is aggravated by increasing failure of the heart to cope with the excessive demands imposed upon it and death follows. Recovery from prolonged shock is often accompanied by acute renal failure.

Treatment or prevention of the 'cycle' lies mainly in replacing the volume of circulating blood by the intravenous infusion of artificially prepared solutions of electrolytes, of simulated or natural plasma or of blood.

Infusion of fluids other than blood

The choice of fluid for infusion depends on careful biochemical monitoring. The laboratory will advise as to the degree of fluid loss, as to the particular electrolytes required and as to the efficacy of treatment. There is no purpose in detailing the methods involved save to say that they are complicated and ideal surveillance may well be beyond the capabilities of a small hospital; in such circumstances, the control of fluid balance has to depend on clinical judgment aided by a fluid balance chart which must be kept to give some quantitative, albeit rough, guide.

Subsequent problems arise from the possibilities that the infusion given contained the wrong electrolytes or that either electrolytes or fluid were given in inadequate quantity to achieve cure. An equally important error is to use too much fluid so that the heart is embarrassed by hypervolaemia—too *great* a circulating blood volume. More fluid then escapes into the tissues and, in particular, into the lungs—the patient is effectively drowning in his own fluid. This condition of overhydration has been regarded as a *novus actus interveniens*[16].

The transmission of a type of jaundice involving the virus-like particle known as Hepatitis B Antigen (HB_sAg) is a particular hazard of transfusing human plasma. Before the agent was discovered, this dangerous form of liver disease was sufficiently common as to almost eliminate human plasma in fluid replacement. It should now rarely occur because artificial plasma expanders, of which dextran is a typical example, are equally, if not more, effective and all blood donors are screened for being potential carriers of HB_sAg.

---

[16] R. v. Jordan (1956) 40 C. or App. R. 152. But there were unusual aspects in this case which must be regarded as exceptional.

Hazards of blood transfusion

Chapter 18 describes the well-demarcated blood group systems related to the red cell. Each system contains a minimum of two alleles and in most there are considerably more. The chances of transfused blood containing a 'foreign' antigen are, therefore, very high. The concept of rejection of non-self by the formation of antibodies has been discussed in Chapter 1. In general, the strength of the rejection reaction depends on the 'strength' of the antigen; from the point of view of blood transfusion reactions, the antigens of the ABO and Rhesus (CDE) systems are by far the most important. Nevertheless, repetitive exposure to the same foreign antigen of any 'strength' leads, in the end, to antibody production so that the effect of the lesser antigens increases as more transfusions are given; clinically, it becomes increasingly difficult to find donor blood that is compatible with the recipient.

The nature of antibodies must be considered if the hazards of blood transfusion are to be properly appreciated. The antibodies in the ABO system are, as described in Chapter 18, of 'naturally occurring' type and are found antithetically to the antigens. The four basic blood profiles can be summarized.:

Blood Group	Antigen present on cell	Antibodies present in plasma
A	A[17]	Anti-B
B	B	Anti-A
AB	AB	None[17]
O	0	Anti-A and Anti-B

Not only are the antigens and antibodies particularly reactive but, since the antibodies are already present, an incompatible ABO transfusion—for example, transfusing group A blood to a group B recipient—will result in an immediate reaction.

All other blood group antibodies are of simple 'immune' type which come into being only as a result of active stimulation by the specific antigen. The effect, say, of transfusing D+ blood into a D−(dd) person will be to alert the body's defensive mechanism and to lay down the template of antibody production in preparation for a second attack. In all probability, there will be no clinical effect from the first 'incompatible' transfusion. Nevertheless, the body has been sensitized, antibody is now circulating and the next similar transfusion may result in an immediate reaction. The word 'may' is used advisedly, as antibody production is dependent on the capability of the recipient and on the 'strength' of the foreign donor antigen; a number of incompatible transfusions may be required to stimulate sufficient antibody to provoke a reaction to the lesser antigens. Immune antibodies are described by serologists as being either 'complete' or 'incomplete'. There is no clinical difference, but the latter require special methods for laboratory demonstration. In modern circumstances, it would be inexcusable to neglect to search for such antibodies prior to transfusion. In some blood group systems the bearing of a fetus of a different group from the mother is equivalent to a transfusion of similarly different blood[18]. The effects may be additive and it follows that a mismatched transfusion may have a profound effect on a woman's future child-bearing capacity. Accurate matching of blood is, therefore, particularly important in the case of female patients.

---

[17] The complications introduced by subgroups of Group A have been described at page 187. Patients of blood group A_2 and particularly of A_2B may contain anti-A_1 in their plasma.

[18] The basis of haemolytic disease of the newborn (see Chapter 18).

An incompatible transfusion may, as described, give no clinical signs but simply set the scene for the future. A mild antigen/antibody reaction will produce a rise in temperature, a 'rigor' and varying constitutional upset. A severe reaction, and particularly one associated with ABO incompatibility, will result from massive destruction of blood within the vessels, the condition of shock will develop and the patient may die. Recovery from this, as from shock of any origin, may well be followed by acute renal failure.

The prevention of transfusion reactions depends on compatibility testing in the laboratory. The techniques are immaterial here; all are well known to laboratory workers and are within the compass of relatively small departments. The lawyer must, however, understand the general principles.

The cells of the recipient are irrelevant in the context of transfusion reactions— their importance lies in indicating the group of the donor to be chosen. The plasma of the donor is similarly irrelevant because any contained antibodies are rapidly diluted in the recipient's body. Thus it is possible, and reasonable in an emergency, to transfuse group O blood (the so-called universal donor blood) to a male recipient irrespective of his blood group. If the O blood is also D−, it could be used for a female recipient, the calculated risk being the provocation of a transfusion reaction due to the presence in the recipient of an immune antibody other than anti-D. Such emergency practice is rarely undertaken; the delay due to testing offers less risk than does an unmatched transfusion and full compatibility is almost always assured.

This is done in two stages. First, the donor cells are selected as being similar in ABO and CDE groups to those of the recipient. Compatibility of the recipient's plasma is then ensured by 'cross-matching'—the effect of mixing the actual donor cells with the actual recipient plasma (in practice, serum) is studied in the laboratory. The possibility of an immediate transfusion reaction can be excluded provided antibodies of both complete and incomplete type are sought by the most sensitive methods. Each donor unit (i.e. bottle or bag of blood) must be tested separately. This method does not exclude the possibility of sensitizing the recipient to one of the less important blood group antigens but testing for complete similarity of all blood group factors would be technologically impossible; provided cross-matching is undertaken regularly, the danger to the patient approximates to zero.

In practice, transfusions that are given and found to be incompatible by reason of inaccuracy of cross-matching are extremely rare; faults are far more often organizational in nature. The commonest mistakes include errors in transcription—due simply to clerical error or to the introduction of confusing terms such as 'group A serum' rather than 'anti-B serum'. Failure of the nursing staff to check the reference on the bag or bottle against the actual laboratory report on compatibility is another potent source of error which may be of catastrophic proportions. The presence of similarly named patients in the ward may be disastrous if the donor blood is not checked against the patient's notes.

Such errors are compounded by the use of the telephone combined with trusting delivery of messages to intermediates—conditions that commonly obtain in an emergency. A famous instance, probably apocryphal, is quoted concerning a telephone message to the effect, 'We are sending up the blood for the melaena patient'—meaning 'for the patient with bowel haemorrhage'; the blood was transfused into a child with the first name 'Melina'[19].

[19] Quoted by Taylor, J. L. (1970). *The Doctor and the Law*, p. 110. London; Pitman Medical.

Not all reactions are due to antigen/antibody incompatibility. Some are due to infection of the unit of blood. It is most important that the storage cabinet be maintained at constant optimal temperature—cabinets should be fitted with alarm systems that operate if the temperature range is exceeded. Similarly, expiry dates must be scrupulously observed as blood that has degenerated may cause considerable disability in its own right due to leakage of electrolytes from damaged red cells.

Finally, the blood may have contained pathogenic organisms other than HB_sAg in life and these must be excluded before it is used—the best-known diseases transmissible through blood transfusion are malaria and syphilis[20].

The expert witness

Much as in the case of 'anaesthetic' deaths, the investigation of transfusion reactions requires the co-operation of all concerned and, again, the primary object must be to prevent similar mistakes in the future.

Inquiries must be made as to the method of cross-matching, the documentation, and the chain of orders by which the transfusion was given and as to the precise clinical presentation. A full investigation of the remaining blood in the container, including a bacteriological analysis, must be made and correlated with the serum obtained from the patient either while living or, if death occurs, at autopsy.

The anatomic pathological evidence will be directed to demonstrating signs of blood destruction, and these are particularly evident in the kidneys. At the same time, the contribution of the condition requiring transfusion to the death has to be assessed and, of course, the presence of unsuspected disease must be sought. In general, the precise cause of death is likely to be elucidated and suitable remedial measures can be introduced.

[20] The problem of the acquired immune deficiency syndrome (AIDS) has arisen between editions of this book.

A guide to medical terminology

Prepositional prefixes

Prefix	Meaning	Example
A- or An-	Without	Anoxia = without oxygen
Ante-	Before	Ante-mortem = before death
Anti-	Against	Antiseptic = prevents sepsis
Circum-	Around	Circumoral = around the mouth
Contra-	Against, opposite	Contralateral = on the other side
De-	Away from	Dehydrate = remove water
Dia-	Through	Dialyse = to pass through a membrane
Dys-	Abnormal	Dysfunction = abnormal function
En- or Endo-	Within	Endotracheal = within the trachea
Epi-	Outside	Epidermis = outermost part of the skin
Extra- or Exo-	Outside	Extradural = outside the coverings of the brain
		Exogenous = produced from outside
Hetero-	Different	Heterotopic = in the wrong place
Homo-	Similar	Homozygous = similar genes combined
Hyper-	Excessive	Hypertrophy = overgrowth
Hypo-	Too little	Hypotension = low blood pressure
Infra-	Below	Infraorbital = below the eye
Inter-	Between	Intercostal = between the ribs
Intra-	Within	Intrahepatic = within the liver
Juxta-	Beside	Juxtaposition = closeness together
Para-	Close to, around	Paravertebral = near the spine
Per-	Through	Percutaneous = through the skin
Poly-	Many	Polymorphic = many-shaped
Post-	After	Post-traumatic = after injury
Pre-	In front of	Prepatellar = in front of the knee cap
Proto-	First	Prototype = the original of the form
Retro-	Behind	Retrosternal = behind the sternum
Sub-	Beneath	Subcutaneous = beneath the skin
Supra-	Above	Supralabial = above the lip

Prefix	Meaning	Example
Syn-	Together	Syndactyly = web fingers
Trans-	Through, across	Transplacental = across the placenta

Some suffixes

Suffix	Meaning	Example
-aemia	In or of the blood	Anaemia = no (or less than normal) blood
-algia	Pain	Neuralgia = pain in a nerve
-ectomy	Removal	Prostatectomy = removal of the prostate
-genic	Producing	Pathogenic = causing disease
-itis	Inflammation of	Laryngitis = inflammation of the larynx
-logy	Study of	Pathology = study of disease
-megaly	Enlargement of	Splenomegaly = enlargement of the spleen
-oma	Tumour	Adenoma = a tumour of glands
-osis	Abnormal process other than inflammation	Fibrosis = proliferation of fibrous tissue (scarring)
-pathy	Abnormal structure or function of	Myopathy = abnormal muscle
-plasia	Growth	Hyperplasia = excessive growth
-stomy	Making a hole	Tracheostomy = artificial opening in trachea

Anatomic prefixes

Prefix	Relating to	Example
Aden(o)-	Glands	Adenitis = inflammation of glands
Angio-	Blood vessels	Angiospasm = spasm of the arteries
Arthr(o)-	Joints	Arthralgia = pain in the joints
Cardio-	Heart	Cardiomyopathy = abnormality of the heart muscle
Cerebro-	Brain	Cerebrospinal fluid = fluid surrounding the brain and spinal cord
Chol(o)-	Bile	Cholecystitis = inflammation of the gall bladder
Chondro-	Cartilage	Chondroma = a tumour of cartilage
Colo-	Large bowel	Colostomy = making an opening in the colon
Costo-	Ribs	Costochondral = of the rib cartilages
Encephal(o)-	Brain	Encephalitis = inflammation of the brain
Enter(o)-	Intestines	Enteritis = inflammation of the intestine

Prefix	Relating to	Example
Gastr(o)-	Stomach	Gastroenterostomy = making a connecting hole between stomach and intestine
Haem(o)-	Blood	Haemothorax = blood in the thoracic cavity
Hepat(o)-	Liver	Hepatomegaly = enlargement of the liver
My(o)-	Muscle	Myesthenia = wasting of the muscle
Nephr(o)-	Kidney	Nephrosis = an abnormal process in the kidney
Neur(o)-	Nerve	Neurotoxic = poisonous to nerves
Pneumo-	Lung (or simply air)	Pneumoconiosis = an abnormality of the lung associated with dust
		Pneumothorax = free air in the thoracic cavity
Oste(o)-	Bone	Osteology = the study of bones

Note: American medical writing does not usually use diphthongs. Hence anaemia becomes anemia; tumour becomes tumor; oesophagus becomes esophagus.

Reporting deaths to Coroners

In deaths in the following circumstances the doctor is advised to inform the Coroner as soon as possible:

Sudden Deaths
When the cause is not clear or when the doctor cannot give a certificate because of non-attendance in the last illness.
    Not due to natural causes.
Accidents
In any way contributing to the cause of death.
Alcoholism
Chronic or acute.
Anaesthetics or Operations
Where it appears that either has caused or contributed to death, or where performed for any injury.
Drugs
Therapeutic or of addiction.
Foster Children
Industrial Diseases
Any pathological condition arising out of the nature of the deceased's employment, e.g. pneumoconiosis, Weil's disease and all diseases and poisons covered by the Factories Act.
Pensions
Where deceased has been in receipt of a disability pension.
Poisoning
From any cause, occupational, accidental, suicidal, homicidal and also food poisoning.
Stillbirths
Where there is any possibility of the child having been born alive.

To the above (from Camps, F. E. and Purchase, W. B. (1956), *Practical Forensic Medicine;* London; Hutchinson's Medical Publications) might be specifically added:
Deaths Due to Want, Exposure or Neglect
Obscure Infant Deaths

Conclusions of the jury/Coroner as to the death

Killed unlawfully
Killed himself [whilst the balance of his mind was disturbed]
Attempted/Self-induced abortion
Accident/Misadventure[1]
Execution of sentence of death
Killed lawfully
Natural causes*
Industrial disease*
Want of attention at birth*
Dependence on drugs/non-dependent abuse of drugs*
Open verdict

* In these cases, and in no others, the words 'the cause of death was aggravated by lack of care/self neglect' may be added. However, it would seem that 'lack of care' can also be used as a free-standing verdict[2].

(Coroners Rules 1984 (S.I. 1984/552), Sched. 4.)

[1] But this distinction is deprecated. R v. Coroner for City of Portsmouth, *ex parte* Anderson (1987) Times, 6 August.

[2] R v. Southwark Coroner, *ex parte* Hicks (1987) discussed by Dyer, C. (1987). Coroner overruled: time for reform ? *British Medical Journal*, **294,** 564.

Deaths reportable to the Procurator Fiscal

1. Any uncertified death.
2. Any death that was caused by an accident arising out of the use of a vehicle, or that was caused by an aircraft or rail accident.
3. Any death arising out of industrial employment, by accident, industrial disease or industrial poisoning.
4. Any death due to poisoning (coal gas, barbiturate, etc.).
5. Any death where the circumstances would seem to indicate suicide.
6. Any death where there are indications that it occurred under an anaesthetic.
7. Any death resulting from an accident in the home, hospital, institution or any public place.
8. Any death following an abortion.
9. Any death apparently caused by neglect (e.g. malnutrition).
10. Any death occurring in prison or a police cell where deceased was in custody at the time of death.
11. Any death of a newborn child whose body is found.
12. Any death (occurring not in a house) where deceased's residence is unknown.
13. Death by drowning.
14. Death of a child from suffocation (including overlaying).
15. Where the death occurred as the result of smallpox or typhoid.
16. Any death as a result of a fire or explosion.
17. Any sudden death.
18. Any other death due to violent, suspicious or unexplained cause.
19. Deaths of foster children.

Deaths reportable after investigation by the Procurator Fiscal to the Crown Office

1. Where there are any suspicious circumstances.
2. Where death was caused by an accident arising out of the use of a vehicle.
3. Where the circumstances point to suicide.
4. Where the death was caused by an accident, poison or disease, notice of which is required to be given to any Government Department or to any Inspector or other officer of a Government Department under or in pursuance of any Act.
5. Where the death occurred in circumstances continuance of which or possible recurrence of which is prejudicial to the health and safety of the public.
6. Where the death occurred in industrial employment.
7. Where the death occurred in any prison or police cell or where the deceased was in custody at the time of death.
8. Where death occurred under an anaesthetic in unusual circumstances or if there are features that suggest negligence.
9. Where death was due to gas poisoning.
10. Where death was directly or indirectly connected with the actions of a third party whether or not criminal responsibility rests on any person.
11. Where any desire has been expressed that a public inquiry should be held into the circumstances of the death or where the Procurator Fiscal is of the opinion that a public inquiry should be held under the Fatal Accidents and Sudden Deaths Inquiry (Scotland) Act 1976.

Approximate times of appearance of some centres of ossification

Intrauterine

1½ months—clavicle.
2 months—shafts of long bones.
3 months—ischium.
5 months—calcaneus.
6 months—manubrium sterni.
7 months—talus.
8 months—all segments of sternum.
9 months—lower end of femur, cuboid, head of humerus.

After Birth

1 month—head of tibia.
3 months—head of femur, lower end of tibia.
6 months—lower end of fibula.
7 months—lower end of radius, greater tuberosity of humerus.
10 months to 3 years—many of the small bones of hands and feet.
3 years—head of fibula, patella, greater trochanter of femur.
4 years—head of radius.
5 years—lower end of ulna.

Later Life

8 years—olecranon.
9 years—lesser trochanter of femur.
10 years—tibial tuberosity.

Later Life

13 years—anterior spine of ilium, iliac crest.
15 years—ischial tuberosity, medial end of clavicle.

Note: While all these appearances are very variable, females are advanced compared with males throughout.

(Adapted from Krogman, W. M. (1962). *The Human Skeleton in Forensic Medicine.* Springfield; Thomas.)

Union of epiphyses

Union	Earliest age (years)	Latest age (years)
Humerus/lower end	15	18
Ulna/upper end	15	21
Ischial tuberosity	15	25
Radius/upper end	16	20
Scapula/acromion	16	25
Tibia/lower end	17	25
Fibula/lower end	17	25
Iliac crest	17	25
Radius/lower end	18	25
Ulna/lower end	18	25
Femur/head of femur	18	25
Tibia/upper end	18	25
Clavicle	18	25
Femur/lower end	19	24
Fibula/upper end	19	25
Humerus/head	20	25

(Adapted from Krogman, W. M. (1962). *The Human Skeleton in Forensic Medicine*. Springfield; Thomas.)

Notification of infectious disease

The following diseases are notifiable to the Community Health Authorities by virtue of Health Services and Public Health Act 1968, s. 48 (Public Health (Infectious Diseases) Regulations 1968, S.I. No. 1366 as amended):

Acute encephalitis
Anthrax
Cholera
Diphtheria
Dysentery
Erysipelas
Food poisoning
Lassa fever
Leprosy
Leptospiral jaundice
Malaria
Marburg disease
Measles
Meningococcal infection
Ophthalmia neonatorum
Paratyphoid A

Paratyphoid B
Plague
Poliomyelitis, acute paralytic
Poliomyelitis, acute non-paralytic
Rabies
Relapsing fever
Scarlet fever
Smallpox
Tuberculosis, respiratory
Tuberculosis, non-respiratory
Typhoid fever
Typhus fever
Viral haemorrhagic fever
Viral hepatitis
Whooping cough
Yellow fever

Local authorities may add to this list by virtue of Public Health (Control of Diseases) Act 1984, s. 16 and National Health Service (Scotland) Act 1972, s. 53. Rubella (German measles) is a fairly common addition.

Prescribed diseases

Prescribed disease or injury	Occupation
A. *Conditions due to physical agents*	Any occupation involving:
A1. Inflammation, ulceration or malignant disease of the skin or subcutaneous tissues or of the bones, or blood dyscrasia, or cataract, due to electromagnetic radiations (other than resident (*see*) heat), or to ionizing particles	Exposure to electromagnetic radiations (other than radiant heat) or to ionizing particles
A2. Heat cataract	Frequent or prolonged exposure to rays from molten or red-hot material
A3. Dysbarism, including decompression sickness, barotrauma and osteonecrosis	Subjection to compressed or rarefied air or other respirable gases or gaseous mixtures
A4. Cramp of the hand or forearm due to repetitive movements	Prolonged periods of handwriting, typing or other repetitive movements of the fingers, hand or arm
A5. Subcutaneous cellulitis of the hand (beat hand)	Manual labour causing severe or prolonged friction or pressure on the hand
A6. Bursitis or subcutaneous cellulitis arising at or about the knee due to severe or prolonged external friction or pressure at or about the knee (beat knee)	Manual labour causing severe or prolonged external friction or pressure at or about the knee
A7. Bursitis or subcutaneous cellulitis arising at or about the elbow due to severe or prolonged external friction or pressure at or about the elbow (beat elbow)	Manual labour causing severe or prolonged external friction or pressure at or about the elbow
A8. Traumatic inflammation of the tendons of the hand or forearm, or of the associated tendon sheaths	Manual labour, or frequent or repeated movements of the hand or wrist
A9. Miner's nystagmus	Work in or about a mine:
A10. Substantial sensorineural hearing loss amounting to at least 50dB in each ear, being due in the case of at least one ear to occupational noise, and being the average of pure tone losses measured by audiometry	(*a*) The use of, or work wholly or mainly in the immediate vicinity of, pneumatic percussive tools or high-speed grinding tools, in the cleaning, dressing or finishing of cast metal or of ingots, billets or blooms

Prescribed disease or injury	Occupation
over the 1, 2, and 3 kHz frequencies (occupational deafness)	(b) The use of, or work wholly or mainly in the immediate vicinity of, pneumatic percussive tools on metal in the shipbuilding or ship repairing industries

Any occupation involving:

(c) The use of, or work in the immediate vicinity of, pneumatic percussive tools on metal, or for drilling rock in quarries or underground, or in mining coal, for at least an average of one hour per working day

(d) Work wholly or mainly in the immediate vicinity of drop-forging plant (including plant for drop-stamping or drop-hammering) or forging press plant engaged in the shaping of metal

(e) Work wholly or mainly in rooms or sheds where there are machines engaged in weaving man-made or natural (including mineral) fibres or in the bulking up of fibres in textile manufacturing

(f) The use of, or work wholly or mainly in the immediate vicinity of, machines engaged in cutting, shaping or cleaning metals nails

(g) The use of, or work wholly or mainly in the immediate vicinity of, plasma spray guns engaged in the deposition of metal

(h) The use of, or work wholly or mainly in the immediate vicinity of, any of the following machines engaged in the working of wood or material composed partly of wood, that is to say: multi-cutter moulding machines, planing machines, automatic or semi-automatic lathes, multiple cross-cut machines, automatic shaping machines, double-end tenoning machines, vertical spindle moulding machines (including high speed routing machines), edge banding

Prescribed disease or injury	Occupation
	machines, bandsawing machines with a blade width of not less than 75 millimetres and circular sawing machines in the operation of which the blade is moved towards the material being cut
	(*i*) The use of chain saws in forestry
A11. Episodic blanching, occurring throughout the year, affecting the middle or proximal phalanges or in the case of a thumb the proximal phalanx, of	(*a*) The use of hand-held chain saws in forestry
(*a*) In the case of a person with 5 fingers (including thumb) on one hand, any 3 of those fingers	(*b*) The use of hand-held rotary tools in grinding or in the sanding or polishing of metal, or the holding of material being ground, or metal being sanded or polished, by rotary tools
(*b*) In the case of a person with only 4 such fingers, any 2 of those fingers	Any occupation involving:
(*c*) In the case of a person with less than 4 such fingers, any one of those fingers or, as the case may be, the one remaining finger (vibration white finger)	(*c*) The use of hand-held percussive metal-working tools, or the holding of metal being worked upon by percussive tools in riveting, caulking, chipping, hammering, fettling or swaging
	(*d*) The use of hand-held powered percussive drills or hand-held powered percussive hammers in mining, quarrying, demolition, or on roads or footpaths, including road construction
	(*e*) The holding of material being worked upon by pounding machines in shoe manufacture
B. *Conditions due to biological agents*	
B1. Anthrax	Contact with animals infected with anthrax or the handling (including the loading or unloading or transport) of animal products or residues
B2. Glanders	Contact with equine animals or their carcases
B3. Infection by *leptospira*	(*a*) Work in places which are, or are liable to be, infested by rats, field mice or voles, or other small mammals
	(*b*) Work at dog kennels or the care or handling of dogs

Prescribed disease or injury	Occupation
	(c) Contact with bovine animals or their meat products or pigs or their meat products
B4. Ankylostomiasis	Work in or about a mine
B5. Tuberculosis	Contact with a source of tuberculous infection
B6. Extrinsic allergic alveolitis (including farmer's lung)	Exposure to moulds or fungal spores or heterologous proteins by reason of employment in:
	(a) Agriculture, horticulture, forestry, cultivation of edible fungi or malt-working
	(b) Loading or unloading or handling in storage mouldy vegetable matter or edible fungi
	(c) Caring for or handling birds
	(d) Handling bagasse
B7. Infection by organisms of the genus *Brucella*	Contact with:
	(a) Animals infected by *Brucella*, or their carcases or parts thereof, or their untreated products
	(b) Laboratory specimens of vaccines of or containing *Brucella*
B8. Viral hepatitis	Any occupation involving: Contact with—
	(a) Human blood or human blood products
	(b) A source of viral hepatitis
B9. Infection by *Streptococcus suis*	Contact with pigs infected by *Streptococcus suis*, or with the carcases, products or residues of pigs so infected

C. *Conditions due to chemical agents*

C1. Poisoning by lead or a compound of lead	The use or handling of, or exposure to the fumes, dust or vapour of, lead or a compound of lead, or a substance containing lead
C2. Poisoning by manganese or a compound of manganese	The use or handling of, or exposure to the fumes, dust or vapour of, manganese

Prescribed disease or injury	Occupation
	or a compound of manganese, or a substance containing manganese
C3. Poisoning by phosphorus or an inorganic compound of phosphorus or poisoning due to the anticholinesterase or pseudo anticholinesterase action of organic phosphorus compounds	The use or handling of, or exposure to the fumes, dust or vapour of, phosphorus or a compound of phosphorus, or a substance containing phosphorus
C4. Poisoning by arsenic or a compound of arsenic	The use or handling of, or exposure to the fumes, dust or vapour of, arsenic or a compound of arsenic, or a substance containing arsenic
C5. Poisoning by mercury or a compound of mercury	The use or handling of, or exposure to the fumes, dust or vapour of, mercury or a compound of mercury, or a substance containing mercury
C6. Poisoning by carbon disulphide	The use or handling of, or exposure to the fumes or vapour of, carbon disulphide or a compound of carbon disulphide, or a substance containing carbon disulphide
C7. Poisoning by benzene or a homologue of benzene	The use or handling of, or exposure to the fumes of, or vapour containing benzene or any of its homologues
C8. Poisoning by nitro- or amino- or chloro-derivative of benzene or of a homologue of benzene, or poisoning by nitrochlorobenzene	The use or handling of, or exposure to the fumes of, or vapour containing, a nitro- or amino- or chloro- derivative of benzene, or of a homologue of benzene, or nitrochlorobenzene
C9. Poisoning by dinitrophenol or a homologue of dinitrophenol or by substituted dinitrophenols or by the salts of such substances	The use or handling of, or exposure to the fumes of, or vapour containing, dinitrophenol or a homologue or substituted dinitrophenols or the salts of such substances
C10. Poisoning by tetrachloroethane	Any occupation involving: The use or handling of, or exposure to the fumes of, or vapour containing, tetrachloroethane
C11. Poisoning by diethylene dioxide (dioxan)	The use or handling of, or exposure to the fumes of, or vapour containing, diethylene dioxide (dioxan)
C12. Poisoning by methyl bromide	The use or handling of, or exposure to the fumes of, or vapour containing, methylbromide

Prescribed disease or injury	Occupation
C13. Poisoning by chlorinated naphthalene	The use or handling of, or exposure to the fumes of, or dust or vapour containing, chlorinated naphthalene
C14. Poisoning by nickel carbonyl	Exposure to nickel carbonyl gas
C15. Poisoning by oxides of nitrogen	Exposure to oxides of nitrogen
C16. Poisoning by gonioma kamassi (African boxwood)	The manipulation of gonioma kamassi or any process in or incidental to the manufacture of articles therefrom
C17. Poisoning by beryllium or a compound of beryllium	The use or handling of, or exposure to the fumes, dust or vapour of, beryllium or a compound of beryllium, or a substance containing beryllium
C18. Poisoning by cadmium	Exposure to cadmium dust or fumes
C19. Poisoning by acrylamide monomer	The use or handling of, or exposure to, acrylamide monomer:
C20. Dystrophy of the cornea (including ulceration of the corneal surface) or the eye	(a) The use or handling of, or exposure to, arsenic, tar, pitch, bitumen, mineral oil (including paraffin), soot or any compound, product or residue of any of these substances, except quinone or hydroquinone (b) Exposure to quinone or hydroquinone during their manufacture
C21. (a) Localized new growth of the skin, papillomatous or keratotic (b) Squamous-celled carcinoma of the skin	The use or handling of, or exposure to, arsenic, tar, pitch, bitumen, mineral oil (including paraffin), soot or any compound, product or residue of any of these substances, except quinone or hydroquinone
C22. (a) Carcinoma of the mucous membrane of the nose or associated air sinuses (b) Primary carcinoma of a bronchus or of a lung	Work in a factory where nickel is produced by decomposition of a gaseous nickel compound which necessitates working in or about a building or buildings where that process or any other industrial process ancillary or incidental thereto is carried on
C23. Primary neoplasm (including papilloma, carcinoma in-situ and invasive carcinoma) of the epithelial lining of the urinary tract (renal pelvis, ureter, bladder and urethra)	Any occupation involving: (a) Work in a building in which any of the following substances is produced for commercial purposes: (i) α-Naphthylamine, β-naphthyla-

Prescribed disease or injury	*Occupation*
	mine or methylene-bis-orthochloroaniline
	(ii) Diphenyl substituted by at least one nitro or primary amino group or by at least one nitro and primary amino group (including benzidine)
	(iii) Any of the substances mentioned in (ii) above if further ring substituted by halogeno, methyl or methoxy groups, but not by other groups
	(iv) The salts of any of the substances mentioned in (i)–(iii) above
	(v) Auramine or magenta
	(b) The use or handling of any of the substances mentioned in (a) (i)–(iv), or work in a process in which any such substance is used, handled or liberated
	(c) The maintenance or cleaning of any plant or machinery used in any such process as is mentioned in (b), or the cleaning of clothing used in any such building as is mentioned in (a) if such clothing is cleaned within the works of which the building forms a part or in a laundry maintained and used solely in connection with such works
C24. (a) Angiosarcoma of the liver (b) Osteolysis of the terminal phalanges of the fingers (c) Non-cirrhotic portal fibrosis	(a) Work in or about machinery or apparatus used for the polymerization of vinyl chloride monomer, a process which, for the purposes of this provision, comprises all operations up to and including the drying of the slurry produced by the polymerization and the packaging of the dried product (b) Work in a building or structure in which any part of that process takes place
C25. Occupational vitiligo	The use or handling of, or exposure to, para-tertiary-butylphenol, para-tertiary-

Prescribed disease or injury	Occupation
	butylcatechol, para-amylphenol, hydroquinone or the monobenzyl or monobutyl ether of hydroquinone

D. *Miscellaneous conditions*

D1. Pneumoconiosis	Any occupation: (*a*) Set out in Part II of this Schedule (*b*) Specified in regulation 2 (*b*) (ii)
D2. Byssinosis	Any occupation involving: Work in any room where any process up to and including the weaving process is performed in a factory in which the spinning or manipulation of raw or waste cotton or of flax, or the weaving of cotton or flax, is carried on
D3. Diffuse mesothelioma (primary neoplasm of the mesothelium of the pleura or of the pericardium or of the peritoneum)	(*a*) The working or handling of asbestos or any admixture of asbestos (*b*) The manufacture or repair of asbestos textiles or other articles containing or composed of asbestos (*c*) The cleaning of any machinery or plant used in any of the foregoing operations and any chambers, fixtures and appliances for the collection of asbestos dust (*d*) Substantial exposure to the dust arising from any of the foregoing operations
D4. Inflammation or ulceration of the mucous membrane of the upper respiratory passages or mouth produced by dust, liquid or vapour	Exposure to dust, liquid or vapour
D5. Non-infective dermatitis of external origin (including chrome ulceration of the skin but excluding dermatitis due to ionizing particles or electromagnetic radiations other than radiant heat)	Exposure to dust, liquid or vapour or any other external agent capable of irritating the skin (including friction or heat but excluding ionizing particles or electromagnetic radiations other than radiant heat)
D6. Carcinoma of the nasal cavity or associated air sinuses (nasal carcinoma)	(*a*) Attendance for work in or about a building where wooden goods are manufactured or repaired

Prescribed disease or injury	*Occupation*
	(*b*) Attendance for work in a building used for the manufacture of footwear or components of footwear made wholly or partly of leather or fibre board
	(*c*) Attendance for work at a place used wholly or mainly for the repair of footwear made wholly or partly of leather or fibre board
D7. Asthma which is due to exposure to any of the following agents:	Any occupation involving: Exposure to any of the agents set out in column 1 of this paragraph
(*a*) Isocyanates	
(*b*) Platinum salts (*c*) Fumes or dusts arising from the manufacture, transport or use of hardening agents (including epoxy resin curing agents) based on phthalic anhydride, tetrachloro-phthalic anhydride, trimellitic anhydride or triethylene-tetramine	
(*d*) Fumes arising from the use of rosin as a soldering flux	
(*e*) Proteolytic enzymes	
(*f*) Animals or insects used for the purposes of research or education or in laboratories	
(*g*) Dusts arising from the sowing, cultivation, harvesting, drying, handling, milling, transport or storage of barley, oats, rye, wheat or maize, or the handling, milling, transport or storage of meal or flour made therefrom	
(Occupational asthma)	
D8. Primary carcinoma of the lung where there is accompanying evidence of one or both of the following: (*a*) Asbestosis	(*a*) The working or handling of asbestos or any admixture of asbestos (*b*) The manufacture or repair of asbestos textiles or other articles containing or composed of asbestos

Prescribed disease or injury	Occupation
(b) Bilateral diffuse pleural thickening	(c) The cleaning of any machinery or plant used in any of the foregoing operations and of any chambers, fixtures and appliances for the collection of asbestos dust
	(d) Substantial exposure to the dust arising from any of the foregoing operations
D9. Bilateral diffuse pleural thickening	(a) The working or handling of asbestos or any admixture of asbestos
	(b) The manufacture or repair of asbestos textiles or other articles containing or composed of asbestos
	(c) The cleaning of any machinery or plant used in any of the foregoing operations and of any chambers, fixtures and appliances for the collection of asbestos dust
	Any occupation involving:
	(d) Substantial exposure to the dust arising from any of the foregoing operations

Social Security (Industrial Benefit) (Prescribed Diseases) Regulations 1985 (S.I. 1985/967), Sched. 1, Part I.

Prescribed occupations

Pneumoconiosis

1. Any occupation involving:
   (i) the mining, quarrying or working of silica rock or the working of dried quartzose sand or any dry deposit or dry residue of silica or any dry admixture containing such materials (including any occupation in which any of the aforesaid operations are carried out incidentally to the mining or quarrying of other minerals or to the manufacture of articles containing crushed or ground silica rock);
   (ii) the handling of any of the materials specified in the foregoing subparagraph in or incidental to any of the operations mentioned therein, or substantial exposure to the dust arising from such operations.

2. Any occupation involving the breaking, crushing or grinding of flint or the working or handling of broken, crushed or ground flint or materials containing such flint, or substantial exposure to the dust arising from such operations.

3. Any occupation involving sand blasting by means of compressed air with the use of quartzose sand or crushed silica rock or flint, or substantial exposure to the dust arising from sand and blasting.

4. Any occupation involving work in a foundry or the performance of, or substantial exposure to the dust arising from, any of the following operations:
   (i) the freeing of steel castings from adherent siliceous substance;
   (ii) the freeing of metal castings from adherent siliceous substance;
      (a) by blasting with an abrasive propelled by compressed air, by steam or by a wheel; or
      (b) by the use of power-driven tools.

5. Any occupation in or incidental to the manufacture of china or earthenware (including sanitary earthenware, electrical earthenware and earthenware tiles) and any occupation involving substantial exposure to the dust arising therefrom.

6. Any occupation involving the grinding of mineral graphite, or substantial exposure to the dust arising from such grinding.

7. Any occupation involving the dressing of granite or any igneous rock by masons or the crushing of such materials, or substantial exposure to the dust arising from such operations.

8. Any occupation involving the use, or preparation for use, of a grindstone, or substantial exposure to the dust arising therefrom.

9. Any occupation involving:
  (i) the working or handling of asbestos or any admixture of asbestos;
  (ii) the manufacture or repair of asbestos textiles or other articles containing or composed of asbestos;
  (iii) the cleaning of any machinery or plant used in any of the foregoing operations and of any chambers, fixtures and appliances for the collection of asbestos dust;
  (iv) substantial exposure to the dust arising from any of the foregoing operations.

10. Any occupation involving:
  (i) work underground in any mine in which one of the objects of the mining operations is the getting of any mineral;
  (ii) the working or handling above ground at any coal or tin mine of any minerals extracted therefrom, or any operation incidental thereto;
  (iii) the trimming of coal in any ship, barge, or lighter, or in any dock or harbour or at any wharf or quay;
  (iv) the sawing, splitting or dressing of slate, or any operation incidental thereto.

11. Any occupation in or incidental to the manufacture of carbon electrodes by an industrial undertaking for use in the electrolytic extraction of aluminium from aluminium oxide, and any occupation involving substantial exposure to the dust arising therefrom.

12. Any occupation involving boiler scaling or substantial exposure to the dust arising therefrom.

(Social Security (Industrial Benefit) (Prescribed Diseases) Regulations 1985 (S.I. 1985/967), Sched. 1, Part II.)

Diseases notifiable to the Health and Safety Executive

The following industrial diseases, when contracted in a factory, are notifiable to the Health and Safety Executive:

Beryllium poisoning
Cadmium poisoning
Lead poisoning
Phosphorus poisoning
Arsenical poisoning
Mercurial poisoning
Compressed-air illness
Chrome ulceration
Toxic jaundice
Aniline poisoning
Chronic benzene poisoning
Epitheliomatous ulceration
Manganese poisoning
Toxic anaemia
Carbon disulphide poisoning
Poisoning by organic compounds of lead, arsenic and mercury
Poisoning by organophosphorous compounds

(Factories Act 1961, s. 82 amended by Factories Act 1961 etc. (Repeals and Modifications) Regulations 1974 (S.I. 1974/1971) Sched. 2)

Form of consent for amniocentesis

We, the undersigned have requested that amniocentesis should be carried out. The risks and limitations of this procedure have been explained to us by . . . . and we appreciate that the procedure may have to be repeated. We understand that the birth of a normal child cannot be guaranteed from the results of studies on amniotic fluid and its contained cells.

Signed . . . .

. . . .

Date . . . .

Hospital . . . .

Case No. . . . .

Appendix M

Some useful equivalents of weight, capacity, length and temperature

Standard measurements in the form of SI units are described in Appendix P. Many reports will, however, refer to more colloquial terms and the following may be found useful as an aid to conversion of these.

Weight
1 gram (g)   = 15.4 grains
1 kilogram (kg)   = 35.3 ounces (avoirdupois)
1 grain   = 64.8 milligrams (mg)
1 ounce (avoirdupois) = 28.3 grams (g)
1 pound (avoirdupois) = 453.6 grams (g)

Capacity
1 fluid ounce   = 28.4 millilitres (ml)*
1 gill   = 5 fluid ounces
1 pint   = 568 millilitres (ml)
1 gallon (Imp.) = 4.55 litres (*l*)
1 litre (*l*)   = 1.76 pints
1 litre (*l*)   = 35.2 fluid ounces

Length
1 micron (μm)   = 10^{-6} metre (m)†
1 inch   = 2.54 centimetres (cm)
1 foot   = 30.5 centimetres (cm)
1 Ångstrom unit = 10^{-10} metre (m)

Temperature
An interval of 1 degree Centigrade (°C) corresponds to 1.8 degrees Fahrenheit (°F)
To convert °F to °C:
$$\frac{F-32}{9} = \frac{C}{5}$$

* For all practical purposes 1 millilitre is equivalent to 1 cubic centimetre (cc or cm^3).
† The symbol μ is also still used to express the micron.

Some parts of the Electromagnetic Spectrum (*wavelength*)
Ultraviolet = 100–400 nanometres (nm)
Visible   = 400–800 nm
Infrared   = 800–100 000 nm

Some medical and dental qualifications in the United Kingdom

Primary Medical Qualifications

LMSSA	Licentiate in Medicine and Surgery of the Society of Apothecaries.
MRCS, LRCP	Member of the Royal College of Surgeons of England, Licentiate of the Royal College of Physicians of London.
LRCP, LRCS (Edin. or Irel.)	Licentiate of the Royal Colleges of Physicians and Surgeons of Edinburgh or in Ireland.
LRCPS	Licentiate of the Royal College of Physicians and Surgeons of Glasgow.
MB (or BM), BCh (or BS or ChB)	Bachelor of Medicine and Surgery. Graduating degree awarded by Universities with Medical Schools.

Note. All qualifying degrees refer both to medicine and to surgery but not every doctor practises major surgery. Many doctors are also qualified BA (or subsequently MA) or BSc; these are intermediate University degrees taken before clinical training.

Some Postgraduate Medical Degrees

MD	Doctor of Medicine. Almost always obtained by thesis.
MS (or MCh or ChM)	Master of Surgery. Sometimes taken by thesis, sometimes by general examination.
PhD	Doctor of Philosophy. Obtained by thesis after a period of approved scientific research.
MSc	Master of Science. Obtainable in many scientific subjects related to medicine.

Such degrees indicate research in depth of a particular subject. They imply that there is some specific field in which the holder is an outstanding authority. Other special masterships are offered—e.g., in radiology.

Membership of the Royal Colleges and Faculties
Possession of these higher qualifications is certain evidence of specialization. They
are obtained by means of a searching examination; only very rarely is 'membership'
conferred by virtue of published work or reputation. The Colleges of Physicians in
London, Edinburgh and Glasgow (Physicians and Surgeons) at one time conferred
individual memberships; examinations are now on a United Kingdom basis. In
general, members are elected to be fellows of individual colleges after a delineated
period; the main exceptions are the Royal Colleges of Surgeons which confer
fellowship by examination.

FRCS	Fellow of the Royal College of Surgeons.
MRCP	Member of the Royal College of Physicians.
MRCOG	Member of the Royal College of Obstetricians and Gynaecologists.
MRCPath	Member of the Royal College of Pathologists.
MRCPsych	Member of the Royal College of Psychiatrists.
MRCGP	Member of the Royal College of General Practitioners.
MRCR	Members of the Royal College of Radiologists
FFA RCS	Fellow of the Faculty of Anaesthetists.
FFCM	Fellow of the Faculty of Community Medicine.

Postgraduate Medical Diplomas
The Universities and the Royal Colleges issue diplomas on the basis of
examination. The role of the diploma in indicating the narrower field of interest
and expertise of the holder has been somewhat reduced by the growth of
increasingly specialized Royal Colleges; in many cases, however, they are the sole
indication of a particular proficiency while others may be looked upon as
'stepping-stones' to membership.
    The following list is certainly not exhaustive.

DA	Diploma in Anaesthetics
DAvMed	Diploma in Aviation Medicine
DipBact	Diploma in Bacteriology
DCH	Diploma in Child Health
DIH	Diploma in Industrial Health
DLO	Diploma in Laryngology and Otology
DMJ	Diploma in Medical Jurisprudence
DO	Diploma in Ophthalmology
DObstRCOG	Diploma in Obstetrics of the Royal College of Obstetricians and Gynaecologists
BAO	Bachelor of the Art of Obstetrics (given in Ireland)
DPath	Diploma in Pathology
DRCPath	Diploma of the Royal College of Pathologists
DPhysMed	Diploma in Physical Medicine
DPM	Diploma in Psychiatric Medicine
DPH	Diploma in Public Health
DMRD or T	Diploma in Radiological Diagnosis or Therapy
DipSocMed	Diploma in Social Medicine
DTM & H	Diploma in Tropical Medicine and Hygiene
DTPH	Diploma in Tropical Public Health
DTCD	Diploma in Tuberculosis and Chest Diseases

Primary Dental Qualifications
LDS   Licentiate in Dental Surgery of the Royal Colleges
BDS or BChD   Bachelor of Dental Surgery. Graduating degree awarded by
                              most Universities with Dental Schools.

Some Postgraduate Dental Degrees
MDS or MChD   Master of Dental Surgery. Generally only available in
                              Universitites that do not offer a DDS.
MDentSc   Master in Dental Science.
MCDH   Master of Community Dental Health
DDS   Doctor of Dental Surgery
DDSc   Doctor of Dental Science.

Membership of the Royal Colleges and Faculties
MGDS RCS   Membership in General Dental Surgery
FDS RCS   Fellowship in Dental Surgery
Dental pathologists may also qualify as Members or Fellows of the Royal College
of Pathologists. Many dentists are also medically qualified and may proceed to higher
medical qualifications; these may be specialized—e.g. FRCS in faciomaxillary
surgery.

Some Postgraduate Dental Diplomas
DDH   Diploma in Dental Health
DDO or DDOrth   Diploma in Dental Orthopaedics
DDPH   Diploma in Dental Public Health
DOrth   Diploma in Orthodontics
DPD   Diploma in Public Dentistry
DRD   Diploma in Restorative Dentistry
HDD   Higher Dental Diploma

Report to Procurator Fiscal of death associated with anaesthesia and/or operation

Sir,

We hereby report the death of ....

at .... (Hospital, Nursing Home, etc.) on ..... date

which was associated with anaesthesia and/or operation. (See Note 1.)

1. Full Name .... Age ..... Ward .....

   Home Address ....

2. Date admitted to Hospital, and time ....

3. Nature of Disease, Injury or Ailment for which operation was advised.

4. Was formal consent for operation and administration of anaesthetic obtained?

5. Was the operation of an Elective or Emergency nature? ....

6. Note on clinical findings of examination of Heart, Lungs and Urine.

7. Note on any concurrent pathological condition or ailment present, or other relevant pre-operative details.

8. What precautions and medicaments were used in preparing the patient for anaesthesia and the surgical or other procedures? Where applicable give quantities and times.

9. Anaesthetic:

   Date and Time: Administration started .... Stopped ....

   Details of agents and techniques used, including sequences and quantities.

   Remarks

   Anaesthetist

10. Operations:
    Date and Time: Started .... Finished ....
    Nature of operation proposed, performed, or in progress:

    Remarks

    Operator
11. Date, Time and Place of Death (*i.e.,* Theatre, Ward, etc.).
12. Details in chronological order of events immediately preceding death and of resuscitative measures undertaken.

13. Opinion as to Cause of Death, and any other general observations on the case:

    Date ....   Signature ....(Operator)
                                   Signature .... (Anaesthetist)
The Procurator Fiscal,
       ....

Notes:
1. Only deaths, the circumstances of which fulfil any one or more of the following conditions, should be reported on this form, *viz:*
    (*a*) Deaths which occur during the actual administration of a general or local anaesthetic, or during operation performed under a general or local anaesthetic, or
    (*b*) Deaths which are considered to be clinically due to the anaesthetic, or
    (*c*) Deaths which occur in the immediate postoperative period ordinarily not exceeding 12 hours following a general anaesthetic from which consciousness has not been regained.
2. Wherever practicable this form should be completed in consultation with any other Medical Practitioner specially concerned or specifically mentioned and forwarded to the Procurator Fiscal as soon as possible.
3. The Death Certificate must not be issued until instructions have been received from the Procurator Fiscal or his representative.
4. The completion of Question 13 is a matter of discretion; while it is to assist the Procurator Fiscal and his Medical Adviser to arrive at a certifiable cause of death, it is not in itself the certified cause of death.

Notes on the International System of Units (SI Units)

There is a general move to report laboratory results, etc., in terms of SI units (*Système Internationale d'Unités*), many of which will be unfamiliar. The following notes are not exhaustive but may be found useful.

The independent base units of SI are (physical quantity, name of unit, and symbol):

length	metre	m
mass	kilogram	kg
time	second	s
electric current	ampere	A
thermodynamic temperature	kelvin	K
luminous intensity	candela	cd
amount of substance	mole	mol

Decimal multiples and fractions of the units are formed by prefixes, with appropriate symbols (*see also* Appendix M):

10^{12}	tera	T	10^{-1}	deci	d
10^9	giga	G	10^{-2}	centi	c
10^6	mega	M	10^{-3}	milli	m
10^3	kilo	k	10^{-6}	micro	μ
10^2	hecto	h	10^{-9}	nano	n
10	deca	da	10^{-12}	pico	p
			10^{-15}	femto	f
			10^{-18}	atto	a

Other units can be derived from these—e.g. the SI unit of area is the square metre (m^2) and of volume the cubic metre (m^3). When there is a combination, the divider ('per') is shown by the use of negative powers. Thus:

speed = metres per second = $m\,s^{-1}$

acceleration = metres per second per second = $m\,s^{-2}$.

Several derived SI units have been given new and special names. Few of these are of great medical interest save, perhaps:

unit of force = newton = $N = kg\,m\,s^{-2}$ (i.e. mass × acceleration)

unit of pressure = pascal = $Pa = N\,m^{-2}$ (i.e. force per square metre).

Despite this, the common unit of weight (gram = g) and of volume (litre = *l*) will continue in use.

Slowly, therefore, reports will include less well-known terms—e.g.:

Blood pressure = 150/75 mmHg = 20/10 kPa

Amount of phenobarbitone = 10 mg/100 ml = 430 μmol·l^{-1}.

It is even conceivable that a blood alcohol of 80 mg/100 ml will be reported as 17.4 mmol · l^{-1}.

Temperature on the clinical scale is now preferably referred to in terms of degrees Celsius (°C). The units are identical with degrees centigrade.

Organ weights at various ages in grams*

Age	Lungs Men	Lungs Women	Brain Men	Brain Women	Heart Men	Heart Women	Kidneys Men	Kidneys Women	Liver Men	Liver Women	Spleen Men	Spleen Women
Newborn	51.7	50.9	353	347	19	20	24	24	124	125	8	6
0–3 mth	68.8	63.6	435	411	—	—	—	—	—	—	—	—
3–6 mth	94.1	93.4	600	534	—	—	—	—	—	—	—	—
6–9 mth	128.5	114.7	877	726	41	36	60	52	300	240	26	25
9–12 mth	142.4	142.1										
1–2 yr	170.3	175.3	971	894	54	48	72	65	400	390	35	34
2–3 yr	245.9	244.3	1076	1012	63	62	85	75	460	450	42	41
3–4 yr	304.7	265.5	1179	1076	73	71	93	84	510	500	48	47
4–5 yr	314.2	311.7	1290	1156	83	80	100	93	555	550	53	52
5–6 yr	360.6	319.9	1275	1206	95	90	106	102	595	595	58	57
6–7 yr	399.5	357.5	1313	1225	103	100	112	112	630	635	62	62
7–8 yr	365.4	404.4	1338	1265	110	113	120	123	665	685	64	67
8–9 yr	405.0	382.1	1294	1208	122	126	128	135	715	745	68	71
9–10 yr	376.4	358.4	1360	1226	132	140	138	148	770	810	73	77
10–11 yr	474.5	571.2	1378	1247	144	154	150	163	850	880	82	85
11–12 yr	465.6	535.0	1348	1259	157	168	164	180	950	950	91	93
12–13 yr	458.8	681.7	1383	1256	180	188	178	195	1050	1080	101	103
13–14 yr	504.5	602.3	1382	1243	202	207	196	210	1150	1180	111	112
14–15 yr	692.8	517.0	1356	1318	238	226	212	222	1240	1270	121	120
15–16 yr	691.7	708.8	1407	1271	258	238	229	230	1315	1330	135	127
16–17 yr	743.3	626.5	1419	1300	282	243	244	236	1380	1360	145	134
17–18 yr	776.9	649.5	1409	1254	300	247	260	240	1450	1380	152	140
18–19 yr	874.7	654.9	1426	1312	310	250	270	244	1510	1395	157	146
19–20 yr	1035.6	785.2	1430	1294	318	251	282	247	1580	1405	160	151
20–21 yr	953.0	792.8	—	—	322	252	290	248	1630	1415	162	155

*From Boyd, E. (1962). In *Growth, Including Reproduction and Morphological Development*. Ed. by Altman and Dittmer, pp. 346–348. Biological Handbooks, Federation of American Societies for Experimental Biology; Washington. Reproduced by permission of the publishers.

Weights of the organs

Table of Statutes

List of cases

Bibliography

The first edition of this book was virtually unreferenced as a matter of policy. As time has gone on, however, it has seemed more and more desirable to quote sources and there is a definite increase in the number of footnotes. In deference to my reviewers, I have included a table of statutes and a list of cases but these should be read as a form of index only; there is no suggestion that the annotations are complete. Again, I have limited my medical references in the main to review articles or to papers that are easily obtainable.

The lawyer wishing to improve his knowledge of specialist pathology should consult the many textbooks that are written primarily for doctors. Those that I would suggest as being particularly useful in this context include:

Gradwohl's Legal Medicine, 3rd edn. (1976), Ed. by F. E. Camps, A. E. Robinson and B. G. B. Lucas (Bristol; Wright). This multi-author book corresponds most closely to my concept of the range of forensic medicine.

Essentials of Forensic Medicine, 4th edn. (1985), by C. J. Polson, D. J. Gee and B. Knight (Oxford; Pergamon). An authoritative work which is particularly well referenced. It includes no toxicology.

Forensic Medicine, 9th edn. (1985), by K. Simpson and B. Knight (London; Edward Arnold). A classic work which compresses an amazing amount of information into a slim volume.

Glaister's Medical Jurisprudence and Toxicology, 13th edn. (1973), Ed. by E. Rentoul and H. Smith (Edinburgh; Churchill Livingstone). This is the only other extant work that presents the subject with due regard to Scots practice. It has, however, little else to commend it in its current form.

Legal Aspects of Medical Practice, 3rd edn. (1982), by B. Knight (Edinburgh; Churchill Livingstone). A highly informative little book but one that is essentially written for general medical practitioners.

The Pathology of Violent Injury (1978), Ed. by J. K. Mason (London; Edward Arnold). One hesitates to include a work of one's own but many of the contributions are authoritative. An attempt to up-date forensic pathology.

Medicolegal Investigation of Death, 2nd edn. (1980), Ed. by W. U. Spitz and R. S. Fisher (Springfield; C. C. Thomas). An American book that would be my 'Desert Island' choice.

Ethics, Legal Medicine and Forensic Pathology (1983), by V. D. Plueckhahn (Melbourne University Press). A valuable Antipodean contribution which incorporates my views on the importance of medical jurisprudence to the subject.

I have also drawn heavily on the following monographs in relation to medical jurisprudence:

The Human Body and the Law (1970), by D. W. Meyers (Edinburgh University Press). A PhD thesis concerned with the law as it applies to selected problems in medical ethics.
Law of Doctor and Patient (1973), by S. R. Speller (London; H. K. Lewis). An authoritative work on the subject.
The Doctor and the Law (1970), by J. L. Taylor (London; Pitman Medical). A short and easy-to-read account of the doctor's medico-legal responsibilities.
Law Relating to Medical Practice, 2nd edn. (1979), by C. R. A. Martin. Authoritative and by a doubly qualified author.

The following are interesting recent additions to the list:

Decision Making in Medicine (1979), Ed. by G. Scorer and A. Wing (London; Edward Arnold). A very Christian-orientated but useful series of essays.
Dictionary of Medical Ethics, 2nd edn. (1981), Ed. by A. S. Duncan, G. R. Dunstan and R. B. Welbourn (London; Darton Longman and Todd). A wide-ranging guide.
Legal Issues in Medicine (1981), Ed. by S. A. M. McLean (Aldershot; Gower). Very much for and by the lawyer.
The Unmasking of Medicine (1981), by I. Kennedy (London; George Allen and Unwin). Essential reading of the 'alternative view'.

My preference among books on forensic odontology is for:

Dental Identification and Forensic Odontology (1976), by W. Harvey (London; Kimpton).

It goes without saying that this list is highly personalized and is by no means exhaustive.

Index

Italicized page numbers refer to illustrations